Emerging Bariatric Surgical Procedures

Editor

SHANU N. KOTHARI

SURGICAL CLINICS OF NORTH AMERICA

www.surgical.theclinics.com

Consulting Editor
RONALD F. MARTIN

April 2021 • Volume 101 • Number 2

ELSEVIER

1600 John F. Kennedy Boulevard ● Suite 1800 ● Philadelphia, Pennsylvania, 19103-2899

http://www.surgical.theclinics.com

SURGICAL CLINICS OF NORTH AMERICA Volume 101, Number 2
April 2021 ISSN 0039-6109, ISBN-13: 978-0-323-77840-4

Editor: John Vassallo, j.vassallo@elsevier.com

Developmental Editor: Arlene Campos

Surgical Clinics of North America (ISSN 0039-6109) is published bimonthly by Elsevier Inc., 360 Park Avenue South, New York, NY 10010-1710. Months of publication are February, April, June, August, October, and December. Business and Editorial Offices: 1600 John F. Kennedy Blvd., Suite 1800, Philadelphia, PA 19103-2899. Periodicals postage paid at New York, NY and additional mailing offices. Subscription prices are $443.00 per year for US individuals, $1198.00 per year for US institutions, $100.00 per year for US & Canadian students and residents, $547.00 per year for Canadian individuals, $1270.00 per year for Canadian institutions, $536.00 for international individuals, $1270.00 per year for international institutions and $250.00 per year for foreign students/residents. To receive student/resident rate, orders must be accompanied by name of affiliated institution, date of term, and the *signature* of program/residency coordinator on institution letterhead. Orders will be billed at individual rate until proof of status is received. Foreign air speed delivery is included in all *Clinics* subscription prices. All prices are subject to change without notice. POSTMASTER: Send address changes to *Surgical Clinics*, Elsevier Health Sciences Division, Subscription Customer Service, 3251 Riverport Lane, Maryland Heights, MO 63043. **Customer Service (orders, claims, online, change of address): Telephone: 1-800-654-2452 (U.S. and Canada); 314-447-8871 (outside U.S. and Canada). Fax: 314-447-8029. E-mail: journalscustomerservice-usa@elsevier.com (for print support); journalsonlinesupport-usa@elsevier.com (for online support)**.

Reprints. For copies of 100 or more, of articles in this publication, please contact the Commercial Reprints Department, Elsevier Inc., 360 Park Avenue South, New York, New York 10010-1710. Tel. 212-633-3874, Fax: 212-633-3820, E-mail: reprints@elsevier.com.

The Surgical Clinics of North America is also published in Spanish by McGraw-Hill Interamericana Editores S.A., P.O. Box 5-237 06500 Mexico D.F. Mexico; and in Portuguese by Interlivros Edicoes Ltda., Rua Comandante Coelho 1085, CEP 21250, Rio de Janeiro, Brazil; and in Greek by Paschalidis Medical Publications, Athens Greece.

The Surgical Clinics of North America is covered in *MEDLINE/PubMed (Index Medicus)*, *EMBASE/Excerpta Medica*, *Current Contents/Clinical Medicine*, *Current Contents/Life Sciences*, *Science Citation Index*, and *ISI/BIOMED*.

Contributors

CONSULTING EDITOR

RONALD F. MARTIN, MD, FACS
Colonel (Retired), United States Army Reserve, General and HPB Surgeon, Department of
General Surgery and Surgical Oncology, Madigan Army Medical Center, JBLM , Tacoma,
Washington, USA

EDITOR

SHANU N. KOTHARI, MD, FACS, FASMBS
Vice Chair of Medical Staff Affairs, Department of Surgery, Prisma Health, Greenville,
South Carolina, President-Elect, American Society for Metabolic & Bariatric Surgery,
Gainesville, Florida, USA

AUTHORS

ERIC AHNFELDT, DO, FACS, FASMBS
General, Bariatric, and Metabolic Surgery Department, William Beaumont Army Medical
Center, El Paso, Texas, USA

VANCE L. ALBAUGH, MD, PhD
Department of General Surgery, Bariatric and Metabolic Institute, Cleveland Clinic,
Cleveland, Ohio, USA

VAMSI V. ALLI, MD
Assistant Professor, Minimally Invasive and Bariatric Surgery, Penn State Hershey Medical
Center

GRETCHEN AMES, PhD, ABPP
Clinical Health Psychologist, Mayo Clinic, Jacksonville, Florida, USA

ALI AMINIAN, MD
Department of General Surgery, Bariatric and Metabolic Institute, Cleveland Clinic,
Cleveland, Ohio, USA

MEHRAN ANVARI, MB, BS, PhD, FRCSC, FACS
Department of Surgery, Centre for Minimal Access Surgery, McMaster University, St.
Joseph's Healthcare, Hamilton, Ontario, Canada

MOHIT BHANDARI, MS
Mohak Bariatrics and Robotics Center, SAIMS Campus, Indore, Madhya Pradesh, India

VANESSA BOUDREAU, MD, MSc
Department of Surgery, Centre for Minimal Access Surgery, Department of Health
Research Methods, Evidence and Impact, Faculty of Health Sciences, McMaster
University, Hamilton, Ontario, Canada

KEVIN CLIMACO, MD
General, Bariatric, and Metabolic Surgery Department, William Beaumont Army Medical Center, El Paso, Texas, USA

DANIEL COTTAM, MD
Bariatric Medicine Institute, Salt Lake City, Utah, USA

SAMUEL COTTAM, BS
Bariatric Medicine Institute, Salt Lake City, Utah City, Utah, USA

ARISTITHES G. DOUMOURAS, MD, MPH
Department of Surgery, Centre for Minimal Access Surgery, McMaster University, Hamilton, Ontario, Canada

MATHIAS FOBI, MD FACS, FACN, FICS
Mohak Bariatrics and Robotics Center, SAIMS Campus, Indore-Ujjain Highway, Indore, Madhya Pradesh, India

RACHEL E. GOETZE, PhD
Clinical Psychologist, VA Maine Healthcare System-Togus, VA Center, Augusta, Maine, USA

BRANDON T. GROVER, DO, FACS, FASMBS
Department of Surgery, Gundersen Health System, La Crosse, Wisconsin, USA

KAREN BARLOW, HonsBSc
Department of Surgery, Centre for Minimal Access Surgery, McMaster University, St. Joseph's Healthcare, Hamilton, Ontario, Canada

JASON M. JOHNSON, DO, FACS, FASMBS
Program Director, General Surgery Residency, Chair, General and Trauma Surgery, Saint Joseph Hospital, Denver, Colorado, USA

MARTA KARPINSKI, MSc, BHSc
Department of Health Research Methods, Evidence and Impact, Faculty of Health Sciences, McMaster University, Maple, Ontario, Canada

MANOJ KHURANA, MS
Mohak Bariatrics and Robotics Center, SAIMS Campus, Indore, Madhya Pradesh, India

TAMMY L. KINDEL, MD, PhD
Department of Surgery, Medical College of Wisconsin, Milwaukee, Wisconsin, USA

MICHAEL J. KLINGLER, MD
Cleveland Clinic, Cleveland, Ohio, USA

AFTON M. KOBALL, PhD, ABPP
Clinical Health Psychologist, Behavioral Medicine, Gundersen Health System, La Crosse, Wisconsin, USA

SUSMIT KOSTA, PhD
Mohak Bariatrics and Robotics Center, SAIMS Campus, Indore, Madhya Pradesh, India

MATTHEW KROH, MD
Cleveland Clinic Abu Dhabi, Abu Dhabi, United Arab Emirates

YUNG LEE, MD
Department of Surgery and Centre for Minimal Access Surgery, McMaster University, Hamilton, Ontario, Canada

JAMES N. LUO, MD
Laboratory for Surgical and Metabolic Research, Department of Surgery, Brigham and Women's Hospital, Harvard Medical School, Boston, Massachusetts, USA

WILLIAM CAMERON MACLELLAN, MD, MBA
Surgery Residency, Saint Joseph Hospital, Denver, Colorado, USA

ROSHAN S. MALHAN, BHSc
Department of Health Research Methods, Evidence and Impact, Faculty of Health Sciences, McMaster University, Hamilton, Ontario, Canada

PETER R.A. MALIK, BHSc
Department of Surgery, Centre for Minimal Access Surgery, Department of Health Research Methods, Evidence and Impact, Faculty of Health Sciences, McMaster University, St. Catharines, Ontario, Canada

WINNI MATHUR, BPT, MBA(HA)
Mohak Bariatrics and Robotics Center, SAIMS Campus, Indore, Madhya Pradesh, India

KATELYN M. MELLION, MD
Department of Medical Education, Advanced Gastrointestinal Minimally Invasive Surgery and Bariatric Fellowship, Gundersen Health System, La Crosse, Wisconsin, USA

KATELIN MIRKIN, MD
Instructor, Minimally Invasive and Bariatric Surgery, Penn State Hershey Medical Center

STEVEN E. NISSEN, MD
Department of Cardiovascular Medicine, Heart and Vascular Institute, Cleveland Clinic, Cleveland, Ohio, USA

SEAN C. O'CONNOR, MD
Department of Surgery, Division of Minimal Access and Bariatric Surgery, Prisma Health, Greenville, South Carolina, USA

DIANA E. PETERMAN, MD
Resident Physician, Department of Surgery, Prisma Health-Upstate, Greenville, South Carolina, USA

JANEY S.A. PRATT, MD, FACS, FASMBS
Clinical Associate Professor, Department of Surgery, Division of Pediatric Surgery, Stanford University School of Medicine, Lucille Packard Children's Hospital, Stanford, California, USA

MANOJ KUMAR REDDY, MS
Mohak Bariatrics and Robotics Center, SAIMS Campus, Indore-Ujjain Highway, Indore, Madhya Pradesh, India

JOHN H. RODRIGUEZ, MD, FACS
Assistant Professor of Surgery, Cleveland Clinic Lerner College of Medicine, Director of Surgical Endoscopy, Cleveland, Ohio, USA

ANN M. ROGERS, MD, FACS, FASMBS
Professor, Minimally Invasive and Bariatric Surgery, Penn State Hershey Medical Center

JOHN D. SCOTT, MD
Clinical Professor, Department of Surgery, Division of Minimal Access and Bariatric Surgery, Prisma Health, Greenville, South Carolina, USA

ADI STEINHART, BS, BA
Assistant Clinical Research Coordinator, Department of Pediatrics, Stanford University School of Medicine, Palo Alto, California, USA

AMIT SURVE, MD
Bariatric Medicine Institute, Salt Lake City, Utah, USA

ALI TAVAKKOLI, MD
Chief, Division of General and Gastrointestinal Surgery, Laboratory for Surgical and Metabolic Research, Department of Surgery, Brigham and Women's Hospital, Harvard Medical School, Boston, Massachusetts, USA

DEBORAH TSAO, BS
Medical Student, Stanford University School of Medicine, Stanford, California, USA

JEREMY A. WARREN, MD
Associate Professor, Department of Surgery, Division of Minimal Access and Bariatric Surgery, Prisma Health-Upstate, University of South Carolina School of Medicine Greenville, Greenville South Carolina, USA

JOSHUA S. WINDER, MD
Clinical Fellow, Surgical Endoscopy, Cleveland Clinic, Cleveland, Ohio, USA

Contents

Roux-en-Y gastric bypass has been considered the gold standard bariatric procedure for decades. The surgical technique for Roux-en-Y gastric bypass and perioperative management for patients who undergo the procedure are still being improved for better clinical outcomes, shorter hospitalization, and faster return to normal activity. In the past 15 years there have been similar improvements and further development of novel surgical weight loss procedures. As data on other surgical alternatives emerge, the data need to be compared with Roux-en-Y gastric bypass to determine noninferiority. Further long-term investigations are needed to determine superiority of one bariatric procedure over another.

Bariatric surgery has emerged as the most effective means of achieving weight loss. Obesity surgery is a quickly expanding field. Laparoscopic vertical sleeve gastrectomy is a great option for patients because it is simple, exceedingly safe, has a fairly defined postoperative complication profile, and is as effective as more complex bariatric surgery options. Specific consideration of patients' comorbidities, assessment of surgeon's skill, and knowledge of preoperative, perioperative, and postoperative course is a must for all surgeons who wish to perform this procedure. If properly used, vertical sleeve gastrectomy is a powerful tool in combating obesity and its deleterious effects.

Single-anastomosis duodenal ileostomy with sleeve gastrectomy (SADI-S) is an important emerging procedure in bariatric surgery as an alternative to performing the Roux-en-Y gastric bypass (RYGB) or the Roux-en-Y duodenal switch. With this significant weight loss and low weight regain, SADI-S has low complication rates. SADI-S, because of its anatomic configuration, also does not increase ulcer risk in patients, with almost no ulcers observed. Because of the short common channel, malnutrition is a risk. Diabetes resolution is higher than with RYGB. Overall SADI-S is a safe and effective procedure for patients with higher body mass index and patients with diabetes.

Childhood obesity can lead to comorbidities that cause significant decrease in health-related quality of life and early mortality. Recognition of obesity as a disease of polygenic etiology can help deter implicit bias. Current guidelines for treating severe obesity in children recommend referral to a multidisciplinary treatment center that offers metabolic and bariatric surgery at any age when a child develops a body mass index that is greater than 120% of the 95th percentile. Obesity medications and lifestyle counseling about diet and exercise are not adequate treatment for severe childhood obesity. Early referral can significantly improve quality and quantity of life.

Revisional bariatric surgery is a growing subset of all bariatric procedures. Although revisions can be associated with higher morbidity rates and less optimal outcomes than those seen with primary procedures, they can be safely performed, with excellent outcomes and improved quality of life for patients. Facility and familiarity with revisional principles and techniques are necessary components of bariatric surgical practice.

Bariatric and metabolic surgery has evolved from simple experimental procedures for a chronic problem associated with significant morbidity into a sophisticated multidisciplinary treatment modality rooted in biology and physiology. Although the complete mechanistic narrative of bariatric surgery cannot yet be written, significant advance in knowledge has been made in the past 2 decades. This article provides a brief overview of the most studied hypotheses and their supporting evidence. Ongoing research, especially in frontier areas, such as the microbiome, will continue to refine, and perhaps even revise, current mechanistic understanding.

The prevalence of noncommunicable diseases has increased dramatically in North America and throughout the world and is expected to continue increasing in coming years. Obesity has been linked to several types of cancers and is associated with increased morbidity and mortality following cancer diagnosis. Bariatric surgery has emerged as the prominent model to evaluate the effects of intentional weight loss on cancer incidence and outcomes. Current literature, comprising prospective cohort investigations, indicates site-specific reductions in cancer risk with select bariatric procedures. Future research is required to establish evidence-based indications for bariatric surgery in the context of cancer prevention.

Type 2 diabetes mellitus (T2D) and associated comorbid medical conditions are leading causes of strain on the American health care system. There has been a synchronous rise of obesity to epidemic proportions. If poorly treated, T2D is a scourge for patients, leading to end-organ damage and early mortality. Although T2D is considered best managed with lifestyle modification, medical management, and pharmacotherapy, recent studies have confirmed the superiority of metabolic surgery to conventional treatment algorithms as a path to remission. Increasing access to metabolic surgery will continue to yield benefits to patient health and improve the macroeconomic health of the world.

Cardiovascular disease (CVD) remains a leading cause of morbidity and mortality in developed countries, with worsening pandemics of type 2 diabetes mellitus and obesity as major cardiovascular (CV) risk factors. Clinical trials of nonsurgical obesity treatments have not shown benefits in CVD, although recent diabetes trials have demonstrated major CV benefits. In many retrospective and prospective cohort studies, however, metabolic (bariatric) surgery is associated with substantial and reproducible CVD benefits. Despite a lack of prospective, randomized clinical trials, data suggest metabolic surgery may be the most effective modality for CVD risk reduction, likely through weight loss and weight loss–independent mechanisms.

Obesity is an independent risk factor for osteoarthritis due to mechanical and inflammatory factors. The gold-standard treatment of end-stage knee and hip osteoarthritis is total joint arthroplasty (TJA). Weight loss decreases progression of osteoarthritis and complications following TJA in patients with obesity. Bariatric surgery allows significant, sustained weight loss and comorbidity resolution in patients with morbid obesity. Existing data describing bariatric surgery on TJA outcomes are limited but suggest a benefit to bariatric surgery prior to TJA. Further studies are needed to determine optimal risk stratification, bariatric procedure selection, and timing of bariatric surgery relative to TJA.

Ventral and incisional hernias in obese patients are particularly challenging. Suboptimal outcomes are reported for elective repair in this population. Preoperative weight loss is ideal but is not achievable in all patients

safer, and results have been reproducible across the world. Despite these efforts, a limited number of patients have access to high quality surgical care and pursue these interventions. Endoscopic bariatric interventions have been designed to offer safer interventions despite decreased effectiveness and durability, when compared to current metabolic operations. Multiple devices and techniques dedicated to weight management are being developed and have either been approved for use or are undergoing clinical trial. This article reviews many of these endoscopic interventions in bariatric surgery, including gastric aspiration devices, incisionless magnetic anastomotic systems, endoluminal, bypass barrier sleeves, primary surgery obesity endoluminal, endoscopic sleeve gastroplasty, and duodenal mucosal resurfacing. These effective techniques may serve either as a primary therapy or as a bridge to bariatric surgery.

SURGICAL CLINICS
OF NORTH AMERICA

SERIES OF RELATED INTEREST

Advances in Surgery
https://www.advancessurgery.com/
Surgical Oncology Clinics
https://www.surgonc.theclinics.com/
Thoracic Surgery Clinics
http://www.thoracic.theclinics.com/

Foreword

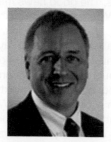

Ronald F. Martin, MD, FACS
Consulting Editor

As I write this foreword, I am nagged by a question of an epistemic nature: are we living in a post–fact world, and if so, how would we know it? I full-well realize that as we age it is common to become more circumspect as to the relative certainty of ideas that we once held as matters of great importance. I also realize that many people choose the opposite tack and double-down on stupid. With that acknowledged, however, I am intellectually plagued by the cognitive dissonance that abounds at this time. I am even more concerned that the particular challenge posed to us also thwarts our conventional approach to resolution since opposing view-holders simply refuse to accept the other's data.

The past year or so has been as collectively trying as any period I can recall. I know of no one who could fully escape the circumstances. To be sure, there have been greatly inequitable distributions of misery. So many have died. So many have been alone. So many have lost opportunities that money cannot regain. So many have been heard, and so many more have not been heard. The pandemic has pervaded all aspects of life, and all aspects of life have had to factor in the pandemic. Social and political situations made their demands for large gatherings, and large gatherings made it easier to spread disease. Here in the United States, elections came and went and, as of this writing, we do not have a collective agreement to how they ended. Furthermore, it does not appear that we can agree on how we could find a way to agree. Not only have rules, laws, conventions, norms, and other matters of historical civility evaded us for now but also they appear as if they may not return any time soon, if at all.

We humans have always had a waxing and waning comfort level with collectivism. Cultures vary greatly on their willingness to tolerate or shun individualism. Some collective efforts when the chips are down have frequently been useful. An overinsistence on conformity and collectivism (especially groupthink style) can lead to catastrophic conflict or persecution. From a sociopolitical standpoint, leveraging that collectivist/anti-collectivist tension has made and broken fortunes on both personal and national levels. The low-hanging fruit for abusers in either camp is to tap into those beliefs that are neither readily proved nor disproved.

Surg Clin N Am 101 (2021) xiii–xiv
https://doi.org/10.1016/j.suc.2021.01.002
0039-6109/21/© 2021 Published by Elsevier Inc.

For quite a long time I have been of the belief that despite the tremendous temptations that may exist for some to exploit fear and confusion, that when confronted with a problem that had scientific roots, a large majority of us would be able to turn to an agreed upon set of facts for our solutions. At present, it is not clear to me that that majority, who could supplant desire to facts and reason, still exists. The good news may be that it will not likely rely on "all of us" to agree on anything. What will matter in the short term will be for enough agreement to forge a sustainable path for survival. In the longer run, whether any of us agree or not may not be that relevant at all: reality always prevails given enough time independent of whether we are cognitively onboard or not.

The *Surgical Clinics* is dedicated to giving a platform to help our readers understand the facts as best we can. As I have stated before, we strive to "put content in context." That is one of the reasons we come back to certain topics on a periodic basis. We don't do it because we are looking for a mulligan on the last attempt to educate but because we realize that new information comes to light and our ability to analyze also evolves. We expect it to. And as such, we must revisit our facts, thoughts, and conclusions to consider whether or not we need to incur a revision of belief.

To do that, we must turn to those we trust, fallible though we all are. In this case, we are fortunate to have Dr Kothari and his colleagues to help guide us. The evolution of bariatric and metabolic surgery, including the evaluation, procedures, medical management, and behavioral care, have evolved and will continue to do so. Our contributors have provided us with facts, analysis, references, and perspectives. At the end of the day, we can use this material to inform ourselves and inform others. We can be grateful we have it for our needs and be hopeful that we can transmit it to those who need this knowledge in a manner they can understand and accept.

As we were taught in math when we were young, we need definitions and axioms in order to have a foundation upon which to build higher-level mathematical constructs. In surgery, we need fundamental scientific data and dispassionate analysis in order to build the artistic and human aspects of our profession. I thank our colleagues for providing us with this excellent foundation. I can only hope that this learning process that we have revered for so many centuries can find its way back into society writ large with the efficiency of a virus.

Be well and stay safe.

Ronald F. Martin, MD, FACS
Colonel (retired), United States Army Reserve
Department of General Surgery and Surgical Oncology
Madigan Army Medical Center
9040 Jackson Avenue
Tacoma, WA 98431, USA

E-mail address:
rfmcescna@gmail.com

Preface

Metabolic and Bariatric Surgery: Continual Advances and Challenges

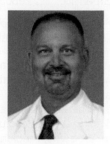

Shanu N. Kothari, MD, FACS, FASMBS
Editor

As President-Elect of the American Society for Metabolic and Bariatric Surgery and a practicing bariatric surgeon who has dedicated the last 20 years to caring for patients with the disease of obesity, it is an honor to be invited to guest edit another issue of the *Surgical Clinics* dedicated to metabolic and bariatric surgery.

I had the opportunity to guest edit the 2011 issue. Since then, the rise in the obesity epidemic in the United States and abroad continues. In conjunction with this is the staggering prediction that by the year 2050 there will be an estimated 30 million patients with type 2 diabetes in the United States alone.

Over this same time frame, along with several advances in the field, we have seen vertical sleeve gastrectomy emerge as the most commonly performed bariatric surgical procedure in the United States. We have also seen the development of endoluminal therapies as well as a variety of emerging procedures, including single anastomosis duodenoileostomy with sleeve gastrectomy. These interventions and more are highlighted in this issue.

This year has also brought challenges related to the COVID-19 pandemic. It is clear that patients suffering from the disease of obesity are at increased risk of morbidity and mortality with COVID-19 infection. This vulnerable population should have increased access to life-changing and life-saving metabolic and bariatric surgery.

Surg Clin N Am 101 (2021) xv–xvi
https://doi.org/10.1016/j.suc.2021.01.001
0039-6109/21/© 2021 Published by Elsevier Inc.

I hope that this issue improves your knowledge base and ability to care for this population as much as it has for me.

Shanu N. Kothari, MD, FACS, FASMBS
Vice Chair, Medical Staff Affairs
Department of Surgery
Prisma Health
701 Grove Road
Support Tower 3rd Floor
Greenville, SC 29605, USA

E-mail address:
Shanu.Kothari@prismahealth.org

Laparoscopic Gastric Bypass
Still the Gold Standard?

William Cameron Maclellan, MD, MBA, Jason M. Johnson, DO*

KEYWORDS

- Gastric bypass • Gold standard • Weight loss • Bariatric

KEY POINTS

- Gastric bypass is the gold standard with which all other bariatric procedures should be compared.
- Gastric bypass has excellent weight loss and improvement of comorbidities, which comes at the cost of a slight increase in frequency of complications compared with other weight loss procedures.
- Further long-term data are needed to clarify the superiority of one bariatric procedure over another.

INTRODUCTION

Roux-en-Y gastric bypass (RNYGB) has been the gold standard of weight loss procedures for more than 20 years. After Pories and coworkers[1] published their sentinel paper on weight loss, and more importantly remission of diabetes in long-term follow-up, surgeons have been collecting data that have showed the long-term clinical efficacy of RNYGB. Evidence has shown clear benefit over medical management in terms of weight loss, quality of life, and remission of comorbidities.[2,3] Even after more than 25 years, the surgical technique for RNYGB and perioperative management for patients who undergo the procedure are still being improved on for better clinical outcomes, shorter hospitalization, and faster return to normal activity. In the past 15 years there have been similar improvements and further development of novel surgical weight loss procedures. To date, there is no clear answer to which weight loss surgery is best.[4] Thus, it is imperative to define the advantages and drawbacks of various surgical treatments of obesity and in conjunction with patients identify which may be the most appropriate surgical approach for weight loss. Using the RNYGB as the gold standard ensures other weight loss procedures produce at least equivalent short- and long-term outcomes.

Saint Joseph Hospital, 1375 East 19th Avenue, Denver, CO 80218, USA
* Corresponding author.
E-mail address: Jason.johnson@sclhealth.org

Surg Clin N Am 101 (2021) 161–175
https://doi.org/10.1016/j.suc.2020.12.013
0039-6109/21/© 2020 Elsevier Inc. All rights reserved.

surgical.theclinics.com

PATIENT EVALUATION OVERVIEW

The preoperative evaluation and work-up of potential candidates for bariatric surgery is crucial to successful outcomes. Regardless of procedure chosen a multidisciplinary preoperative work-up ensures appropriate patient selection, education, and risk mitigation. Patient compliance and postoperative behavior is essential to achieving desirable outcomes and can only be assessed by a comprehensive, multidisciplinary evaluation. The indications for bariatric surgery are widely accepted and do not vary based on surgical procedure done[5]:

- Body mass index (BMI) ≥40, or more than 100 lb overweight
- BMI ≥35 and at least one or more obesity-related comorbidity
- Inability to achieve a healthy weight loss sustained for a period of time with prior weight loss efforts

The comorbid conditions related to obesity that serve as indications for surgical intervention in patients with BMI 35 to 40 include the following[4]:

- Type 2 diabetes
- Hypertension (HTN)
- Hyperlipidemia
- Obstructive sleep apnea (OSA)
- Obesity hypoventilation syndrome
- Pickwickian syndrome
- Nonalcoholic fatty liver disease and steatohepatitis
- Idiopathic intracranial HTN
- Asthma
- Venous stasis disease
- Severe urinary incontinence
- Debilitating arthritis
- Gastroesophageal reflux disease (GERD)

Although this set of criteria seems simple, the decision as to which procedure is the best for a patient remains debatable. When choosing the most appropriate procedure for the patient it is imperative to compare long-term outcomes in not only weight loss but remission and improvement of comorbid conditions with a set of standards. The set standards are RNYGB because this procedure has the most robust and long-term outcome and follow-up data of any of the weight loss procedures.

GASTRIC BYPASS AND ITS ALTERNATIVE SURGICAL OPTIONS
Roux-en-Y Gastric Bypass

The essential steps of the gastric bypass procedure include creation of an approximate 20- to 30-mL gastric pouch, creation of a gastrojejunal anastomosis, and creation of a jejunojejunostomy between the Roux and the biliopancreatic limb **(Fig. 1)**. Desired length of the Roux limb and the biliopancreatic limb varies, but most agree on lengths of 75 to 150 cm and 40 to 50 cm, respectively. A meta-analysis showed an optimal combined Roux and biliopancreatic limb length of 100 to 200 cm.[6] A variety of anastomotic techniques are also used for the gastrojejunostomy including hand-sewn, linear stapled, and circular stapled. There is no evidence supporting hand-sewing as opposed to stapling of the gastrojejunostomy. Several studies have shown higher rates of postoperative bleeding, infection, and need for endoscopic dilation for patients who have a circular stapled gastrojejunostomy.[7–9]

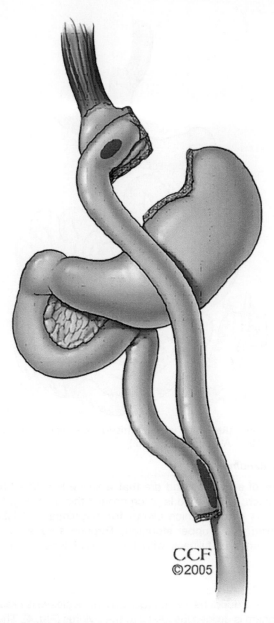

CCF
©2005

Fig. 1. Gastric bypass. (Reprinted with permission, Cleveland Clinic Center for Medical Art & Photography ©2021. All Rights Reserved.)

Vertical Sleeve Gastrectomy

The essential steps of the sleeve gastrectomy (SG) include mobilization of the greater curvature (**Fig. 2**) and creation of a "sleeve" by using a bougie adjacent to the lesser curve and then resecting a large portion of the stomach. The patient is left with a cylindrical stomach. Data have shown that there are restrictive and hormonal changes that occur after one undergoes SG.

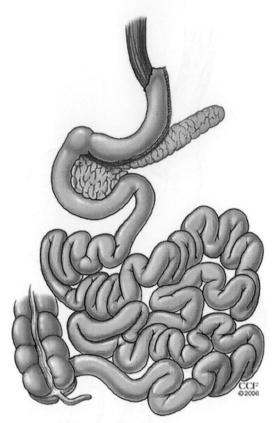

Fig. 2. Sleeve gastrectomy. (Reprinted with permission, Cleveland Clinic Center for Medical Art & Photography ©2021. All Rights Reserved.)

Adjustable Gastric Banding

The essential steps of a gastric band are that a space is created behind the upper portion of the stomach, and a band is place around this area (**Fig. 3**). Additionally, a subcutaneous port is placed, which allows for sequential instillations of saline to constrict the opening to the upper stomach. Through a variety of feedback loops the patient has a sense of fullness with the goal of limiting the amount of food consumed.

Duodenal Switch

The essential steps of a duodenal switch (DS) are that a sleeve is created much like an SG, and the duodenum is divided just distal to the pylorus (**Fig. 4**). The ileum is divided at a set measurement back from the ileocecal valve and anastomosed to the duodenal stump. The biliary limb is then reimplanted at a specific distance from the ileocecal valve.

SHORT-TERM OUTCOMES
Mortality

Elective weight loss procedures should optimize perioperative mortality and increase long-term life expectancy. The 30-day mortality for all procedures is less than 1%.[10] Mortality has been shown to be slightly higher for RNYGB when compared with SG

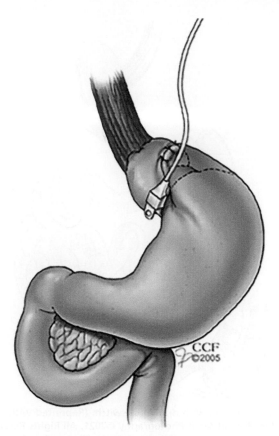

Fig. 3. Adjustable gastric band. (Reprinted with permission, Cleveland Clinic Center for Medical Art & Photography ©2021. All Rights Reserved.)

(0.14%–0.20% vs 0.10%).[11,12] Mortality following adjustable gastric band (AGB) is 0.05%.[11] Mortality following DS ranges from 0% to 1.1%.[13,14]

Bleeding

Postoperative bleeding in bariatric surgery can occur in several locations including intraluminal, intra-abdominal, or at the port sites. It most commonly occurs at staple lines when larger staples are unable to provide adequate compression of smaller vessels. It presents with tachycardia, melena, or hematemesis, and potentially hypotension. Laboratory values show a reduced hemoglobin and hematocrit. Bleeding is treated via correction of coagulopathy; transfusions; endoscopic therapy; and if all else fails, return to surgery. RNYGB has a postoperative hemorrhage rate of 1.11%, compared with 2.5% for SG and 2.1% for DS. Bleeding following AGB is low (0.05%).[11,15–18]

Leak

Anastomotic leak is a life-threatening complication that must be identified and managed immediately. In general leaks present in the first few days up to several weeks after surgery and are hailed by tachycardia, abdominal pain, and fever. Risk factors for postoperative leaks for all procedures include oxygen use, malnutrition, OSA, HTN, and diabetes. Unique to RNYGB leaks are such factors as open surgery, revisional surgery,

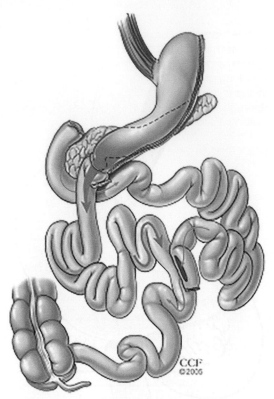

Fig. 4. Biliopancreatic diversion with duodenal switch. (Reprinted with permission, Cleveland Clinic Center for Medical Art & Photography ©2021. All Rights Reserved.)

and routine drain placement.[12,19,20] Using MBSAQIP data, leak rates of RNYGB were found to be 1.2%.[21] Leak rate after SG ranges from 0.1% to 2.4%.[12,22,23] Leak rate after DS ranges from 1.6% to 5%.[20,24] As an analogous measure of leak for Laparoscopic Adjustable Gastric Band (LAGB), esophageal/gastric perforation during band placement is incredibly rare with only a few case reports published.

Unique to RNYGB and DS are leaks at the jejunojejunostomy. Jejunojejunostomy leaks account for 10% of the total presenting postoperative leaks in the larger series looking at post–weight loss surgery leaks.[25] In general, leaks at the jejunojejunostomy are associated with a higher mortality (up to 40%) than leaks at the gastro/duodenojejunostomy and this is thought to be caused by the slow progression of the symptoms and the often delayed diagnosis.[25]

Venous Thromboembolic Events

Deep venous thrombosis and pulmonary embolism are commonly shared entities among all weight loss surgery procedures. These events are estimated to occur at a rate of 0.42% within 90 days postoperatively and are more likely to occur in RNYGB.[26] Venous thromboembolism was also associated with open approach, age, male sex, and greater preoperative BMI.

Additionally, mesenteric venous thrombosis, mainly superior mesenteric vein thrombosis, can occur with SG. Rates are generally reported at 0.37% to 1%, but some authors believe this is underreported because patients may not seek medical attention for mild abdominal pain following SG.[27,28]

Bowel Obstruction

Immediate postoperative bowel obstructions following weight loss surgery are generally technical issues. The most common reason for early bowel obstruction after RNYGB is an early internal hernia, stricture of the mesocolic closure if the Roux limb is retrocolic, or kinking of the jejunostomy. Likewise, for DS the cause is an early internal hernia or kinking of the jejunoileostomy. SG and LAGB have low rates of postoperative bowel obstruction and they are related to port site hernias or hernias involving the band tubing. Rates of early bowel obstruction for RNYGB are reported between 0.017% and 1.7%.[29-31] Early bowel obstruction is so rare for SG and AGB that no substantial data exist to define precise frequency.

Readmission

Reasons for readmission following weight loss surgery can vary from dehydration to more serious complications, such as leak, pulmonary embolism, or cardiac reasons. Readmissions are closely tracked and trended among most weight loss programs and are a general subject of performance improvement programs. Decreasing Readmissions Through Opportunities Provided (DROP) was a program developed by the Metabolic and Bariatric Surgery Quality Improvement Program (MBSAQIP). The DROP program focused on preventable readmissions, such as nausea, vomiting, and dehydration, and laid a foundation for programs to proactively manage these issues and prevent readmission. Reported overall rates of 30-day readmission for each procedure are 6.47% to 7.17% for RNYGB, 4.25% to 5.4% for SG, 3% to 5% for biliopancreatic diversion (BPD), and 1.71% to 3.05% for AGB.[11,32-34]

Reoperation

Reoperations following weight loss surgery have several causes. Bleeding and leak remain two of the most common reasons patient need to return to the operating room. Other common reasons are bowel obstruction, wound complication, slipped band, and many other complications. Reoperation rates for RNYGB range from 0.7% to 5.02%.[11,20,35] Reoperation rate for SG is 2.97%, AGB is 0.9%, and DS is 3.3%.[11,16,20]

LONG-TERM OUTCOMES
Weight Loss

One essential metric for success of a bariatric procedure is the amount of weight lost and whether or not that weight loss is sustained. The standardized method for measuring weight loss is percentage of excess body weight lost (EWL). The magnitude of postoperative weight loss is multifactorial and sustaining weight loss is a common problem. The current available literature reports outcomes for long-term follow-up (more than 10 years) for the major weight loss procedures. RNYGB remains the gold standard for comparison because of the sheer number of patients combined with the number of patients with prospectively collected long-term follow-up. Ten-year EWL for RNYGB ranges from 52% to 56%.[36,37] SG boasts a 10-year EWL of 53.2%.[37,38] Long-term follow-up studies for patients with LAGB show EWL as 27%.[39] Ten-year weight loss after DS remains around 68%.[14]

Survival

Long-term survival benefits are seen in patients who have opted for surgical management of obesity when compared with medical treatment and lifestyle changes. There is no clear-cut weight loss procedure that accounts for a better survival advantage. Most studies have focused on populations of patients who undergo weight loss surgery and not individual procedures. Overall remission of comorbidities, such as HTN and diabetes, seems to be the best predictor of longer-term survival, but reduction in cancer rates may be caused by actual weight loss and decrease in inflammation.[40]

Remission of Comorbidities (Diabetes Mellitus, Gastroesophageal Reflux Disease, Obstructive Sleep Apnea, Hypertension)

Diabetes is almost six times more prevalent among obese patients than normal-weight individuals.[41] Patients with BMI greater than 40 have coexisting diabetes at a rate of 25% to 27%.[42] Rates of complete diabetes remission in RNYGB are 83% for people with diabetes who are not dependent on insulin.[1] The rates of remission and improvement are based on the severity of the diabetes, and in general the amount of insulin patients consume. The most robust long-term follow-up, remissions rates, and discontinuance rates of insulin are found in patients who undergo RNYGB. Schauer and colleagues[43] published a randomized controlled trial of RNYGB or vertical SG (VSG) versus medical management for treatment of diabetes. They found that 29% of patients who underwent RNYGB and 23% who had VSG had glycated hemoglobin of less than 6.0 versus 5% in the medical treatment arm.[43] This paper has been one of the few papers to date that has compared treatment in a head-to-head randomized manner of surgical versus medical management of diabetes. Comparing the diabetes remission rates among RNYGB, DS, VSG, and AGB and which one is superior remains a challenge because little data exist on quality head-to-head trials comparing one with the other. As such, RNYGB is considered the gold standard for weight loss surgery because other procedures are compared with it to ensure the match up (noninferiority) to the remission and improvement rates seen in RNYGB.

GERD is an interesting disease to study in the context of bariatric surgery because it is improved by some procedures and exacerbated by others. Bypass procedures that create small gastric pouches remove most acid-producing parietal cells and divert flow from the pylorus, which reduces backpressure in the stomach. Conversely, the VSG retains an amount of parietal cell mass and reduces the volume in the stomach while preserving the pylorus, creating a high-pressure cylinder. With RNYGB, 50% to 70% of patients experience resolution of GERD.[11,44] After LAGB, GERD remission is shown to be 64%.[11] However, 50% to 84% of patients with preoperative GERD continue to experience symptoms after SG and 8.6% of patients without GERD preoperatively go on to develop it after SG.[11,45]

OSA is a disorder heavily associated with obesity, such that a 10% gain in weight conferred a six-fold increase in the odds of developing OSA.[46] In a retrospective study of patients undergoing bariatric surgery, routine screening identified an additional 25% of patients having previously undiagnosed OSA.[47] A 2013 meta-analysis showed remission rates of OSA after RNYGB, LSG, BPD, and LAGB to be 66% to 73%, 62% to 72%, 82.3%, and 38% to 70.5%, respectively.[11,48]

Obese patients are almost three times as likely to have HTN than normal-weight individuals.[41] HTN is present in approximately 49% to 51% of patients with BMI greater than 40.[42] After RNYGB, 46% to 79% of patients have remission of HTN, and this was achieved within the first month postoperatively.[11,49] After SG and LAGB, remission of HTN was achieved in 38.8% to 68% and 44% of patients, respectively.[11,50] In a single-center, BPD was shown to reduce SBP by a mean of 14% as compared with 9% by RNYGB.[51]

Marginal Ulcer

Marginal ulcers are complications that occur in RNYGB and DS patients. They arise secondary to acidic injury to the jejunal side of the gastro/duodenojejunostomy

(1.2%–2.3%).[52,53] One retrospective review found the risk of marginal ulcer in RNYGB to be higher than that of DS, 1.2% versus 0.3%, respectively.[20] Patients with marginal ulcers present with post-prandial abdominal pain, nausea, vomiting, gastrointestinal bleeding, or perforation. Modifiable risk factors for the development of ulcers include smoking, steroid use, nonsteroidal anti-inflammatory drug use, and *Helicobacter pylori* infection. Mean time after surgery to diagnose marginal ulcers is 15 months.[53] Without routine proton pump inhibitor use, ulcer rate can rise to 3.5% to 4%.[54,55] Diagnosis is generally made based on symptoms along with endoscopic screening. Treatment includes cessation of the offending agenda and medical treatment with proton pump inhibitor and *H pylori* eradication if indicated. In cases of perforation or persistent pain or bleeding refractory to medical management, surgical revision is indicated.

Anastomotic Stricture

Anastomotic stenosis is a complication defined by an inability to tolerate oral intake in the setting of anastomotic narrowing, usually to the extent of less than 10 mm.[56] The cause is likely multifactorial, relating to tissue ischemia and inflammation and anastomotic tension and even chronic ulcer disease. The rates of anastomotic stenosis following RNYGB has been reported to be anywhere between 2.6% and 20%, and is dependent on many factors to include type and size of anastomosis performed.[8,57,58] Clinically a stricture presents weeks to months after surgery with nausea, vomiting, dysphagia, and oral intolerance. It is diagnosed and treated with endoscopy and serial balloon dilations. However, if these are not successful, the anastomosis requires surgical revision. Strictures do occur following VSG and DS, but rates are difficult to determine because of the lower incidence and the ill-defined nature of the terminology. Often times stricture of a VSG is reported as dysphagia and not as a technical problem, such as stricture of the sleeve.

Internal Hernia

Internal hernias are a complication of particular interest in RNYGB and DS patients. Controversy exists among the best route of the Roux limb in an RNYGB. Some surgeons perform a retrocolic Roux limb, whereas others an antecolic. Meta-analysis found that 1.4% of patients with an antecolic Roux limb experienced bowel obstructions compared with 5.2% of patients with a retrocolic Roux limb.[59] This finding is substantiated by a retrospective study that found the transverse mesocolon defect to be the most common site of internal herniation.[60]

The new anatomy established by the procedure creates two or three new defects through which herniation can occur depending on whether the Roux limb is placed antecolic or retrocolic. These include:

1. Defect in the mesentery of the jejunojejunostomy
2. Petersen defect, the space between the transverse colon and Roux limb
3. If the retrocolic approach is taken in RNYGB, an additional defect is created in the transverse mesocolon

In a multicenter, randomized trial investigating mesenteric closure, incidence of reoperation because of small bowel obstruction was significantly reduced in the mesenteric closure group.[61] However, closure of the defects increased the risk of postoperative complications likely caused by kinking of the jejunojejunostomy and narrowing of mesocolon around the retrocolic Roux limb.[61] Internal hernias are usually diagnosed by history and physical examination. When the history and physical are not revealing, a computed tomography scan with oral and intravenous contrast is done as an adjunct to aid in the diagnosis. Patients with suspicion or confirmed diagnosis of internal hernia should be taken to the operating room for reduction of the hernia and repair of the defects.

Nutritional Deficiencies

Because of the malabsorptive nature of RNYGB and BPD, patients undergoing these procedures are at risk for nutritional deficiencies. Specifically, patients have difficulty maintaining adequate levels of iron, vitamins B_{12} and D, folate, and thiamine.[62–71] Macronutrient deficiencies are rare following RNYGB. RNYGB patients develop nutritional complications at a rate of 2.1%.[20] DS has low vitamin complications (4%) but can have protein malnutrition rates of 20%.[63] SG and LAGB are purely restrictive procedures and thereby harbor minimal inherent risk of malnourishment; however, this complication is still a possibility depending on the patient's eating habits and food choices. Correction of nutritional deficiencies in RNYGB patients is generally limited to vitamin and protein supplementation (**Table 1**).

DISCUSSION

Over the past 40 years RNYGB has become the gold standard for weight loss surgery. It should still be considered the gold standard because of the vast amount of data regarding outcomes. When other procedures are developed and studied, they should be compared with RNYGB. When contemplating best approaches for patients, the baseline RNYGB data should be quoted because of the vast data available. Patients should be presented other procedures in light of the RNYGB and allowed to make educated choices regarding best procedure for them based on all available data. Surgeons should also compare their own personal outcomes with that of the published RNYGB outcomes.

Table 1
Summary of outcomes

	Bariatric Procedure (%)			
	RNYGB	SG	BPD	LAGB
Short-term outcomes				
Mortality	0.14–0.2	0.1–0.11	0–1.1	0.05
Bleeding	0.4–1.11	0.6–2.5	0.4–2.1	0–0.05
Leak	1–1.6	0.1–2.4	1.5–5	Rare
Readmission	6.47–7.17	4.25–5.4	3–5	1.71–3.05
Reoperation	0.7–5.02	2.97	0.9–0.92	3.30
Long-term outcomes				
Weight loss	52–56	52.30	67.90	27
Marginal ulcer	1.2–2.3	—	0.30	—
Nutritional deficiencies	2.10	—	4.10	—
Effect on comorbidities				
GERD	5–70	16–50	—	64
OSA	66–73	62–72	82.30	38–70.5
HTN	46–79	38.8–68	—	44

CLINICS CARE POINTS

- RNYGB has been the gold standard bariatric procedure for more than 20 years.
- Surgical alternatives to the bypass include SG, BPD with duodenal switch, and adjustable gastric band.
- RNYGB and BPD have higher perioperative complication rates than SG and LAGB.
- Some complications are specific to RNYGB and BPD as compared with SG and LAGB, such as internal hernia, marginal ulcer, and anastomotic stricture/stenosis.
- RNYGB and BPD have higher percentage of EWL compared with SG and LAGB.
- There is no clear evidence to suggest long-term survival benefit of one bariatric procedure over the others.
- All bariatric surgeries provide improvement in comorbidities to varying degrees except in the case of GERD, in which SG can worsen or even hasten symptoms.
- RNYGB continues to be the gold standard by which all bariatric procedures should be compared.

DISCLOSURE

None.

REFERENCES

1. Pories WJ, Swanson MS, MacDonald KG, et al. Who would have thought it? An operation proves to be the most effective therapy for adult-onset diabetes mellitus. Ann Surg 1995;222(3):339–52.
2. Sjöström L, Narbro K, Sjöström CD, et al. Effects of bariatric surgery on mortality in Swedish obese subjects. N Engl J Med 2007;357(8):741–52.
3. Colquitt JL, Pickett K, Loveman E, et al. Surgery for weight loss in adults. Cochrane Database Syst Rev 2014;(8):CD003641.
4. Mechanick JI, Youdim A, Jones DB, et al. Clinical practice guidelines for the perioperative nutritional, metabolic, and nonsurgical support of the bariatric surgery patient–2013 update: cosponsored by American Association of Clinical Endocrinologists, The Obesity Society, and American Society for Metabolic & Bariatric Surgery. Obesity (Silver Spring) 2013;21(Suppl 1 0 1):S1–27.
5. Who is a Candidate for Bariatric Surgery?: American Society for Metabolic and Bariatric Surgery. 2020. Available at: https://asmbs.org/patients/who-is-a-candidate-for-bariatric-surgery. Accessed October 1, 2020.
6. Mahawar KK, Kumar P, Parmar C, et al. Small bowel limb lengths and Roux-en-Y gastric bypass: a systematic review. Obes Surg 2016;26(3):660–71.
7. Giordano S, Salminen P, Biancari F, et al. Linear stapler technique may be safer than circular in gastrojejunal anastomosis for laparoscopic Roux-en-Y gastric bypass: a meta-analysis of comparative studies. Obes Surg 2011;21(12):1958–64.
8. Lee S, Davies AR, Bahal S, et al. Comparison of gastrojejunal anastomosis techniques in laparoscopic Roux-en-Y gastric bypass: gastrojejunal stricture rate and effect on subsequent weight loss. Obes Surg 2014;24(9):1425–9.
9. Jiang HP, Lin LL, Jiang X, et al. Meta-analysis of hand-sewn versus mechanical gastrojejunal anastomosis during laparoscopic Roux-en-Y gastric bypass for morbid obesity. Int J Surg 2016;32:150–7.

10. DeMaria EJ, Pate V, Warthen M, et al. Baseline data from American Society for Metabolic and Bariatric surgery-designated bariatric surgery centers of excellence using the bariatric outcomes longitudinal database. Surg Obes Relat Dis 2010;6(4):347–55.

11. Hutter MM, Schirmer BD, Jones DB, et al. First report from the American College of Surgeons Bariatric Surgery Center Network: laparoscopic sleeve gastrectomy has morbidity and effectiveness positioned between the band and the bypass. Ann Surg 2011;254(3):410–22.

12. Kumar SB, Hamilton BC, Wood SG, et al. Is laparoscopic sleeve gastrectomy safer than laparoscopic gastric bypass? A comparison of 30-day complications using the MBSAQIP data registry. Surg Obes Relat Dis 2018;14(3):264–9.

13. Buchwald H, Avidor Y, Braunwald E, et al. Bariatric surgery: a systematic review and meta-analysis. JAMA 2004;292(14):1724–37 [published correction appears in JAMA. 2005 Apr 13;293(14):1728].

14. Sethi M, Chau E, Youn A, et al. Long-term outcomes after biliopancreatic diversion with and without duodenal switch: 2-, 5-, and 10-year data. Surg Obes Relat Dis 2016;12(9):1697–705.

15. Mocanu V, Dang J, Ladak F, et al. Predictors and outcomes of bleed after sleeve gastrectomy: an analysis of the MBSAQIP data registry. Surg Obes Relat Dis 2019;15(10):1675–81.

16. Lancaster RT, Hutter MM. Bands and bypasses: 30-day morbidity and mortality of bariatric surgical procedures as assessed by prospective, multi-center, risk-adjusted ACS-NSQIP data. Surg Endosc 2008;22(12):2554–63.

17. Biertho L, Simon-Hould F, Marceau S, et al. Current outcomes of laparoscopic duodenal switch. Ann Surg Innov Res 2016;10:1.

18. Zilberstein B, Santo MA, Carvalho MH. Critical analysis of surgical treatment techniques of morbid obesity. Arq Bras Cir Dig 2019;32(3):e1450.

19. Smith MD, Adeniji A, Wahed AS, et al. Technical factors associated with anastomotic leak after Roux-en-Y gastric bypass. Surg Obes Relat Dis 2015;11(2): 313–20.

20. Nelson DW, Blair KS, Martin MJ. Analysis of obesity-related outcomes and bariatric failure rates with the duodenal switch vs gastric bypass for morbid obesity. Arch Surg 2012;147(9):847–54.

21. Alizadeh RF, Li S, Inaba C, et al. Risk factors for gastrointestinal leak after bariatric surgery: MBASQIP Analysis. J Am Coll Surg 2018;227(1):135–41.

22. Alvarenga ES, Lo Menzo E, Szomstein S, et al. Safety and efficacy of 1020 consecutive laparoscopic sleeve gastrectomies performed as a primary treatment modality for morbid obesity. A single-center experience from the metabolic and bariatric surgical accreditation quality and improvement program. Surg Endosc 2016;30(7):2673–8.

23. Aurora AR, Khaitan L, Saber AA. Sleeve gastrectomy and the risk of leak: a systematic analysis of 4,888 patients. Surg Endosc 2012;26(6):1509–15.

24. Hedberg J, Sundström J, Sundbom M. Duodenal switch versus Roux-en-Y gastric bypass for morbid obesity: systematic review and meta-analysis of weight results, diabetes resolution and early complications in single-centre comparisons. Obes Rev 2014;15(7):555–63.

25. Lee S, Carmody B, Wolfe L, et al. Effect of location and speed of diagnosis on anastomotic leak outcomes in 3828 gastric bypass cases. J Gastrointest Surg 2007;11(6):708–13.

26. Winegar DA, Sherif B, Pate V, et al. Venous thromboembolism after bariatric surgery performed by bariatric surgery center of excellence participants: analysis of

the bariatric outcomes longitudinal database. Surg Obes Relat Dis 2011;7(2): 181–8.

27. Shaheen O, Siejka J, Thatigotla B, et al. A systematic review of portomesenteric vein thrombosis after sleeve gastrectomy. Surg Obes Relat Dis 2017;13(8): 1422–31.

28. Shoar S, Saber AA, Rubenstein R, et al. Portomesentric and splenic vein thrombosis (PMSVT) after bariatric surgery: a systematic review of 110 patients. Surg Obes Relat Dis 2018;14(1):47–59.

29. Shimizu H, Maia M, Kroh M, et al. Surgical management of early small bowel obstruction after laparoscopic Roux-en-Y gastric bypass. Surg Obes Relat Dis 2013;9(5):718–24.

30. Podnos YD, Jimenez JC, Wilson SE, et al. Complications after laparoscopic gastric bypass: a review of 3464 cases. Arch Surg 2003;138(9):957–61.

31. Khoraki J, Mazzini GS, Shah AS, et al. Early small bowel obstruction after laparoscopic gastric bypass: a surgical emergency. Surg Obes Relat Dis 2018;14(8): 1118–25.

32. Garg T, Rosas U, Rogan D, et al. Characterizing readmissions after bariatric surgery. J Gastrointest Surg 2016;20(11):1797–801.

33. Antanavicius G, Katsichtis T, Alswealmeen W, et al. Three hundred four robotically assisted biliopancreatic diversion with duodenal switch operations with gradual robotic approach implementation: short-term outcomes, complication profile, and lessons learned. Obes Surg 2020;30(10):3961–7.

34. Polega JR, Barreto TW, Kemmeter KD, et al. A matched cohort study of laparoscopic biliopancreatic diversion with duodenal switch and sleeve gastrectomy performed by one surgeon. Surg Obes Relat Dis 2017;13(3):411–4.

35. Jones KB Jr, Afram JD, Benotti PN, et al. Open versus laparoscopic Roux-en-Y gastric bypass: a comparative study of over 25,000 open cases and the major laparoscopic bariatric reported series. Obes Surg 2006;16(6):721–7.

36. Mehaffey JH, LaPar DJ, Clement KC, et al. 10-year outcomes after Roux-en-Y gastric bypass. Ann Surg 2016;264(1):121–6.

37. Jiménez A, Ibarzabal A, Moizé V, et al. Ten-year outcomes after Roux-en-Y gastric bypass and sleeve gastrectomy: an observational nonrandomized cohort study. Surg Obes Relat Dis 2019;15(3):382–8.

38. Bohdjalian A, Langer FB, Shakeri-Leidenmühler S, et al. Sleeve gastrectomy as sole and definitive bariatric procedure: 5-year results for weight loss and ghrelin. Obes Surg 2010;20(5):535–40.

39. Kowalewski PK, Olszewski R, Kwiatkowski A, et al. Life with a gastric band. long-term outcomes of laparoscopic adjustable gastric banding-a retrospective study. Obes Surg 2017;27(5):1250–3.

40. Kim J, Eisenberg D, Azagury D, et al. American Society for Metabolic and Bariatric Surgery position statement on long-term survival benefit after metabolic and bariatric surgery. Surg Obes Relat Dis 2016;12(3):453–9.

41. Nguyen NT, Magno CP, Lane KT, et al. Association of hypertension, diabetes, dyslipidemia, and metabolic syndrome with obesity: findings from the National Health and Nutrition Examination Survey, 1999 to 2004. J Am Coll Surg 2008; 207(6):928–34.

42. Bays HE, Chapman RH, Grandy S, SHIELD Investigators' Group. The relationship of body mass index to diabetes mellitus, hypertension and dyslipidaemia: comparison of data from two national surveys. Int J Clin Pract 2007;61(5):737–47 [published correction appears in Int J Clin Pract. 2007 Oct;61(10):1777-8].

43. Schauer PR, Kashyap SR, Wolski K, et al. Bariatric surgery versus intensive medical therapy in obese patients with diabetes. N Engl J Med 2012;366(17): 1567–76.

44. Madalosso CA, Gurski RR, Callegari-Jacques SM, et al. The impact of gastric bypass on gastroesophageal reflux disease in morbidly obese patients. Ann Surg 2016;263(1):110–6.

45. DuPree CE, Blair K, Steele SR, et al. Laparoscopic sleeve gastrectomy in patients with preexisting gastroesophageal reflux disease: a national analysis. JAMA Surg 2014;149(4):328–34.

46. Peppard PE, Young T, Palta M, et al. Longitudinal study of moderate weight change and sleep-disordered breathing. JAMA 2000;284(23):3015–21.

47. Nepomnayshy D, Hesham W, Erickson B, et al. Sleep apnea: is routine preoperative screening necessary? Obes Surg 2013;23(3):287–91.

48. Sarkhosh K, Switzer NJ, El-Hadi M, et al. The impact of bariatric surgery on obstructive sleep apnea: a systematic review. Obes Surg 2013;23(3):414–23.

49. Schiavon CA, Bersch-Ferreira AC, Santucci EV, et al. Effects of bariatric surgery in obese patients with hypertension: the GATEWAY randomized trial (gastric bypass to treat obese patients with steady hypertension). Circulation 2018; 137(11):1132–42 [published correction appears in circulation. 2019;140(14): e718].

50. Zhang N, Maffei A, Cerabona T, et al. Reduction in obesity-related comorbidities: is gastric bypass better than sleeve gastrectomy? Surg Endosc 2013;27(4): 1273–80.

51. Mingrone G, Panunzi S, De Gaetano A, et al. Bariatric surgery versus conventional medical therapy for type 2 diabetes. N Engl J Med 2012;366(17):1577–85.

52. Bekhali Z, Sundbom M. Low risk for marginal ulcers in duodenal switch and gastric bypass in a well-defined cohort of 472 patients. Obes Surg 2020; 30(11):4422–7.

53. Moon RC, Teixeira AF, Goldbach M, et al. Management and treatment outcomes of marginal ulcers after Roux-en-Y gastric bypass at a single high volume bariatric center. Surg Obes Relat Dis 2014;10(2):229–34.

54. Dallal RM, Bailey LA. Ulcer disease after gastric bypass surgery. Surg Obes Relat Dis 2006;2(4):455–9.

55. Gumbs AA, Duffy AJ, Bell RL. Incidence and management of marginal ulceration after laparoscopic Roux-Y gastric bypass. Surg Obes Relat Dis 2006;2(4):460–3.

56. Ukleja A, Afonso BB, Pimentel R, et al. Outcome of endoscopic balloon dilation of strictures after laparoscopic gastric bypass. Surg Endosc 2008;22(8):1746–50.

57. Schneider BE, Villegas L, Blackburn GL, et al. Laparoscopic gastric bypass surgery: outcomes. J Laparoendosc Adv Surg Tech A 2003;13(4):247–55.

58. Nguyen NT, Goldman C, Rosenquist CJ, et al. Laparoscopic versus open gastric bypass: a randomized study of outcomes, quality of life, and costs. Ann Surg 2001;234(3):279–91.

59. Al Harakeh AB, Kallies KJ, Borgert AJ, et al. Bowel obstruction rates in antecolic/antegastric versus retrocolic/retrogastric Roux limb gastric bypass: a meta-analysis. Surg Obes Relat Dis 2016;12(1):194–8.

60. Higa KD, Ho T, Boone KB. Internal hernias after laparoscopic Roux-en-Y gastric bypass: incidence, treatment and prevention. Obes Surg 2003;13(3):350–4.

61. Stenberg E, Szabo E, Ågren G, et al. Closure of mesenteric defects in laparoscopic gastric bypass: a multicentre, randomised, parallel, open-label trial. Lancet 2016;387(10026):1397–404.

62. Tucker O, Szomstein S, Rosenthal R. Nutritional consequences of weight-loss surgery. Med Clin North Am 2007;91(3):499.
63. Lupoli R, Lembo E, Saldalamacchia G, et al. Bariatric surgery and long-term nutritional issues. World J Diabetes 2017;8(11):464–74.
64. Faria GR. A brief history of bariatric surgery. Porto Biomed J 2017;2(3):90–2.
65. Pratt JSA, Browne A, Browne NT, et al. ASMBS pediatric metabolic and bariatric surgery guidelines. Surg Obes Relat Dis 2018;14(7):882–901.
66. Doraiswamy A, Rasmussen JJ, Pierce J, et al. The utility of routine postoperative upper GI series following laparoscopic gastric bypass. Surg Endosc 2007; 21(12):2159–62.
67. White S, Han SH, Lewis C, et al. Selective approach to use of upper gastroesophageal imaging study after laparoscopic Roux-en-Y gastric bypass. Surg Obes Relat Dis 2008;4(2):122–5.
68. Nguyen NT, Huerta S, Gelfand D, et al. Bowel obstruction after laparoscopic Roux-en-Y gastric bypass. Obes Surg 2004;14(2):190–6.
69. Escalona A, Devaud N, Pérez G, et al. Antecolic versus retrocolic alimentary limb in laparoscopic Roux-en-Y gastric bypass: a comparative study. Surg Obes Relat Dis 2007;3(4):423–7.
70. Courcoulas AP, Goodpaster BH, Eagleton JK, et al. Surgical vs medical treatments for type 2 diabetes mellitus: a randomized clinical trial. JAMA Surg 2014;149(7):707–15.
71. Hickey MS, Pories WJ, MacDonald KG Jr, et al. A new paradigm for type 2 diabetes mellitus: could it be a disease of the foregut? Ann Surg 1998;227(5): 637–44.

Laparoscopic Vertical Sleeve Gastrectomy

Kevin Climaco, MD*, Eric Ahnfeldt, DO

KEYWORDS

• Sleeve • Gastrectomy • Background • Evidence • Technique • Pearls • Pitfalls

KEY POINTS

• Vertical sleeve gastrectomy is a simple, safe, and effective surgical option for obesity.
• Risk of GERD, portal vein thrombosis, strictures, leak, and bleeding are specific considerations in VSG.
• There are key preoperative, perioperative, and postoperative aspects to VSG that every surgeon must know.

OBESITY AND SURGERY

Bariatric surgery has emerged as the most effective means of achieving weight loss, and all of its associated health benefits.[1] According to an obesity expert panel from the American College of Cardiology and American Heart Association, intensive lifestyle changes, such as a reduced-calorie diet, increased physical activity, and behavior therapy, led to an average weight loss of 8 kg at 1 year, whereas commercial-based lifestyle interventions averaged 6.6 to 10 kg at 1 year. Only 35% to 60% of the people who underwent such lifestyle changes maintained a weight loss of greater than 5% of their initial weight at 2 years.[2] Bariatric surgery produces more medically significant and long-lasting weight loss.[1,3,4]

Today, the most commonly performed primary bariatric surgery in the United States is the laparoscopic vertical sleeve gastrectomy (VSG), which accounted for 61.4% of bariatric surgeries in 2018. This number was up from 17.8% in 2011. The second most commonly performed surgery is the laparoscopic Roux-en-Y gastric bypass (RYGB), which accounted for 17% of surgeries in 2018, down from 36.7% in 2011.[5] Other surgical options include the duodenal switch, single anastomosis duodenoileal bypass (SADI), gastric band, gastric balloon, and multiple endoluminal procedures.[1,2,6]

William Beaumont Army Medical Center, General Surgery Department, 18511 Highlander Medics Street, Fort Bliss, TX 79918, USA
* Corresponding author.
E-mail address: Kevin.a.climaco@gmail.com
Twitter: @docKJ57 (K.C.); @AhnfeldtEric (E.A.)

Surg Clin N Am 101 (2021) 177–188
https://doi.org/10.1016/j.suc.2020.12.015
0039-6109/21/Published by Elsevier Inc.

LAPAROSCOPIC VERTICAL SLEEVE GASTRECTOMY

VSG was initially part of the biliopancreatic diversion with duodenal switch procedure that Douglas Hess devised in 1988.[7] It was not until 11 years later that De Csepel and coworkers[8] performed the duodenal switch laparoscopically. Unfortunately, the laparoscopic duodenal switch was associated with significant complications, especially in patients with high body mass index.[9,10] Thus, Gagner chose to perform a staged duodenal switch, with the VSG being the first step of the procedure. His modification was met with good results, resulting in a 33% average excess body weight loss from this first stage alone. These findings, coupled with promising findings from the Magenstrasse and Mill operation (the decreasing of gastric volume without resection),[11] demonstrated that sleeve gastrectomies may be a viable option as a stand-alone bariatric procedure.[12] In 2012, the American Society for Metabolic and Bariatric Surgery (ASMBS) published a position statement that recognized VSG as an acceptable primary bariatric procedure.[3]

Mechanism of Action

Removing 70% to 80% of the stomach in VSG decreases gastric capacity and caloric intake, making satiety easier to achieve.[13] This restrictive mechanism was initially thought to be the only mechanism of action for VSG. However, emerging literature has shown that the procedure also has several hormonal effects. Decreased ghrelin production from removal of the fundus is one such hormonal reaction implicated with weight loss.[4,14,15] Ghrelin has been found to increase hunger via action on the hypothalamus,[13] and it has also been implicated in the inhibition of insulin.[16–18] VSG is also believed to affect glucagon-like-peptide-1 production. This hormone has antiorexigenic effects and delays gastric emptying.[19,20] VSG has been found to increase the expression of glucagon-like-peptide-1 in the jejunum and ileum.[21,22] Additionally, peptide YY and pancreatic polypeptide are exaggerated after sleeve gastrectomies, leading to decreased hunger and food intake (**Fig. 1**).[23–28]

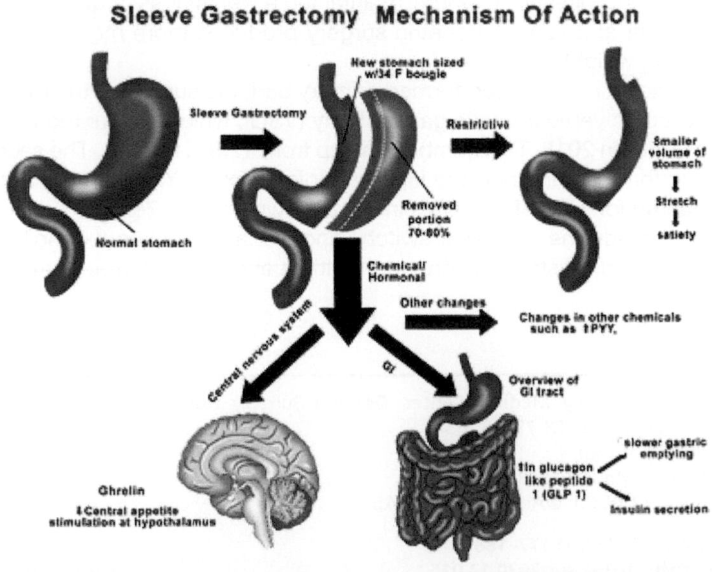

Fig. 1. Overview of VSG mechanisms of action. GI, gastrointestinal.

Weight Loss After Surgery

VSG leads to an average excess body weight loss of about 60% at 5 years and beyond, showing effectiveness and sustainability.[10–12] These same studies have demonstrated that VSG and RYGB have similar weight loss at 1, 4, and 5 years.

Comorbidities

Bariatric surgery is associated with a 19.5% risk difference (that is the relative risk difference between surgical therapy and medical management alone) for hypertension remission. The risk difference for diabetes remission was measured at 42.7%.[29] With specific regards to diabetes, the STAMPEDE trial by Schauer and colleagues[30] showed that the primary end goal of hemoglobulin A_{1c} of less than 6.0 was achieved in only 5% of patients undergoing medical therapy. Twenty-three percent of patients undergoing RYGB and 19% of those undergoing VSG reached this same end point. Several other well-designed, large retrospective studies (which combined looked at thousands of bariatric surgery patients) further support bariatric surgery's positive effects on comorbidities to a significant degree. These findings were reproduced for dyslipidemias, renal function, arthralgia, obstructive sleep apnea, hyperuricemia, depression, and quality-of-life scores.[31–33]

Vertical Sleeve Gastrectomy Versus Roux-en-Y Gastric Bypass

The benefits of VSG have been well-established in the literature. VSG is much simpler relative to an RYGB from a technical aspect, has decreased operative time, and is associated with significantly fewer major complications within 30 days of surgery.[34] A look at the National Surgical Quality Improvement Program data shows that mean operative times (101 vs 131 minutes; $P<.01$), blood loss requiring transfusion (0.6% vs 1.5%; $P = .05$), serious morbidity rate (3.8% vs 5.8%; $P<.01$), and 30-day reoperation rate (1.6% vs 2.5%; $P<.01$) were all significantly lower in VSG than in RYGB.[35] The overall mortality associated with VSG ranged from 0% to 1.2%.[35]

A meta-analysis of long-term and midterm outcomes published in 2017 looked at 14 studies with more than 5000 patients and showed no statistical difference between a VSG and RYGB with regards to resolution of type 2 diabetes, hypertension, hyperlipidemia, and hypertriglyceridemia.[36]

Risks Associated with Vertical Sleeve Gastrectomy

Increased gastroesophageal reflux

The rate of gastroesophageal reflux disease (GERD) development and degree of postoperative severity in the VSG setting is difficult to quantify. The rate of de novo GERD ranged from 7.4% to 26.7%.[37,38] The exact degree of clinical significance varied, with some studies showing that most resolved with proton pump inhibitors alone.[33] Although some studies showed resolution of preexisting GERD symptoms with VSG in up to 15.9% to 64.7% of patients,[38,39] other patients demonstrated worsening symptoms and the need for revisional surgery given the severity of reflux.[40] Thus, it may be prudent to be more liberal in using preoperative manometry, especially if underlying esophageal dysfunction is a concern.

The ASMBS put out a position statement asserting that severe GERD symptoms and Barrett esophagus are relative contraindications to VSG.[3] As always, surgeons should thoroughly evaluate their own comfort with and ability to perform the procedure, and discuss the overall risks and benefits with the patient.

Portal vein thrombosis

Portal vein thrombosis is a known complication linked to laparoscopic VSG that is associated with mortality of 40%.[41] A study that looked at 5706 bariatric surgery patients found that 17 patients (0.29%) developed portal vein thrombosis. Sixteen of these 17 patients had undergone VSG.[42] Another retrospective study that looked at 5951 patients who underwent VSG demonstrated that 18 patients (0.3%) developed portal vein thrombosis.[43] Portal vein thrombosis is typically diagnosed with a computed tomography scan, and it is generally treated with anticoagulation.[41,43] However, the condition can also result in intra-abdominal catastrophe, requiring emergent laparotomy and bowel resection.

The exact action mechanism is complex, but it is attributed to a multitude of factors. The patient's baseline hypercoagulable state given their obesity, and endothelial injury with recent surgery (two of the three elements of Virchow triad) are contributing factors. Other proposed factors include CO_2 insufflation and anesthetics increasing intra-abdominal pressure, causing hemodynamic changes (specifically, decreased splanchnic and portal venous flow). Thermal effects during energy dissection of the gastroepiploic arcade possibly also contribute to this disease process.[44]

Weight regain

Weight regain can occur in all postoperative bariatric patients, including VSG patients. Five important factors identified in weight regain include

1. Nutritional noncompliance[45,46]
2. Hormonal/metabolic imbalance[45,47,48]
3. Mental health[45,47,49]
4. Physical inactivity[45,47,49]
5. Anatomic/surgical factors[45]

A study published in 2016 showed that removal of less than 500 mL of stomach is a predictor of treatment failure/early weight regain.[45] The size of the bougie used, incomplete resection of the fundus, and dilatation of the antrum are also surgical factors associated with weight regain after surgery.[45] Adequate follow-up after surgery, nutrition, and psychiatry, coupled with appropriate surgical technique, could help mitigate all of the previously mentioned factors.[47]

Leak

A systematic analysis of 4888 patients showed that the leak rate associated with VSG was 2.4%.[50] A meta-analysis looking at 40,653 VSG patients identified an overall leak rate of 1.5%,[51] with their reviewed papers citing a leak rate of 0.7% to 2.7%.

Expert opinion from the international VSG consensus conference in 2011 indicated that 77% of surgeons deemed buttressing as an acceptable adjunct[52]; however, the overall utility of buttressing for the specific purpose of decreasing leak rate is still under debate. Typical reinforcement adjuncts used include oversewing, nonabsorbable bovine pericardial strips, tissue sealant, and absorbable polymer membrane. A meta-analysis of 40,653 patients found that, of these adjuncts, the lowest leak rate occurred with absorbable polymer membrane (0.7%; $P<.007$).[51]

Bleeding

A meta-analysis published in 2015 looked at 41,864 postoperative gastrointestinal surgery patients for bleeding complications and identified a bleeding risk of 1.28% (bovine pericardium reinforcement) to 3.45% (no staple line reinforcement).[53] A separate study reviewed 98,142 patients and found that 623 of them had a postop hemorrhage (0.63%) with 181 needing reoperation (0.18%).[54] In this same paper, oversewing, or buttressing the staple line, was found to decrease the rate of postoperative hemorrhage by up to 30%. Risk factors associated with increased rates of hemorrhage were inexperience in bariatric surgery (odds ratio, 2.85) and lack of staple line reinforcement (odds ratio, 3.34). Decreased risk rates were identified in patients without obstructive sleep apnea (odds ratio, 0.22) and lack of hypertension (0.38).[55]

Stricture

Stricture rates ranged from 0% clinical stenosis[56] to 3.5%.[57] Stenosis is anatomic, via inflammation or aggressive surgical narrowing; or functional, via technique error (gastric twisting or incorrect angulation).[58] Management options for stenosis include endoscopic balloon dilation, stenting, and conversion to RYGB, depending on the cause.[56–58]

CONDUCT OF THE OPERATION (PREOPERATIVE, OPERATION, AND POSTOPERATIVE)
Preoperative and Postoperative Considerations

In 2016, ASMBS developed a comprehensive care pathway for laparoscopic sleeve gastrectomy.[59] Their routine recommendations are summarized in **Fig. 2**. Of note, other select considerations may be important based on specific patient factors.

Operative

Although many techniques have been described, we describe the technique used at our institution. The patient is positioned in the supine, arms-out position. Padding is

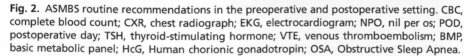

Routine Recommendations

Pre-operative:

- Routine Labs (CBC, BMP, A1c, Vitamins, HcG, TSH, Coag panel)
- OSA, age/gender appropriate malignancy screening), functional status, smoking, substance abuse
- Nutrition and Psychology Consult
- CXR and EKG
- Pre-operative liquid diet

Post-Operative:

- VTE and nausea prophylaxis
- NPO/ Clears on POD0, Bariatric Fulls on POD1
- Multimodal pain management
- Routine post-op visits
- Routine vitals, strict I/Os, +/- telemetry
- Proton Pump Inhibitor, Multivitamins
- Early Ambulation

Fig. 2. ASMBS routine recommendations in the preoperative and postoperative setting. CBC, complete blood count; CXR, chest radiograph; EKG, electrocardiogram; NPO, nil per os; POD, postoperative day; TSH, thyroid-stimulating hormone; VTE, venous thromboembolism; BMP, basic metabolic panel; HcG, Human chorionic gonadotropin; OSA, Obstructive Sleep Apnea.

placed over all pressure points and areas where nerve entrapment can occur (axilla, elbows, lateral knee). The patient is given antibiotic and deep venous thrombosis chemoprophylaxis before incision. Sequential Compression Devices (SCDs) are also placed before induction. Our typical trocar placement is presented in **Fig. 3**.

The liver is usually retracted, although that is not a necessity. This retraction is accomplished via a Nathanson retractor; a fan; a paddle; or through more novel means, such as magnets and suture. The patient is then placed in reverse Trendelenburg position. A suction bougie, measuring at least 34F catheter, is placed. This size is important, because smaller bougies, although with higher theoretic percent of removed stomach, have been associated with higher leak rates.[50,60–62]

The pylorus is then identified by pinpointing an area of muscular thickening in the distal stomach or by visualizing the prepyloric vein of Mayo (**Fig. 4**). An area 2 to 6 cm proximal to the pylorus is identified, so as to allow for proper gastric emptying and to avoid stenosis. The lesser sac is entered by dividing the vascular attachments (left gastroepiploics, short gastrics) along the greater curve using an energy device (**Fig. 5**).

The dissection is taken up to the level of the left crus. The hiatus is assessed and hiatal hernias are repaired.[60,63] The left crus must be cleared of all adherent stomach to reveal any hiatal hernia, and the angle of His clearly identified. Typically, hiatal hernias are missed posterior to the esophagus because of inadequate dissection of the left crus.

Using a laparoscopic stapler, gastric transection begins 2 to 6 cm from the pylorus and moves toward the angle of His. Buttressing the staple line has been shown to increase burst pressure and decrease bleeding risk, but it has not been shown to decrease leak rates.[64,65] Staples, their heights, and buttressing are evolving topics of discussion. At our institution, we use 4.1 mm/2 mm (open/closed height) buttressed

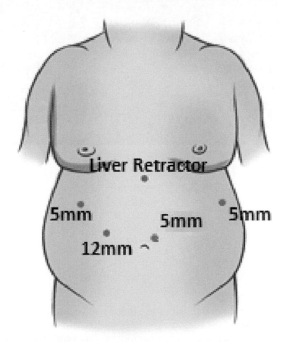

Fig. 3. Trocar placement and their respective sizes.

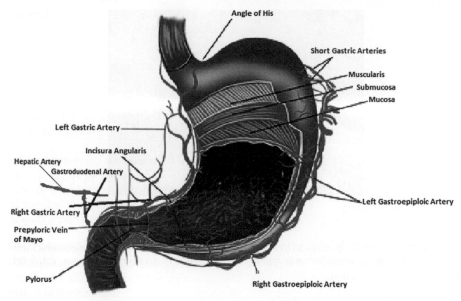

Fig. 4. Stomach anatomy.

staple loads near the pylorus, 3.8 mm/1.8 mm buttressed staple loads over the gastric body, and a 3.5 mm/1.5 mm unbuttressed load over the fundus (**Fig. 6**).

Although no correlation between leak testing and postoperative complications of a leak[66,67] has been identified, a leak test is a simple adjunct that can identify gross surgical errors/equipment failure at time of surgery. Endoscopy, methylene blue, and a suction bougie can all be used to perform a leak test.

The specimen is then extracted in a protected manner, the fascia is closed over the site of extraction, and the port sites are closed.

ROBOTIC VERTICAL SLEEVE GASTRECTOMY

Evidence or data regarding robotic VSG and how it compares with VSG are limited. The current thought is that, given the straightforward nature of VSG, the robot's

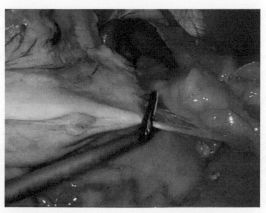

Fig. 5. Taking down of gastroepiploics using an energy device.

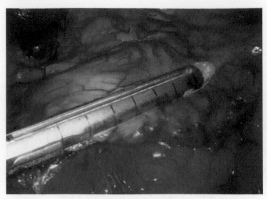

Fig. 6. Stomach stapling.

advantages are not truly realized in terms of increased room times and increased cost. However, as greater experience is gained on the platform and more data are obtained, this thought may change.

FUTURE STEPS/REVISIONAL SURGERY

VSG has proven to be an important surgical tool in the battle against obesity and its associated comorbidities. However, it is not without its issues. Refractory reflux and unintended weight regain are some problems that may warrant reoperation. In fact, the rate of reoperative bariatric surgery is increasing. A systematic review by the ASMBS shows that VSG to RYGB can be performed for patients who are good candidates for additional weight loss surgery.[68] Another emerging surgical technique is the SADI with sleeve gastrectomy. This surgery, as its name implies, involves a sleeve gastrectomy, division of the duodenum post-pylorically, and bringing up an ileal loop. A recent study published shows that the SADI with sleeve gastrectomy is safe and effective in the short term and midterm.[69] Additionally, SADI with sleeve gastrectomy has outperformed the RYGB with regards to weight loss, comorbidity resolution, and potential long-term issues.[70]

SUMMARY

VSG is a great weight loss surgery option. It is exceedingly safe and extremely effective for weight loss, it improves comorbidities, and it is technically straightforward. Still, several factors surrounding the surgery are important considerations for the surgeon and the patient. If properly used, VSG is a powerful tool in combating obesity and its deleterious effects.

CLINICS CARE POINTS

- A key consideration when stapling the stomach is to ensure that the stomach remains in one plane and that the staple line is truly lateral. This measure prevents spiraling around the sizing bougie, which would create a problematic helical sleeve. Such sleeves can lead to a functional stenosis and reflux.
- Two other important considerations include making sure that the stapler is not impinging on the incisura and that the bougie is not distorting the stomach in such a way that it

unnaturally stretches the stomach. This measure can prevent an obstruction/stenosis in the future.

- Finally, when working at the fundus, it is important to have appropriate lateral traction so that the posterior wall of the stomach does not bowl down. Taking this action lowers the incidence of a retained fundus and thus helps decrease reflux rates.

DISCLOSURE

No author has any competing or conflicting interests to disclose. The views expressed here reflect those of the authors and do not necessarily reflect the views of the US Army, Department of Defense, or the US Government.

REFERENCES

1. Wolfe BM, Kvach E, Eckel RH. Treatment of obesity: weight loss and bariatric surgery. Circ Res 2016;118:1844–55.
2. Jensen MD, Ryan DH, Donato KA, et al. Executive Summary: guidelines (2013) for the management of overweight and obesity in adults. A Report of the American College of Cardiology/American Heart Association Task Force on Practice Guidelines and The Obesity Society. Obesity 2014;22(2):5–39.
3. Ali M, El Chaar M, Ghiassi S, et al. American Society for Metabolic and Bariatric Surgery updated position statement on sleeve gastrectomy as a bariatric procedure. Surg Obes Relat Dis 2017;13(10):1652–7.
4. Diamantis T, Apostolou KG, Alexandrou A, et al. Review of long-term weight loss results after laparoscopic sleeve gastrectomy. Surg Obes Relat Dis 2014;10(1): 177–83.
5. American Society for Metabolic and Bariatric Surgeons. Available at: https:// asmbs.org/. Accessed July 26, 2020.
6. Dakin GF, Eid G, Mikami D, et al. Endoluminal revision of gastric bypass for weight regain: a systematic review. Surg Obes Relat Dis 2013;9(3):335–42.
7. Hess DS, Hess DW. Biliopancreatic diversion with a duodenal switch. Obes Surg 1998;8:267–82.
8. De Csepel J, Burpee S, Jossart G, et al. Laparoscopic biliopancreatic diversion with a duodenal switch for morbid obesity: a feasibility study in pigs. J Laparoendosc Adv Surg Tech A 2001;11(2):79–83.
9. Gumbs AA, Gagner M, Dankin G, et al. Sleeve gastrectomy for morbid obesity. Obes Surg 2007;17(7):962–9.
10. Regan JP, Inabnet WB, Gagner M, et al. Early experience with two-stage laparoscopic Roux-en-Y gastric bypass as an alternative in the super-super obese patient. Obes Surg 2003;13:861–4.
11. Ren CJ, Patterson E, Gagner M. Early results of laparoscopic biliopancreatic diversion with duodenal switch: a case series of 40 consecutive patients. Obes Surg 2000;10:514–23.
12. Faria GR. A brief history of bariatric surgery. Porto Biomed J 2017;2(3):90–2.
13. Huang R, Ding X, Fu H, et al. Potential mechanisms of sleeve gastrectomy for reducing weight and improving metabolism in patients with obesity. Surg Obes Relat Dis 2019;15(10):1861–72.
14. Karamanakos SN, Vagenas K, Kalfarentzos F, et al. Weight loss, appetite suppression, and changes in fasting and postprandial ghrelin and peptide-YY levels after Roux-en-Y gastric bypass and sleeve gastrectomy: a prospective, double

blind   study.   Ann   Surg   2008;247:401–7.   https://doi.org/10.1097/SLA.
0b013e318156f012.

15. Langer FB, Reza Hoda MA, Bohdjalian A, et al. Sleeve gastrectomy and gastric banding: effects on plasma ghrelin levels. Obes Surg 2005;15:1024–9.

16. Dezaki K, Sone H, Koizumi M, et al. Blockade of pancreatic islet-derived ghrelin enhances insulin secretion to prevent high-fat diet-induced glucose intolerance. Diabetes 2006;55(12):3486–93.

17. Zigman JM, Nakano Y, Coppari R, et al. Mice lacking ghrelin receptors resist the development of diet-induced obesity. J Clin Invest 2005;115(12):3564–72.

18. Verhulst PJ, Depoortere I. Ghrelin's second life: from appetite stimulator to glucose regulator. World J Gastroenterol 2012;18(25):3183–95.

19. Liu J, Conde J, Zhang P, et al. Enhanced AMPA receptor trafficking mediates the anorexigenic effect of endogenous glucagon-like Peptide-1 in the paraventricular hypothalamus. Neuron 2017;96(4):897–909.

20. Williams DL. Neural integration of satiation and food reward: role of GLP-1 and orexin pathways. Physiol Behav 2014;136:194–9.

21. Ye M, Huang R, Min Z, et al. Comparison of the effect by which gastric plication and sleeve gastrectomy procedures alter metabolic and physical parameters in an obese type 2 diabetes rodent model. Surg Obes Relat Dis 2017;13(11): 1819–28.

22. Li L, Wang X, Bai L, et al. The effects of sleeve gastrectomy on glucose metabolism and glucagon-like peptide 1 in Goto-Kakizaki rats. J Diabetes Res 2018;2018:1–11.

23. Dimitriadis E, Daskalakis M, Marilena K, et al. Alterations in gut hormones after laparoscopic sleeve gastrectomy: a prospective clinical and laboratory investigational study. Ann Surg 2013;257(4):647–54.

24. Van de Laar A, van Rijswijk AS, Kakar H, et al. Sensitivity and specificity of 50% excess weight loss (50%EWL) and twelve other bariatric criteria for weight loss success. Obes Surg 2018;28:2297–304.

25. Pai MP, Paloucek FP. The origin of the "ideal" body weight equations. Ann Pharmacol 2000;34(9):1066–9.

26. Peterli R, Borbely Y, Kern B, et al. Early results of the Swiss Multicentre Bypass or Sleeve Study (SM-BOSS): a prospective randomized trial comparing laparoscopic sleeve gastrectomy and Roux-en-Y gastric bypass. Ann Surg 2013; 258(5):690–5.

27. Vidal P, Ramón JM, Goday A, et al. Laparoscopic gastric bypass versus laparoscopic sleeve gastrectomy as a definitive surgical procedure for morbid obesity. Mid-term results. Obes Surg 2013;23(3):292–9.

28. Leyba JL, Llopis SN, Aulestia SN. Laparoscopic Roux-en-Y gastric bypass versus laparoscopic sleeve gastrectomy for the treatment of morbid obesity. A prospective study with 5 years of follow-up. Obes Surg 2014;24(12):2094–8.

29. Jakobsen GS, Smastuen MC, Sandu R, et al. Association of bariatric surgery vs medical obesity treatment with long term medical complications and obesity-related comorbidities. J Am Med Assoc 2018;319(3):291–301.

30. Schauer PR, Kashyap SR, Wolski K, et al. Bariatric surgery versus intensive medical therapy in obese patients with diabetes. N Engl J Med 2012;366(17): 1567–76.

31. Schauer PR, Bhatt DL, Kirwan JP, et al. Bariatric surgery versus intensive medical therapy for diabetes: 3-year outcomes. N Engl J Med 2014;370(21):2002–13.

32. Colquitt JL, Pickett K, Loveman E, et al. Surgery for weight loss in adults. Cochrane Database Syst Rev 2014;8:1–184.

33. Peterli R, Wolnerhanssen BK, Vetter D, et al. Laparoscopic sleeve gastrectomy versus Roux-Y-gastric bypass for morbid obesity: 3 year outcomes of the Prospective Randomized Swiss Multicenter Bypass or Sleeve Study (SM-BOSS). Ann Surg 2017;265(3):466–73.
34. Osland E, Yunus RM, Khan S, et al. Postoperative early major and minor complications in laparoscopic vertical sleeve gastrectomy (LVSG) versus laparoscopic Roux-en-Y gastric bypass (LRYGB) procedures: a meta-analysis and systematic review. Obes Surg 2016;26(10):2273–84.
35. Young MT, Gebhart A, Phelan MJ, et al. Use and outcomes of laparoscopic sleeve gastrectomy vs laparoscopic gastric bypass: analysis of the American College of Surgeons NSQIP. J Am Coll Surg 2015;220(5):880–5.
36. Shoar S, Saber AA. Long-term and midterm outcomes of laparoscopic sleeve gastrectomy versus Roux-en-Y gastric bypass: a systematic review and meta-analysis of comparative studies. Surg Obes Relat Dis 2017;13(2):170–80.
37. Rawlins L, Rawlins MP, Brown CC, et al. Sleeve gastrectomy: 5-year outcomes of a single institution. Surg Obes Relat Dis 2013;9(1):21–5.
38. Boza C, Daroch D, Barros D, et al. Long-term outcomes of laparoscopic sleeve gastrectomy as a primary bariatric procedure. Surg Obes Relat Dis 2014;10(6): 1129–33.
39. DuPree CE, Blair K, Steele SR, et al. Laparoscopic sleeve gastrectomy in patients with preexisting gastroesophageal reflux disease: a national analysis. JAMA Surg 2014;149(4):328–34.
40. Felsenreich DM, Kefurt R, Schermann M, et al. Reflux, sleeve dilation, and Barrett's esophagus after laparoscopic sleeve gastrectomy: long-term follow-up. Obes Surg 2017;27:3092–101.
41. Belnap L, Rodgers GM, Cottam D, et al. Portal vein thrombosis after laparoscopic sleeve gastrectomy: presentation and management. Surg Obes Relat Dis 2016; 12(10):1787–94.
42. Goitein D, Matter I, Raziel A, et al. Portomesenteric thrombosis following laparoscopic bariatric surgery: incidence, patterns of clinical presentation, and etiology in a bariatric patient population. JAMA Surg 2013;148(4):340–6.
43. Tan SBM, Greenslade J, Martin D, et al. Portomesenteric vein thrombosis in sleeve gastrectomy: a 10-year review. Surg Obes Relat Dis 2018;14(3):271–5.
44. Salinas J, Barros D, Salgado N, et al. Portomesenteric vein thrombosis after laparoscopic sleeve gastrectomy. Surg Endosc 2014;28:1083–9.
45. Lauti M, Kularatna M, Hill AG, et al. Weight regain following sleeve gastrectomy: a systematic review. Obes Surg 2016;26:1326–34.
46. Faria SL, Kelly EO, Lins RD, et al. Nutritional management of weight regain after bariatric surgery. Obes Surg 2010;20:135–9.
47. Himpens J, Dobbeleir J, Peeters G. Long-term results of laparoscopic sleeve gastrectomy for obesity. Ann Surg 2010;252(2):319–24.
48. Magro DO, Geloneze B, Delfini R, et al. Long term weight regain after gastric bypass: a 5 year prospective study. Obes Surg 2008;18:648–51.
49. Odom J, Zalesin KC, Washington TL, et al. Behavioral predictors of weight regain after bariatric surgery. Obes Surg 2010;20:349–56.
50. Aurora AR, Khaitan L, Saber AA. Sleeve gastrectomy and the risk of leak: a systematic analysis of 4,888 patients. Surg Endosc 2012;26(6):1509–15.
51. Gagner M, Kemmeter P. Comparison of laparoscopic sleeve gastrectomy leak rates in five staple-line reinforcement options: a systematic review. Surg Endosc 2019;34:396–407.

52. Rosenthal RJ, International Sleeve Gastrectomy Expert Panel. International sleeve gastrectomy expert panel consensus statement: best practice guidelines based on experience of > 12,000 cases. Surg Obes Relat Dis 2012;8(1):8–19.
53. Shikora SA, Mahoney CB. Clinical benefit of gastric staple line reinforcement in gastrointestinal surgery: a meta-analysis. Obes Surg 2015;25:1133–41.
54. Zafar SN, Felton J, Miller K, et al. Staple line treatment and bleeding after laparoscopic sleeve gastrectomy. JSLS 2018;22(4):1–10.
55. Janik MR, Walędziak M, Brągoszewski J, et al. Prediction model for hemorrhagic complications after laparoscopic sleeve gastrectomy: development of SLEEVE BLEED Calculator. Obes Surg 2017;27(4):968–72.
56. Deslauriers V, Beauchamp A, Garofalo F, et al. Endoscopic management of post-laparoscopic sleeve gastrectomy stenosis. Surg Endosc 2018;32:601–9.
57. Parikh A, Alley JB, Peterson RM, et al. Management options for symptomatic stenosis after laparoscopic vertical sleeve gastrectomy in the morbidly obese. Surg Endosc 2012;26(3):738–46.
58. Rebibo L, Hakim S, Dhahri A, et al. Gastric stenosis after laparoscopic sleeve gastrectomy: diagnosis and management. Obes Surg 2016;26:995–1001.
59. Telem DA, Gould J, Pesta C, et al. American Society for Metabolic and Bariatric Surgery: a care pathway development for laparoscopic sleeve gastrectomy. Surg Obes Relat Dis 2017;13(5):742–9.
60. Gagner M, Hutchinson C, Rosenthal R. Fifth International Consensus Conference: Current status of sleeve gastrectomy. Surg Obes Relat Dis 2016;12(4):750–6.
61. Yuval JB, Mintz Y, Cohen MJ, et al. The effects of bougie caliber on leaks and excess weight loss following laparoscopic sleeve gastrectomy. Is there an ideal bougie size? Obes Surg 2013;23(10):1685–91.
62. Parikh M, Issa R, McCrillis A, et al. Surgical strategies that may decrease leak after laparoscopic sleeve gastrectomy: a systematic review and meta-analysis of 9991 cases. Ann Surg 2013;257(2):231–7.
63. Che F, Nguyen B, Cohen A, et al. Prevalence of hiatal hernia in the morbidly obese. Surg Obes Relat Dis 2013;9(6):920–4.
64. Aydin MT, Aras O, Karip B, et al. Staple line reinforcement methods in laparoscopic sleeve gastrectomy: comparison of burst pressures and leaks. JSLS 2015;19(3). https://doi.org/10.4293/JSLS.2015.00040.
65. Berger ER, Clements RH, Morton JM, et al. The impact of different surgical techniques on outcomes in laparoscopic sleeve gastrectomies: the first report from the Metabolic and Bariatric Surgery Accreditation and Quality Improvement Program (MBSAQIP). Ann Surg 2016;264(3):464–73.
66. Sethi M, Zagzag J, Patel K, et al. Intraoperative leak testing has no correlation with leak after laparoscopic sleeve gastrectomy. Surg Endosc 2016;30(3):883–91.
67. Bingham J, Lallemand M, Barron M, et al. Routine intraoperative leak testing for sleeve gastrectomy: is the leak test full of hot air? Am J Surg 2016;211(5):943–7.
68. Brethauer SA, Kothari S, Sudan R, et al. Systematic review on reoperative bariatric surgery: American Society for Metabolic and Bariatric Surgery Revision Task Force. Surg Obes Relat Dis 2014;10(5):952–72.
69. Zaveri H, Surve A, Cottam D, et al. Mid-term 4 year outcomes with single anastomosis duodenal-ileal bypass with sleeve gastrectomy surgery at single US center. Obes Surg 2018;28:3062–72.
70. Ceha C, Wezenbeek M, Versteegden D, et al. Matched short-term results of SADI versus GBP after sleeve gastrectomy. Obes Surg 2018;28:3809–14.

Single-Anastomosis Duodenal Ileostomy with Sleeve Gastrectomy "Continued Innovation of the Duodenal Switch"

Daniel Cottam, MD*, Samuel Cottam, BS, Amit Surve, MD

KEYWORDS

- SADI-S • Bile acids • Weight loss • Review • Malnutrition • Complications

KEY POINTS

- Single-anastomosis duodenal ileostomy with sleeve gastrectomy (SADI-S) has high weight loss (>80% excess weight loss).
- SADI-S has a low reoperation and complication rate without the risk of ulceration seen after Roux-en-Y gastric bypass.
- SADI-S malnutrition is a serious and important complication to monitor, but with correct postoperative dietary supplements, risk is minimized.

INTRODUCTION/HISTORY/DEFINITIONS/BACKGROUND

Bariatric surgery began gaining great popularity in the late 1990s and early 2000s with nationwide procedures increasing nearly 10-fold. During this time, the most popular procedures were the vertical banded gastroplasty (VBG) and the Roux-en-Y gastric bypass (RYGB). These procedures, although innovative and more effective than previous attempts at bariatric surgery, had their limitations.

The VBG, initially hailed as easier to perform with fewer nutritional complications, was found to cause horrific strictures from the band or inadequate weight loss if the stoma dilated. The Mayo Clinic found that fewer than 25% of VBG patients were satisfied with the outcome of the procedure.[1]

On the other hand, the RYGB was effective at weight loss and had less weight regain. However, it carried a much higher complication profile, especially long-term marginal ulceration. When longer-term studies were done, the ulceration risk over 5 years was as high as 11.4%, with the risk not limited to the immediate postoperative period.[2]

Bariatric Medicine Institute, 1046 East 100 South, Salt Lake City, UT 84102, USA
* Corresponding author.
E-mail address: drdanielcottam@yahoo.com

The popularity of the VGB eventually dwindled and by the early 2000s was not done in large volumes anywhere in the world. Into this void, the sleeve gastrectomy (SG) was introduced in 2004. The increase of laparoscopy combined with the decline of laparoscopic bands and the realization that RGBP had a high complication profile allowed the SG to quickly become the most popular procedure worldwide because of the ease of the operation, similar weight loss (when compared with RGBP), and its low complication profile.

Despite these advances in weight loss surgery, patients often were unlikely to succeed following SG.[3] Rather than perform the RYGB on all these patients, surgeons looked for an operation that might have lower complication rates and similar high weight loss with low weight regain. One such possible procedure was introduced by Sánchez-Pernaute and colleagues[4] in 2007, now called the single-anastomosis duodenal ileostomy with sleeve gastrectomy (SADI-S).

Dr Torres' group sought to simplify the traditional Roux-en-Y duodenal switch (RYDS). They accomplished this by eliminating the Roux limb and not dividing the omentum, theorizing that the pylorus would eliminate the problems of bile reflux seen in one-anastomosis gastric bypass and that they could keep a long biliopancreatic limb for weight maintenance. Through a series of landmark papers,[5–7] Dr Torres showed that the procedure in their center had better weight loss and diabetes resolution than RYDS with a complication rate that was not inferior to RYDS.

These outcomes spurred Dr Roslin's group in New York City and Dr Cottam's group in Salt Lake City to collaborate to publish a series of comparison articles with both RYGBP and RYDS demonstrating that the technique seemingly carried fewer complications than RYDS and RYGBP, especially ulcers, internal hernias, and bowel obstructions.[8] Other investigators have reinforced these findings.[9–11]

ANATOMY AND SURGICAL TECHNIQUE

The principles of SG surgery are the foundation of understanding the SADI-S. Indeed, the first principle of doing no harm to the vessels on the lesser curve of the stomach to maintain the vascular supply to the stomach is very important to the SADI-S procedure. Following this principle allows surgeons to transect the duodenum safely.

The next principle is that the dissection of the duodenum is facilitated by first taking down all the gastroepiploic perforating vessels. This dissection, although not the traditional way to perform RYDS, allows easy dissection around the head of the pancreas. Once a surgeon lifts the stomach and removes the thin filmy attachments to the pancreas, developing a space to divide the duodenum becomes easier. This dissection is continued to where the pancreas and the duodenum become fused. This dissection is almost always past the pylorus and superior to the gastroduodenal artery. Indeed, most of the time, using these techniques, the gastroduodenal artery is not visualized.

Additional important landmarks include the pancreatic-duodenal vessels, which run on the posterior side of the duodenum and parallel with the duodenum from the head of the pancreas and end at the pylorus. These vessels are almost always present and are different from vessels from the right gastric artery that run perpendicular to the duodenum.

Once that dissection is finished, a window is created toward the liver from the undersurface of the duodenum toward the liver. Using this approach, the surgeon keeps the portal triad below the level of dissection and avoids major vessel injury.[12] Not following these principles and attempting to dissect from above the duodenum toward the lesser sac can result in major vessel injury, as the vessels are usually encased in a fatty layer and cannot easily be seen.[13]

The loop small bowel anastomosis configuration of the SADI-S is seemingly much easier to perform than Roux limbs. Loop limbs have inherently less tension than Roux limbs. When combined with the technique described here, the antrum of the sleeve becomes mobile, making the stomach change from a right-angled organ to a straight organ. The resulting duodenoileostomy takes place below the edge of the liver thereby reducing tension on the anastomosis. This maneuver obviates splitting the omentum and avoids complications associated with jejunojejunostomies and Roux limbs, such as internal hernias, hematomas, intussusceptions, and obstructions.

PREOPERATIVE/PREPROCEDURE PLANNING

The SADI-S shares the same concerns for vitamin and protein malnutrition that all procedures that violate the absorption of the small bowel have. However, with the SADI-S, special concern needs to be paid with the fat-soluble vitamins D, E, A, and K, and copper and zinc. Deficiencies should be treated when found, but surgery does not have to be postponed because of the deficiencies unless they are severe. Almost all deficiencies can be treated with oral supplementation after surgery without affecting outcomes.[14]

In addition, special attention needs to be paid to the education of the preoperative patient about vitamin compliance and testing. Patients should understand that without supplementation, vitamin deficiencies and potential clinical sequelae can occur.

Also, because there is discrepancy in the literature about the appropriate length of common channel in the SADI-S, a basic overview of outcomes versus complications is needed to help the patient understand why a certain length of bowel is chosen and its relative risk of vitamin deficiencies, protein calorie malnutrition, and diarrhea versus beneficial weight loss.[6,15]

PROCEDURAL APPROACH

- Identify the ileocecal valve.
- Measure 250 to 350 cm of small bowel and tack the small bowel to the gastrocolic omentum.
- Place the patient in steep Trendelenburg.
- Perform a standard SG.
- Take down all the gastroepiploic vessels on the greater curvature of the stomach.
- Remove all posterior adhesions down to the head of the pancreas.
- Locate the pancreaticoduodenal vessels posteriorly. The stapler should transect these vessels as they end at the pylorus.
- Dissect toward the liver from underneath the duodenum to break the hepaticogastric ligaments to allow the stapler access to the duodenum.
- Transect the duodenum at the level of the gastroduodenal artery with a linear stapler.
- Pull the marking stitch out of the small bowel and bring the stomach down to the small bowel.
- Connect the proximal duodenum to the distal small bowel using any one of 3 ways: entirely stapled, partially stapled, or all hand sewn. Each can be done well with minimal complications. However, in the literature, most reported all hand-sewn anastomoses (**Fig. 1**).
- Test the anastomosis intraoperatively for leaks with air or liquid contrast.
- Remove the remnant stomach and close the incision sites.

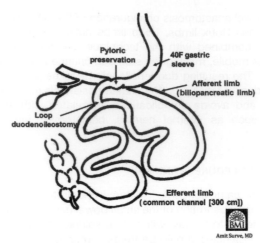

Fig. 1. Final anatomy of a patient following the SADI-S procedure (40F gastric sleeve and 300-cm efferent limb are reference sizes used by the authors, but many sizes of sleeve and efferent limb lengths are appropriate for SADI-S). (*Courtesy of* A. Surve, MD, Salt Lake City, UT.)

RECOVERY AND REHABILITATION

More than 90% of patients are released typically on the first day following surgery. In carefully selected patients with body mass index less than 50 and no comorbidities, SADI-S is safe to perform as an outpatient operation with a hospital or ambulatory surgical center stay of less than 24 hours.[16] Patients are sent home on a full liquid diet for 2 weeks to allow the anastomosis to heal. Then, they have a soft-foods diet for another 2 weeks before resuming a more typical diet. Although this is typical of the authors of this article, a wide variation in postoperative food introduction is seen throughout the world.

Patients are asked to come into the office 2 days and 1 week after surgery to evaluate recovery. They are then also asked to follow up at 1, 3, 6, and 12 months and then yearly thereafter. For patients who received SADI-S in an outpatient setting, they are required to return on postoperative day 1 or 2 for intravenous hydration.

MANAGEMENT

Perhaps the biggest misconception following SADI-S involves dietary management postoperatively. There is a mistaken belief that this procedure is fat malabsorptive, so fat will make the patient have foul-smelling flatulence and oily stools, and thus, fat should be avoided in the diet. This belief is not true, as fat is primarily absorbed in the distal small bowel, and the SADI-S preserves this portion of the small bowel as the common channel. The primary problem is due to carbohydrate malabsorption, as carbohydrates are primarily absorbed in the proximal intestine, and this is entirely bypassed. Thus, when a diet rich in processed carbohydrates is consumed, high levels of carbohydrates are delivered to the colon bacteria, which result in diarrhea, oily stools, and smelly flatulence as a byproduct of bacterial metabolism. This is not entirely unwanted, and it serves as a negative feedback reminder to eat a diet low in processed carbohydrates.

Diarrhea, although extremely rare, does occur after SADI-S and is usually self-limiting. In cases whereby diarrhea is not self-limiting, there are many options. Probiotics are a simple over-the-counter method, which inexpensively helps some patients modify stool frequency and odor. However, there is no literature for this approach nor is there standardization for the kinds of bacteria, amounts of bacteria, or dosages. Patients are also told they can try any over-the-counter antidiarrheal medications, which works in some patients. Bismuth subgallate (Devrom) is the most effective over-the-counter medication. It has proven its efficacy in a randomized double-blinded trial, is inexpensive, and can be mail ordered from anywhere in the world.[17] Rarely, diphenoxylate/atropine (Lomotil) needs to be used, and this is usually for less than 3 months, as the small bowel can and does adapt to shorter intestinal length. Also, activated charcoal taken with simethicone does help a select few patients. When these approaches do not work, operative intervention is called for, and adding 150 cm to the common channel length will alleviate the diarrhea but will result in patient weight gain.[18] This outcome should be discussed in detail with the patient before proceeding to limb lengthening.

The most common complaint following surgery is not diarrhea but constipation. Constipation usually occurs when patients, trying to achieve adequate protein intake, lean heavily on protein drinks to meet protein goals. These drinks, which deliver high levels of beneficial protein, also deliver high levels of calcium, which constipates patients. The treatment is almost always less processed protein.

Smoking and nonsteroidal anti-inflammatory drugs (NSAIDs) are important problems with Roux-based surgical approaches to weight loss. Smoking has known ulcerogenic effects on Roux limbs, although the exact mechanisms are a matter of debate. These concerns are not present in SADI-S and should not be contraindications to surgery. Patients should be informed of the deleterious effects of smoking on blood clots, pneumonia, and surgical site infections, but if smoking cessation cannot be achieved, surgery should not be delayed.[19] Currently, there are no medications that cannot be taken with SADI-S, and patients should be informed of this fact. This alone allows SADI is to be used in a wide variety of medical conditions, whereby NSAIDs are required for thromboembolic prevention, joint pain, menstrual irregularities, and generalized nonnarcotic pain relief.

Vitamin supplementation and access to such supplements vary widely throughout the world. If the patient cannot purchase these vitamins because of expense or unavailability, then SADI-S is not an option for the patient. In all of the developed world and most of the developing world, specialized duodenal switch vitamins high in D, E, A, K, copper, and zinc can be purchased easily and inexpensively over the Internet. All patients should be instructed to take them. However, any vitamin, if combined with appropriate monitoring, can potentially be used.

OUTCOMES

The primary outcome of any bariatric procedure is weight loss, and short-, mid-, and long-term studies are needed to judge success. The SADI-S has many short- and mid-term studies, whereas there are only 2 long-term studies currently (**Table 1**).

Another important outcome of any operation is complication rate. Following SADI-S, the most common complication is nausea, whereas the most common cause for reoperation is diarrhea. Most of the papers focusing on complications following SADI-S have used the Clavien-Dindo scale to classify complications. The 30-day complication rate for class I to IIIa and class IIIb to V is approximately 14.5% and 1%, respectively. This rate is much lower than RYDS and RYGBP. Six-year complication data in a single paper have shown that long-term class I to IIIa and class IIIb to V complication rates are 6.9% and 4.8%, respectively, with a significant portion of those being cholecystectomies and sleeve strictures. Sleeve strictures were part of the early learning curve and were not seen in the last 300 cases.[8,20]

Table 1
Excess weight loss following single-anastomosis duodenal ileostomy with sleeve gastrectomy

Reference, Authors, Year	n	1 y	2 y	3 y	4 y	5 y	6 y
Surve et al,[20] 2020	601	74.5 ± 21.6	84.5 ± 25.3	79 ± 28.1	77.6 ± 25.6	75.1 ± 26.5	80.7 ± 27.9
Sánchez-Pernaute et al,[7] 2015	86	91 ± NA	92 ± NA	85 ± NA	88 ± NA	98 ± NA	NA
Sánchez-Pernaute et al,[5] 2010	50	94.7 ± 19.1	114 ± 9.6	NA	NA	NA	NA
Paul et al,[9] 2020	160	83.3 ± 20.4	88.6 ± 20	NA	NA	NA	NA
Finno et al,[10] 2020	159	79.6 ± NA	74.7 ± 17.1	NA	NA	NA	NA
Neichoy et al,[11] 2018	93	71.5 ± 20.1	88.8 ± 20.2	NA	NA	NA	NA
Lee et al,[15] 2013	26	87.2 ± 14.9	NA	NA	NA	NA	NA
Moon et al,[33] 2018	124	68.1 ± 17	80.8 ± 17	NA	NA	NA	NA
Amit et al,[34] 2020	62	84.5 ± 20.6	94.1 ± 21.2	NA	NA	NA	NA

Abbreviation: NA, not applicable.
Data from Refs.[5,7,9–11,15,20,33,34]

As mentioned earlier, ulcer formation is rare following SADI-S, with just 2 patients in a study of 1328 forming mild ulcers following SADI-S that did not need treatment beyond short-term proton pump inhibitors.[21]

Diabetes resolution rates are especially high following SADI-S. The most recent studies have shown that complete type II diabetes remission occurs in 77% of patients.[20] This is roughly 3 times more effective than an RYGBP and 4 times more effective than an SG.[22]

ADVANTAGES/DISADVANTAGES

One of the main advantages present with the SG and by extension SADI-S is the pylorus preservation. Saving the pylorus slows solid food deposition into the small intestines and so decreases the post–prandial insulin surge. In studies comparing RYDS and RYGB, the mean postprandial glucose change was approximately double that of the RYDS. This same study also found that pre–prandial glucose levels were lower with the RYDS.[23] Decreased post–prandial surges are also tied to increased satiety after a meal, which may increase the long-term anorexia seen after SADI-S and RYDS.

Another advantage of the SADI-S procedure is the lack of a Roux limb. Although the Roux limb was originally introduced to eliminate bile reflux, this is not a common complication following SADI-S because it retains the pylorus. Also, the Roux limb by default is ulcerogenic. This has been known almost since the start of its use as a small intestinal conduit. The SADI-S in contrast is not ulcerogenic, ulcers are extremely rare and mild, and there are no reports in the literature of loop limb perforation following SADI-S. (There are only 2 studies >5 years, which limits the certainty of this statement.)

Another positive association with SADI-S is the high levels of circulating bile acids that happen following surgery. This elevation is driven primarily by the increase in unconjugated bile acids but is seen to some extent for all bile acids. Elevated bile acids have been positively correlated with weight loss results in RYGBP, RYDS, and SADI-S with both forms of the duodenal switch having significantly higher levels than RYGBP. The elevated levels correspond with drops in insulin levels, lower cholesterol levels, and weight loss.[24]

Although the exact mechanism of bile acid increases leading to increased weight loss is not fully evaluated, there is evidence to show it acts through 2 possible pathways. The first is through FGF19 upregulation, which has been observed following RYGB. Although not always observed, FGF19 suppresses hepatic bile acid uptake, increasing circulating bile acids, and can act through receptors in the central nervous system to reduce food intake to improve glucose homeostasis.[25] The second and possibly most important mechanism of action for circulating bile acids is through TGR5 receptors, most importantly in brown adipose tissue. Rodent models and limited human research have shown that circulating bile acids interact with TGR5, increasing type 2 iodothyronine deiodinase expression and spending excess energy as heat. In 1 human study, CDCA (a bile acid) was shown to increase the basal metabolic rate by 5% compared with a control group.[26,27]

Bile acid increase is likely explained through a combination of increased postprandial bile acid release and increased formation and uptake of primary bile acids in the biliopancreatic limb. Although the increased uptake of bile acids in the biliopancreatic limb would likely be fairly immediate following surgery, the increased postprandial release of bile acids seems to be a physiologic response to the new anatomy created in RYGB and is likely to be similar in RYDS and SADI-S. This would explain the delay in circulating bile acid increases following any bariatric procedure.[28]

One main advantage of the SADI-S procedure is the ease of conversion from other popular bariatric procedures, most notably the SG and VBG. Although once quite popular, the VBG left many patients dissatisfied with long-term weight loss. There have been 2 separate studies on conversion from VBG to SADI-S, and both found weight loss greater than 80% EWL (excess weight loss) with 2 year follow-up. The complication rates varied significantly between groups, but both studies had low patient numbers, so complication conclusions are difficult to assess.[29,30] SG is the most commonly performed weight loss surgery in the world. However, weight regain is more common after SG. Because SADI-S is an extension of the sleeve, revision can easily be performed with very low risk as an outpatient procedure. In the 2 currently available studies, patients lost 65% and 79% EWL at 2 years with very minimal complications. All the patients in both studies had failed weight loss with less than 50% EWL following initial SG.[31,32]

A large disadvantage of the SADI-S procedure is the possibility of malnutrition. Malnutrition is always a concern when any segment of the small bowel is bypassed but becomes more likely as the surgeon bypasses more bowel. Originally the SADI-S was proposed with a 200-cm common channel. Although these patients averaged more than 100% EWL, they also had an 8% protein malnutrition rate.[6] This risk of malnutrition is curtailed by making a 300-cm common channel where malnutrition rates have been observed as low as 0.2% in long-term studies.[20]

SUMMARY

The SADI-S with a 300-cm common channel has been shown in short- and mid-term studies to have complication rates lower the both the RYGBP and the RYDS. These findings appear to be repeated in long-term studies, but with only 2 long-term studies, it is far too early to draw a definitive conclusion. SADI-S weight loss is similar to the RYDS and greater than RYGBP and SG. Diabetes, hypertension, and cholesterol resolution mirror RYDS, whereas are clearly superior to SG and RYGBP. Although there is a benefit surrounding SADI-S, there is much more research to be done, elucidating the relative benefits of pyloric preservation and elevated circulating bile acids regarding the long-term outcomes of SADI-S.SADI-S is a safe and effective procedure for weight loss with low complication rates.

CLINICS CARE POINTS

- SADI-S is a safe and effective bariatric procedure.
- SADI-S has a high type II diabetes resolution rate.
- SADI-S shows low weight regain after the first year.
- Malnutrition should be monitored following SADI-S with strict dietary supplementation to minimize risk.

DISCLOSURE

D. Cottam reports personal fees from Medtronic, outside of the submitted work. S. Cottam has nothing to disclose. A. Surve has nothing to disclose.

REFERENCES

1. Balsiger BM, Poggio JL, Mai J, et al. Ten and more years after vertical banded gastroplasty as primary operation for morbid obesity. J Gastrointest Surg 2000; 4(6):598–605.
2. Spaniolas K, Yang J, Crowley S, et al. Association of long-term anastomotic ulceration after Roux-en-Y gastric bypass with tobacco smoking. JAMA Surg 2018; 153(9):862–4.
3. Cottam S, Cottam D, Austin C. Sleeve gastrectomy weight loss and the preoperative and postoperative predictors: a systematic review. Obes Surg 2019;29(4): 1388–96.
4. Sánchez-Pernaute A, Angel Rubio Herrera M, Pérez-Aguirre E, Torres Antonio. Proximal duodenal-ileal end-to-side bypass with sleeve gastrectomy: proposed technique. Obes Surg 2007;17(12):1614–8.
5. Sánchez-Pernaute A, Angel Rubio Herrera M, Pérez-Aguirre ME, et al. Single anastomosis duodeno-ileal bypass with sleeve gastrectomy (SADI-S). One to three-year follow-up. Obes Surg 2010;20(12):1720–6.
6. Sánchez-Pernaute A, Ángel Rubio M, Pérez Aguirre E, et al. Single-anastomosis duodenoileal bypass with sleeve gastrectomy: metabolic improvement and weight loss in first 100 patients. Surg Obes Relat Dis 2013;9(5):731–5.
7. Sánchez-Pernaute A, Rubio MÁ, Cabrerizo L, et al. Single-anastomosis duodenoileal bypass with sleeve gastrectomy (SADI-S) for obese diabetic patients. Surg Obes Relat Dis 2015;11(5):1092–8.
8. Austin C, Cottam D, Zaveri H, et al. An analysis of mid-term complications, weight loss, and type 2 diabetes resolution of stomach intestinal pylorus-sparing surgery (SIPS) versus Roux-en-Y gastric bypass (RYGB) with three-year follow-up. Obes Surg 2018;28(9):2894–902.

9. Paul E, Bull J, Amit S, et al. Comparative analysis of the single-anastomosis duodenal-ileal bypass with sleeve gastrectomy (SADI-S) to established bariatric procedures: an assessment of 2-year postoperative data illustrating weight loss, type 2 diabetes, and nutritional status in a single US center. Surg Obes Relat Dis 2020;16(1):24–33.

10. Finno P, Osorio J, García-Ruiz-de-Gordejuela A, et al. Single versus double-anastomosis duodenal switch: single-site comparative cohort study in 440 consecutive patients. Obes Surg 2020;30(9):3309–16.

11. Neichoy BT, Schniederjan B, Cottam DR, et al. Stomach intestinal pylorus-sparing surgery for morbid obesity. JSLS 2018;22(1). e2017.00063.

12. Amit S, Rao R, Cottam D. Laparoscopic single anastomosis duodeno-ileal bypass with sleeve gastrectomy: surgical technique. Obes Surg 2020. https://doi.org/10.1007/s11695-020-04847-z.

13. Scott S, Amit S, D Cottam, et al. A232 A video of an iatrogenic portal vein injury during duodenal dissection for single anastomosis duodeno-ileal bypass. https://doi.org/10.1016/j.soard.2019.08.177.

14. Cottam D, Mitchell R, Paul E, et al. Single anastomosis duodenal switch: 1-year outcomes. Obes Surg 2020;30(4):1506–14.

15. Lee W-J, Almulaifi AM, Jun-Juin T, et al. Duodenal-jejunal bypass with sleeve gastrectomy versus the sleeve gastrectomy procedure alone: the role of duodenal exclusion. Surg Obes Relat Dis 2015;11(4):765–70.

16. Cottam S, Ng P, Sharp L, et al. Single-anastomosis duodenal ileostomy with sleeve is a safe and effective option for patients in an ambulatory surgical center. Surg Obes Relat Dis 2019;15(11):1990–3.

17. Zaveri H, Amit S, Cottam D, et al. Does bismuth subgallate affect smell and stool character? A randomized double-blinded placebo-controlled trial of bismuth subgallate on loop duodenal switch patients with complaints of smelly stools and diarrhea. Obes Surg 2018;28(11):3511–7.

18. Horsley B, Cottam D, Austin C, et al. Bowel reconstruction to treat chronic diarrhea and hypoproteinemia following single anastomosis duodenal-ileal bypass with sleeve gastrectomy: a single-site experience. Obes Surg 2019;29(8):2387–91.

19. José Signorini F, Polero V, Viscido G, et al. Long-term relationship between tobacco use and weight loss after sleeve gastrectomy. Obes Surg 2018;28(9):2644–9.

20. Surve A, Daniel Cottam D, Medlin W, et al. Long-term outcomes of primary single-anastomosis duodeno-ileal bypass with sleeve gastrectomy (SADI-S). Surg Obes Relat Dis 2020;16(11):1638–46.

21. Amit S, Cottam D, Sanchez-Pernaute A, et al. The incidence of complications associated with loop duodeno-ileostomy after single-anastomosis duodenal switch procedures among 1328 patients: a multicenter experience. Surg Obes Relat Dis 2018;14(5):594–601.

22. Schauer PR, Bhatt DL, Kirwan JP, et al. Bariatric surgery versus intensive medical therapy for diabetes - 5-year outcomes. N Engl J Med 2017;376(7):641–51.

23. Nilsen I, Sundbom M, Abrahamsson N, et al. Comparison of meal pattern and postprandial glucose response in duodenal switch and gastric bypass patients. Obes Surg 2019;29(7):2210–6.

24. Risstad H, Kristinsson JA, Fagerland MW, et al. Bile acid profiles over 5 years after gastric bypass and duodenal switch: results from a randomized clinical trial. Surg Obes Relat Dis 2017;13(9):1544–53.

25. Bozadjieva N, Heppner KM, Seeley RJ. Targeting FXR and FGF19 to treat metabolic diseases-lessons learned from bariatric surgery. Diabetes 2018;67(9):1720–8.
26. Watanabe M, Houten SM, Mataki C, et al. Bile acids induce energy expenditure by promoting intracellular thyroid hormone activation. Nature 2006;439(7075):484–9.
27. Broeders EPM, Nascimento EBM, Havekes B, et al. The bile acid chenodeoxycholic acid increases human brown adipose tissue activity. Cell Metab 2015;22(3):418–26.
28. Yu So SS, Yeung CHC, Mary Schooling C, et al. Targeting bile acid metabolism in obesity reduction: a systematic review and meta-analysis. Obes Rev 2020;21(7):e13017.
29. Wu A, Tian J, Cao L, et al. Single-anastomosis duodeno-ileal bypass with sleeve gastrectomy (SADI-S) as a revisional surgery. Surg Obes Relat Dis 2018;14(11):1686–90.
30. Amit S, Zaveri H, Cottam D, et al. Laparoscopic stomach intestinal pylorus-sparing surgery as a revisional option after failed adjustable gastric banding: a report of 27 cases with 36-month follow-up. Surg Obes Relat Dis 2018;14(8):1139–48.
31. Zaveri H, Amit S, Cottam D, et al. A multi-institutional study on the mid-term outcomes of single anastomosis duodeno-ileal bypass as a surgical revision option after sleeve gastrectomy. Obes Surg 2019;29(10):3165–73.
32. Balibrea JM, Vilallonga R, Hidalgo M, et al. Mid-term results and responsiveness predictors after two-step single-anastomosis duodeno-ileal bypass with sleeve gastrectomy. Obes Surg 2017;27(5):1302–8.
33. Moon RC, Gaskins L, Teixeira AF, et al. Safety and effectiveness of single-anastomosis duodenal switch procedure: 2-year result from a single US institution. Obes Surg 2018;28(6):1571–7.
34. Amit S, Rao R, Cottam D, et al. Early outcomes of primary SADI-S: an Australian experience. Obes Surg 2020;30(4):1429–36.

Pediatric Metabolic and Bariatric Surgery

Adi Steinhart, BS, BA[a], Deborah Tsao, BS[b], Janey S.A. Pratt, MD[c],*

KEYWORDS

- Pediatric • Obesity • Surgery • Bariatric • Adolescent

KEY POINTS

- Metabolic and bariatric surgery is the treatment of choice for children with class III or II obesity with a comorbidity, according to the 2019 American Academy of Pediatrics policy statement.
- Early referral to a multidisciplinary program when a child reaches a body mass index of 120% of the 95th percentile is critical to best outcomes in childhood obesity.
- Lifestyle changes including diet, exercise, and obesity medications cannot be considered adequate treatment for severe pediatric obesity.
- Bias and prejudice surrounding pediatric obesity play a role in the delay and inadequate use of metabolic and bariatric surgery in the treatment of pediatric obesity.
- Both laparoscopic sleeve gastrectomy and Roux-en-Y gastric bypass can be considered standard of care in children with severe obesity as defined by the American Academy of Pediatrics.

INTRODUCTION

Obesity is one of the fastest growing chronic health conditions in the world, presenting with significant comorbidities that affect people of all ages, genders, and ethnicities. The prevalence of obesity in children and adolescents has grown rapidly over the past few decades. Since the 1980s, childhood obesity has tripled, and adolescent obesity has quadrupled.[1,2] Currently, severe obesity affects 7.9% of adolescents aged 12 to 15 years, and 14% of those aged 16 to 19 years, with the latter number having doubled since 1999.[2] Childhood obesity is multifactorial, based strongly on a genetic predisposition that is exacerbated by increased consumption of highly processed foods marketed aggressively toward children and decreased daily activity in

[a] Department of Pediatrics, Stanford University School of Medicine, 1017 Paradise Way, Palo Alto, CA 94306, USA; [b] Stanford University School of Medicine, 227 Ayrshire Farm Ln (Apt 203), Stanford, CA 94305, USA; [c] Division of Pediatric Surgery, Stanford University School of Medicine, Lucille Packard Children's Hospital, M166 Alway Building, 300 Pasteur Drive, Stanford, CA 94305, USA
* Corresponding author.
E-mail address: jsapratt@stanford.edu

Surg Clin N Am 101 (2021) 199–212
https://doi.org/10.1016/j.suc.2020.12.007
0039-6109/21/© 2020 Elsevier Inc. All rights reserved.

an increasingly sedentary lifestyle. In particular, children are susceptible to influence from the behaviors of their parents.[3] If one parent has obesity, the child has a 4 times higher chance of developing obesity, and if both parents have obesity, the child has a 10 times higher chance of developing obesity, confirming the strong genetic contribution to this disease.[4]

Metabolic bariatric surgery (MBS) is an increasingly recognized treatment for childhood obesity.[5] The procedural prevalence has tripled since the early 2000s, from 1000 to 1600 cases each year.[6,7] Many different factors affect the decision and timing for MBS, the most important of which are the body mass index (BMI) and comorbidities.[8] Studies show that early intervention increases the chances of patient reaching a healthy body weight and resolution of comorbidities after MBS.[9]

UNIQUE COMORBIDITIES

Although there are limited data on the specifics of pediatric obesity-associated comorbidities, children with obesity are at higher risk of developing a number of health problems later in life.

Cardiovascular Disease

An increased risk of cardiovascular diseases is strongly correlated with obesity in adults and children. Studies have shown that childhood obesity increases the mortality rate of cardiovascular disease 3 to 5 times by the age of 40.[10] Furthermore, children with severe obesity had a greater left ventricular mass, with reduced systolic and early diastolic tissue compared with normal weight adolescent control subjects.[11,12] Crucially, 3 years after MBS, adolescents show significant decreases in cardiovascular risk factors such as triglycerides, insulin resistance, low-density lipoprotein cholesterol, blood pressure, and C-reactive protein, with earlier intervention favoring better outcomes.[13]

Type 2 Diabetes

Childhood obesity is linked with higher incidence of type 2 diabetes (T2D). In fact, early onset T2D also seems to present more severely. Children with T2D show a decrease in beta cell function at rates 4 times greater than adults with T2D, and children with insulin resistance have twice the fasting insulin levels of adults with the same BMI classification.[14,15] Fortunately, MBS is extremely successful in preventing and reversing T2D progression in children and adolescents. Independent studies have shown that between 86% and 100% of adolescents achieve long-term (>5 years) remission of T2D after laparoscopic Roux-en-Y gastric bypass (RYGB).[16,17] Similar results have been documented after laparoscopic sleeve gastrectomy in children.[18] Finally, the resolution of T2D after MBS is higher in children than in adults, indicating that intervention during childhood is more likely to have a positive long-term effect than delaying to adulthood.[19]

Obstructive Sleep Apnea

Up to one-third of children and adolescents with obesity have obstructive sleep apnea (OSA), and among children undergoing MBS, up to 55% have diagnosed OSA.[20,21] OSA is a significant source of morbidity in childhood, contributing to daytime sleepiness, cardiovascular disease, neurocognitive cognitive impairment, and decreased quality of life. Importantly, pediatric patients after post-MBS weight loss experience a dramatic decrease in hypoxic episodes during sleep and significantly improved nighttime oxygen saturation.[21] In addition, there is some evidence that there are weight-independent factors involved as one study documented a 9-point decrease in the apnea hypopnea index at 3 weeks after MBS in children.[22]

Nonalcoholic Fatty Liver Disease and Nonalcoholic Steatohepatitis

Nonalcoholic fatty liver disease (NAFLD) has a higher incidence in obese children compared with nonobese individuals in the same age group. NAFLD is present in 59% of obese adolescents being treated with MBS, compared with just 9.6% of all children between ages of 2 and 19.[23,24] When NAFLD causes hepatic inflammation, it is referred to as nonalcoholic steatohepatitis. Although lifestyle interventions have proven ineffective in resolving childhood onset nonalcoholic steatohepatitis, adolescent patients after laparoscopic sleeve gastrectomy were found to have complete resolution of nonalcoholic steatohepatitis and up to 90% showed resolution of stage 2 hepatic fibrosis.[25]

Musculoskeletal Disease

Obesity is also a significant risk factor for the development of orthopedic diseases. In particular, Blount's disease and slipped capital femoral epiphysis are associated with childhood obesity and reduced weight-related quality of life.[26] MBS treatment in children results in improved functional mobility, reduced walking-related musculoskeletal pain, and even case reports of resolved Blount's disease.[5,27] Because most lifestyle interventions are unsuccessful in this group of patients, in part owing to their inability to exercise, MBS is an excellent adjunct to orthopedic intervention.[28]

Gastroesophageal Reflux Disease

Gastroesophageal reflux disease (GERD) is commonly associated with both adult and childhood obesity, perhaps owing to both increased intra-abdominal pressure and decreased lower esophageal sphincter tone. Because longstanding GERD is a risk factor for Barrett's esophagus, neoplasia, and esophageal cancer, it is crucial to treat this condition early.[29] In addition to being an effective weight loss intervention, the RYGB is also a good treatment for GERD.[30] In children with GERD and severe obesity, RYGB is preferable to fundoplication because conversion from fundoplication to RYGB is risky and carries significant morbidity.[31,32] After RYGB, the resulting gastric pouch has fewer parietal cells, and the Roux limb itself prevents bile reflux.[31] Although sleeve gastrectomy can cause or worsen underlying GERD, a subset of patients may also improve, and thus it should not be excluded when considering the best operation for a patient with severe obesity and GERD.[5]

Mental Health

Finally, it is necessary to consider the mental health repercussions of obesity in children and adolescents.[33] Obesity has been associated with increased odds of poor mental health in US children and adolescents, because children with obesity are 2 to 4 times more likely to have low self-esteem compared with their normal weight peers.[34,35] Furthermore, among children seeking MBS, 30% meet criteria for clinical depression based on self-reporting and 45% meet criteria based on mother reporting.[36] These facts are unsurprising, because children with obesity are significantly more likely to be bullied, discriminated against, and victimized by their peers. Although MBS and subsequent weight loss do not solve this psychosocial impact, after MBS adolescents do report significantly higher self-esteem compared with baseline.[37]

AMERICAN ACADEMY OF PEDIATRICS POLICY STATEMENT

In October 2019, Armstrong and colleagues[6] released a Policy Statement and Technical Report for the American Academy of Pediatrics defining the eligibility criteria for metabolic and bariatric surgery. They concluded that the medical community should recognize that a BMI of more than 40 or 140% of the 95th percentile, or a BMI greater than 35 or 120% of the 95th percentile, with an obesity-related comorbidity, puts children at risk for severe morbidity and mortality from obesity. They show significant data that children meeting these BMI cut-offs benefit from MBS and are unlikely to be responsive to lifestyle modification or medications alone. The community of physicians should understand the risks and benefits of MBS, particularly in pediatric populations, and improve the process of identifying pediatric patients that meet these criteria for surgery. It is the physician's responsibility to provide patients with referrals to high-quality multidisciplinary care centers. Physicians should coordinate before and after the operation with the multidisciplinary team and monitor patients after MBS for nutrient deficiencies as well as risk taking behaviors and mental health changes.

BARRIERS TO REFERRAL AND CHILDREN GETTING CARE

A significant barrier for pediatric patients receiving MBS and general bariatric care is the stigmatization of obesity – not only among the general public, but also among health care professionals.[38,39] Many physicians are reluctant to refer pediatric patients for MBS because of concerns for impaired nutrition and development and a lack of underlying knowledge about obesity and the available surgical options.[40,41] Problematic psychosocial factors such as family dynamics may also be barriers to providing patient care.[33] Unhealthy communication between the adolescents and their caretakers as well as inadequate involvement by the caretakers are barriers that prevent the involved parties from working together to constructively care for children with severe obesity.[5]

Additionally, inequities in insurance authorization for MBS, exacerbated by race and socioeconomic status, have emerged as significant barriers to treatment. In contrast with the 85% of criteria-passing adults who receive insurance coverage for MBS, fewer than one-half of qualifying adolescent surgical candidates received coverage.[42] Although minority groups are more likely to experience severe obesity and concurrent comorbidities, they are less likely to undergo bariatric surgery owing to these disparities in insurance authorization.[43] This trend is likely most related to the lower socioeconomic status faced by racial minorities, rather than to race and ethnicity themselves.[44,45] However, new data suggest that these inequities may not be explained by insurance alone, because Medicaid increased the likelihood of White adolescents undergoing MBS while decreasing the use of surgery in racial minorities with severe obesity.[46]

Finally, implicit bias by the physicians, families, and children may be responsible for some of the disparities that occur in referral of patients to multidisciplinary obesity treatment programs. Bias can be addressed at all levels by teaching about the genetic, environmental, and social factors that contribute to childhood obesity. We must recognize that children's weight is not under volitional control, but rather regulated by neurohormonal pathways that determine metabolism, hunger, and satiety. MBS is the most effective and safe treatment for severe obesity when compared with both obesity medication and lifestyle modification alone. Combination therapy with MBS, medications and lifestyle counseling is likely to have the greatest success in the long-term treatment of childhood obesity.

PATIENT EVALUATION AND OVERVIEW

A multidisciplinary team of providers is essential to provide the best care for patients undergoing MBS. This team should consist of a psychologist, pediatrician, bariatric and/or pediatric surgeon, dietician, and nurse coordinator.[47] These providers may also choose to include a physiotherapist, social worker, and/or a child life specialist.

Proper patient selection is important to consider before a child undergoes MBS. Obesity in children is defined as a BMI in the 95th percentile or higher.[48] This definition of obesity can be expanded into 3 classes: class I is defined as a BMI between the 95th percentile to 120% of the 95th percentile. Class II is defined as a BMI of 120% of 95th percentile to 140% of 95th percentile. Class III is defined as any BMI greater than 140% of the 95th percentile.[49]

MBS is recommended for children with class III obesity, a BMI of greater than 140% of the 95th percentile or a BMI greater than 40, whichever is lower.[5] It is further recommended for patients with class II with a BMI of 120% of the 95th percentile or a BMI greater than 35 with an obesity-related comorbidity, including hyperlipidemia, T2D, insulin resistance, OSA, GERD, NAFLD, and orthopedic disease, among others.

Contraindications to MBS include active substance abuse, pregnancy, untreated mental illness, or a medical cause of obesity that has not been fully treated (ie, hypothyroid, Cushing syndrome)[8] Patients who have mental illness or substance abuse that have been treated do not have worse outcomes. Patients with developmental delay, autism spectrum disorder, or syndromic obesity can be considered for surgery as long as they are able to tolerate the perioperative diet and cooperate with hospitalization. Ethics committee consults may be considered when risk versus benefit is difficult to determine.[5]

PREOPERATIVE PROGRAM: LIFESTYLE MODIFICATION

Although there are no strict standards for preoperative MBS programs, most will be run by a dietician, psychologist, physical therapist, trainer and/or bariatric nurse coordinator.[47] Many MBS candidates have vitamin B_{12}, folate, iron, and vitamin D deficiencies and may need to start preoperative supplementation.[50] In our experience, a consistent monthly program run in a group format has been very effective at stabilizing weight or initiating weight loss in preoperative pediatric patients. Most insurance companies look for the patient to complete 4 to 6 months of consistent lifestyle intervention before approval for surgery is considered, although there are no data to support this process. Studies show that patients are very unlikely to lose and maintain significant weight through lifestyle interventions alone; however, a multidisciplinary team program may be able to induce mild to moderate weight loss in a small fraction of children with obesity.[51]

The authors' program uses simple mantras to help patients remember their lifestyle goals. The rule of 60s requires 60 g of protein, 60 oz of water, and 60 minutes of exercise every day. Consistently eating more balanced meals while eliminating soda, chips, and fast food is also encouraged (**Table 1**). Patients who follow these simple rules will always decrease their rate of weight gain, which should be the goal for children before surgery. A 2-week preoperative meal replacement or low calorie diet is helpful to shrink the liver and allow for shorter operative times.[52]

SURGICAL TREATMENT OPTIONS

MBS has proven more effective in treating children with severe obesity compared with medical therapy.[53,54] MBS also provides resolution of T2D and OSA, and a more

Table 1		
Lifestyle goals before and after metabolic and bariatric surgery		
Follow the 60–60–60 Rule		
Every Day I Will:		
Eat	Drink	Be Active
60 g of Protein	60 oz of Water	60 min
Eat protein first	Do not drink:	Walk, run, swim, bike, dance
Eat every 3–4 h	1. Sugary drinks	Jump, skip, lift, or play
Do not skip meals	2. For 30 min after eating	For 30 min twice a day

significant improvement in weight-related quality of life than medical therapy alone. Before proceeding with surgical options, patients must demonstrate previous nonsurgical weight loss attempts and behavioral evaluations, although there are still no data to support this process.[8]

Before 2014, the most common operation performed in children was the RYGB (**Fig. 1**). The RYGB has been used to treat obesity since 1967 and has been done laparoscopically (through small incisions) since 1993. In youth, the RYGB has shown significant resolution of comorbidities and increased quality of life. In the Adolescent Morbid Obesity Surgery (AMOS) study 81 MBS-qualifying adolescents were treated

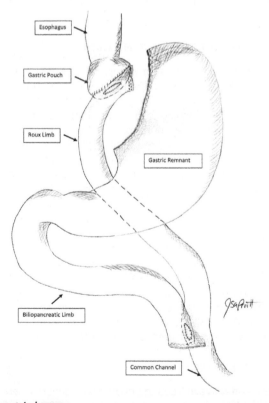

Fig. 1. Roux en Y gastric bypass.

with laparoscopic RYGB, 90% of participants reported achieving and maintaining a 13.1 kg/m² BMI loss or a 29% total body weight loss up to 5 years after surgery, although 25% required reoperation.[17] In the TEEN-Labs cohort from 5 centers in the United States, 181 children who underwent RYGB showed a 28% total body weight loss after 3 years, and were noted to have a 13% reoperation rate.[54] This surgery requires strict medication compliance to ensure that the patients do not develop vitamin deficiencies.[5] RYGB surgery has also been shown to increase sensitivity to alcohol and other drugs, and although insurance databases and surveys have shown an increased prevalence of opioid use after the surgery in adults, there are no data in children.[55,56] Other studies show the prevalence of drug use was decreased in the immediate 6 months after the surgery but overall increased over 7 years in adults.[57,58] RYGB is also a highly effective treatment for GERD, and is recommended over Nissen fundoplication for patients with acid reflux and obesity.

An increasingly popular and preferred choice for MBS in adults and children is the vertical sleeve gastrectomy (VSG, **Fig. 2**). Although the VSG has a slightly lower resolution rate of comorbidities than RYGB, it has similar weight loss (26%–28% total body weight loss at 1 year) and lower risk of complications in youth.[5] Because this is a relatively new procedure (2002), there is a lack of long-term (>10 year) data, particularly in the pediatric population. Based on adult VSG data, VSG is linked to increased cases of GERD after surgery compared with RYGB.[30]

Use of the adjustable gastric band has declined in recent years. Peña and colleagues[59] reported no deaths but high rate of failure and rate of reintervention with adjustable gastric band, concluding that it is not a preferred procedure in adolescents. However, there may be cases where adjustable gastric band is the only option for surgical weight loss in a child and may need to be considered.

TREATMENT RESISTANCE AND COMPLICATIONS

There are cases where, even after MBS, patients show inadequate weight loss. Between 20% and 30% of adult MBS patients experience limited weight loss, but the

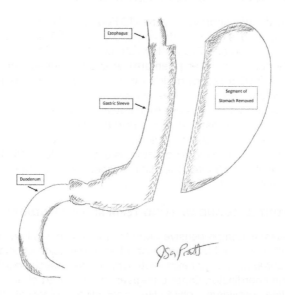

Fig. 2. VSG.

factors that determine weight loss after MBS, specifically in the pediatric population, are not well-understood.[58] In the AMOS study, 11% of patients lost less then 10% of their total body weight at 5 years. One theory for why some patients are unable to lose weight is that they experience loss of control eating after surgery. A higher proportion of adolescents undergoing MBS exhibit eating disorders such as binge eating disorder and loss of control eating; however, these conditions are not associated with worse weight loss outcomes after surgery.[60,61] It is more likely that polygenic- mediated metabolic factors that lead to obesity in childhood may not all be reversed by MBS.[62] Polygenic obesity seems to respond better to MBS than monogenic obesity in several studies; however, most individuals in both groups experience significant weight loss.[63]

Another common complication from RYGB and VSG is micronutrient deficiency.[54] This factor is of particular importance in pediatric populations, because the consequences of nutrient deficiency may impact normal development. These types of MBS require strict medication compliance to ensure proper nutrient intake and avoid deficiencies.[64] Studies have shown a small risk of anemia and bone mass density loss in adolescents after MBS.[65] Although vitamin D deficiency is common in preoperative obese pediatric patients, it does not change significantly after surgery.[54]

In the TEEN-Labs cohort, minor complications were found in 15% and major complications in 8% of participants within 30 days.[9] In the same group, the 30-day rate of reoperation after MBS was similar to that of adults, around 2.7%.[66] Adult patients who undergo VSG are less likely to require reoperation at 5 years or develop alcohol use disorder than those who undergo RYGB.[67,68] Gallstones and kidney stones can occur after rapid weight loss and are more common after RYGB than VSG, so patients should be informed of the symptoms and when to seek medical attention. Reflux (GERD) is a known complication of VSG in some patients; therefore, long-term postoperative screening for both symptomatic and asymptomatic GERD after VSG in children should be standard. Ulcers and internal hernias can occur after RYGB and can require emergency interventions; therefore, abdominal pain in a post-RYGB patient must be evaluated to rule out one of these complications.

PHARMACOLOGIC AND MEDICAL TREATMENT OPTIONS

Currently, the only 2 drugs approved by the US Food and Drug Administration for adolescents with severe obesity are metformin and Orlistat.[69] There are no medications approved by the US Food and Drug Administration for obesity in children less than 12 years old. Other drugs, such as phentermine and topiramate, are prescribed off-label owing to their weight-reducing side effects and safety profile in children. The use of metformin in children has not been shown to produce significant or sustained weight loss. It is important to consider medications in patients who do not respond to MBS as both adult and pediatric data support the synergistic effect of medications after surgery.[70,71] Further the use of medications for obesity in children has not been fully studied, but may become more common as both an adjunct to MBS as well as a stand-alone treatment in the future. Specific monogenic obesity-targeted medications are currently in development.

EVALUATION OF OUTCOME AND/OR LONG-TERM RECOMMENDATIONS

Patients who present to comprehensive pediatric metabolic and bariatric surgery programs are typically evaluated by a pediatric obesity medicine specialist, a pediatric and/or bariatric surgeon, a registered dietician, a child psychologist, and a social worker or program coordinator. Other caregivers may be part of any team, including advanced practice providers, child life specialists, physical therapists, and subspecialists in pulmonary medicine, gastroenterology, endocrine, and cardiology.[47] A multidisciplinary team meeting to share all provider findings and make a plan for the patient's path to surgery is critical.

Lifestyle changes are initiated early in the program and should be continued for 4 to 6 months to assess a patient and their family's compliance with the program. In some cases, the medical risk of delaying surgery will outweigh the risk of proceeding without initial lifestyle interventions and surgery should be pursued as soon as possible. The only measure of compliance with lifestyle modifications is observation of the patient's weight. Perhaps because of the genetic nature of childhood obesity, not all children who are compliant will lose weight, but most can stop gaining or at least stop gaining at the rate that they were before initiating the program.

Patients who proceed to metabolic and bariatric surgery need close postoperative follow-up to measure vitamin levels and adjust vitamin prescriptions, assess weight loss and to monitor for complications. Follow-up at 2 weeks, 6 weeks, and then at 3, 6, 9, 12, 18 and 24 months is standard, with annual follow-up thereafter. Weight loss after sleeve gastrectomy is expected to be 25% to 30% of the total body BMI at 1 year in at least 75% of patients. Patients with inadequate weight loss (<10% total BMI loss) should be reevaluated by the dietician and the psychologist and if needed started on medications to improve weight loss. If medications are not successful a conversion to an RYGB can be considered.

Arguably, the most important outcome measures are quality of life and quantity of life. In children with obesity, health-related quality of life is comparable with patients with cancer, after MBS health-related quality of life is significantly improved.[72,73] Prospective and retrospective studies in adult populations show a clear survival benefit in patients after MBS compared with patients who are treated with lifestyle changes alone.[74,75] It is likely that the improved mortality after MBS is shared by children; however, long term studies are still needed to asses this outcome.

SUMMARY

Despite strong evidence showing that metabolic and bariatric surgery is both safe and effective, it remains underutilized in children. MBS is recommended by the American Academy of Pediatrics for the treatment of severe obesity in children and adolescents. Although many surgical options exist, evidence suggests that the laparoscopic sleeve gastrectomy has the highest benefit to risk ratio in this population and should be considered standard of care at this time. RYGB should also be considered standard of care and considered, especially in children with severe T2D or GERD. The inclusion of lifestyle modification education and physical activity is standard of care. Further study regarding the use of medications, including timing, dosage, and duration, is necessary to maximize the weight loss and improvement of comorbidities afforded by MBS.

Indications for MBS should be based on weight and comorbidities, not age or Tanner stage. The current inclusion criteria for MBS in children are a BMI of 140% of the 95 percentiles (class III obesity) or a BMI of 120% of the 95th percentile (class II obesity) with a comorbidity.

CLINICS CARE POINTS

- VSG and RYGB are both considered Metabolic and Bariatric surgery and should be used in children with class III obesity or class II obesity with a comorbidity.

- Referral to a multidisciplinary pediatric obesity center should be initiated as soon as a child reaches class II obesity, regardless of age or comorbidity status.
- Lifestyle interventions and obesity medications alone cannot, at this time, be considered adequate treatment for class II (BMI >120% of the 95th percentile) obesity in children.
- Children who have undergone MBS for obesity should be followed over the long term for vitamin deficiencies, weight regain, and other common complications of MBS.

DISCLOSURE

Authors have nothing to disclose.

REFERENCES

1. Ogden CL, Carroll MD, Fryar CD, et al. Prevalence of obesity among adults and youth: United States, 2011-2014. NCHS Data Brief 2015;(219):1–8.
2. Skinner AC, Ravanbakht SN, Skelton JA, et al. Prevalence of obesity and severe obesity in US Children, 1999–2016. Pediatrics 2018;141(3):e20173459.
3. Patrick H, Nicklas TA. A review of family and social determinants of children's eating patterns and diet quality. J Am Coll Nutr 2005;24(2):83–92.
4. Reilly JJ, Armstrong J, Dorosty AR, et al. Early life risk factors for obesity in childhood: cohort study. BMJ 2005;330(7504):1357.
5. Pratt JSA, Browne A, Browne NT, et al. ASMBS pediatric metabolic and bariatric surgery guidelines, 2018. Surg Obes Relat Dis 2018;14(7):882–901.
6. Armstrong SC, Bolling CF, Michalsky MP, et al. Pediatric metabolic and bariatric surgery: evidence, barriers, and best practices. Pediatrics 2019;144(6): e20193223.
7. Zwintscher NP, Azarow KS, Horton JD, et al. The increasing incidence of adolescent bariatric surgery. J Pediatr Surg 2013;48(12):2401–7.
8. Bolling CF, Armstrong SC, Reichard KW, et al. Metabolic and bariatric surgery for pediatric patients with severe obesity. Pediatrics 2019;144(6):e20193224.
9. Inge TH, Zeller MH, Jenkins TM, et al. Perioperative outcomes of adolescents undergoing bariatric surgery: the Teen-Longitudinal Assessment of Bariatric Surgery (Teen-LABS) study. JAMA Pediatr 2014;168(1):47–53.
10. Twig G, Yaniv G, Levine H, et al. Body-mass index in 2.3 million adolescents and cardiovascular death in adulthood. N Engl J Med 2016;374(25):2430–40.
11. Michalsky M, Reichard K, Inge T, et al. ASMBS pediatric committee best practice guidelines. Surg Obes Relat Dis 2012;8(1):1–7.
12. Obert P, Gueugnon C, Nottin S, et al. Two-Dimensional Strain And Twist By Vector Velocity Imaging In Adolescents With Severe Obesity. Obesity 2012;20(12): 2397–405.
13. Michalsky MP, Inge TH, Jenkins TM, et al. Cardiovascular risk factors after adolescent bariatric surgery. Pediatrics 2018;141(2):e20172485.
14. Viner R, White B, Christie D. Type 2 diabetes in adolescents: a severe phenotype posing major clinical challenges and public health burden. Lancet 2017; 389(10085):2252–60.
15. Arslanian S, Kim JY, Nasr A, et al. Insulin sensitivity across the lifespan from obese adolescents to obese adults with impaired glucose tolerance: who is worse off? Pediatr Diabetes 2018;19(2):205–11.
16. Inge TH, Courcoulas AP, Jenkins TM, et al. Five-year outcomes of gastric bypass in adolescents as compared with adults. N Engl J Med 2019;380(22):2136–45.

17. Olbers T, Beamish AJ, Gronowitz E, et al. Laparoscopic Roux-en-Y gastric bypass in adolescents with severe obesity (AMOS): a prospective, 5-year, Swedish nationwide study. Lancet Diabetes Endocrinol 2017;5(3):174–83.
18. Jaramillo JD, Snyder E, Farrales S, et al. A multidisciplinary approach to laparoscopic sleeve gastrectomy among multiethnic adolescents in the United States. J Pediatr Surg 2017;52(10):1606–9.
19. Stanford FC, Mushannen T, Cortez P, et al. Comparison of short and long-term outcomes of metabolic and bariatric surgery in adolescents and adults. Front Endocrinol 2020;11:157.
20. Verhulst SL, Van Gaal L, De Backer W, et al. The prevalence, anatomical correlates and treatment of sleep-disordered breathing in obese children and adolescents. Sleep Med Rev 2008;12(5):339–46.
21. Kalra M, Inge T, Garcia V, et al. Obstructive sleep apnea in extremely overweight adolescents undergoing bariatric surgery. Obes Res 2005;13(7):1175–9.
22. Amin R, Simakajornboon N, Szczesniak R, et al. Early improvement in obstructive sleep apnea and increase in orexin levels after bariatric surgery in adolescents and young adults. Surg Obes Relat Dis 2017;13(1):95–100.
23. Duncan M, Zong W, Biank VF, et al. Nonalcoholic fatty liver disease in pediatrics. Pediatr Ann 2016;45(2):e54–8.
24. Xanthakos SA, Jenkins TM, Kleiner DE, et al. High prevalence of nonalcoholic fatty liver disease in adolescents undergoing bariatric surgery. Gastroenterology 2015;149(3):623–34.e8.
25. Manco M, Mosca A, De Peppo F, et al. The benefit of sleeve gastrectomy in obese adolescents on nonalcoholic steatohepatitis and hepatic fibrosis. J Pediatr 2017;180:31–7.e32.
26. Zeller MH, Inge TH, Modi AC, et al. Severe obesity and comorbid condition impact on the weight-related quality of life of the adolescent patient. J Pediatr 2015;166(3):651–9.e4.
27. Ryder JR, Edwards NM, Gupta R, et al. Changes in functional mobility and musculoskeletal pain after bariatric surgery in teens with severe obesity: teen-longitudinal assessment of bariatric surgery (LABS) Study. JAMA Pediatr 2016;170(9):871–7.
28. Griggs CL, Perez NP, Chan MC, et al. Slipped capital femoral epiphysis and Blount disease as indicators for early metabolic surgical intervention. Surg Obes Relat Dis 2019;15(10):1836–41.
29. Shaheen N, Ransohoff DF. Gastroesophageal reflux, Barrett esophagus, and esophageal cancer: scientific review. Jama 2002;287(15):1972–81.
30. Navarini D, Madalosso CAS, Tognon AP, et al. Predictive factors of gastroesophageal reflux disease in bariatric surgery: a controlled trial comparing sleeve gastrectomy with gastric bypass. Obes Surg 2020;30(4):1360–7.
31. Patti MG. An evidence-based approach to the treatment of gastroesophageal reflux disease. JAMA Surg 2016;151(1):73–8.
32. Ibele A, Garren M, Gould J. The impact of previous fundoplication on laparoscopic gastric bypass outcomes: a case-control evaluation. Surg Endosc 2012;26(1):177–81.
33. Sagar R, Gupta T. Psychological aspects of obesity in children and adolescents. Indian J Pediatr 2018;85(7):554–9.
34. Tevie J, Shaya FT. Association between mental health and comorbid obesity and hypertension among children and adolescents in the US. Eur Child Adolesc Psychiatry 2015;24(5):497–502.

35. Franklin J, Denyer G, Steinbeck KS, et al. Obesity and risk of low self-esteem: a statewide survey of Australian children. Pediatrics 2006;118(6):2481–7.
36. Zeller MH, Roehrig HR, Modi AC, et al. Health-related quality of life and depressive symptoms in adolescents with extreme obesity presenting for bariatric surgery. Pediatrics 2006;117(4):1155–61.
37. Järvholm K, Bruze G, Peltonen M, et al. 5-year mental health and eating pattern outcomes following bariatric surgery in adolescents: a prospective cohort study. Lancet Child Adolesc Health 2020;4(3):210–9.
38. Puhl R, Suh Y. Health consequences of weight stigma: implications for obesity prevention and treatment. Curr Obes Rep 2015;4(2):182–90.
39. Garcia JT, Amankwah EK, Hernandez RG. Assessment of weight bias among pediatric nurses and clinical support staff toward obese patients and their caregivers. J Pediatr Nurs 2016;31(4):e244–51.
40. Vanguri P, Lanning D, Wickham EP, et al. Pediatric health care provider perceptions of weight loss surgery in adolescents. Clin Pediatr (Phila) 2014;53(1):60–5.
41. Woolford SJ, Clark SJ, Gebremariam A, et al. To cut or not to cut: physicians' perspectives on referring adolescents for bariatric surgery. Obes Surg 2010;20(7):937–42.
42. Inge TH, Boyce TW, Lee M, et al. Access to care for adolescents seeking weight loss surgery. Obesity (Silver Spring) 2014;22(12):2593–7.
43. Kelleher DC, Merrill CT, Cottrell LT, et al. Recent national trends in the use of adolescent inpatient bariatric surgery: 2000 through 2009. JAMA Pediatr 2013; 167(2):126–32.
44. Stanford FC, Jones DB, Schneider BE, et al. Patient race and the likelihood of undergoing bariatric surgery among patients seeking surgery. Surg Endosc 2015; 29(9):2794–9.
45. Wallace AE, Young-Xu Y, Hartley D, et al. Racial, socioeconomic, and rural-urban disparities in obesity-related bariatric surgery. Obes Surg 2010;20(10):1354–60.
46. Perez NP, Westfal ML, Stapleton SM, et al. Beyond insurance: race-based disparities in the use of metabolic and bariatric surgery for the management of severe pediatric obesity. Surg Obes Relat Dis 2020;16(3):414–9.
47. Pratt JSA, Roque SS, Valera R, et al. Preoperative considerations for the pediatric patient undergoing metabolic and bariatric surgery. Semin Pediatr Surg 2020; 29(1):150890.
48. Kelly AS, Barlow SE, Rao G, et al. Severe obesity in children and adolescents: identification, associated health risks, and treatment approaches: a scientific statement from the American Heart Association. Circulation 2013;128(15): 1689–712.
49. Skinner AC, Skelton JA. Prevalence and trends in obesity and severe obesity among children in the United States, 1999-2012. JAMA Pediatr 2014;168(6): 561–6.
50. Roust LR, DiBaise JK. Nutrient deficiencies prior to bariatric surgery. Curr Opin Clin Nutr Metab Care 2017;20(2):138–44.
51. Mameli C, Krakauer JC, Krakauer NY, et al. Effects of a multidisciplinary weight loss intervention in overweight and obese children and adolescents: 11 years of experience. PLoS One 2017;12(7):e0181095.
52. Ekici U, Ferhatoglu MF. Perioperative and postoperative effects of preoperative low-calorie restrictive diets on patients undergoing laparoscopic sleeve gastrectomy. J Gastrointest Surg 2020;24(2):313–9.

53. Inge TH, Laffel LM, Jenkins TM, et al. Comparison of surgical and medical therapy for type 2 diabetes in severely obese adolescents. JAMA Pediatr 2018; 172(5):452–60.
54. Inge TH, Courcoulas AP, Jenkins TM, et al. Weight loss and health status 3 years after bariatric surgery in adolescents. N Engl J Med 2015;374(2):113–23.
55. Smith KE, Engel SG, Steffen KJ, et al. Problematic alcohol use and associated characteristics following bariatric surgery. Obes Surg 2018;28(5):1248–54.
56. Amalie HS, Louise L, Lona LC, et al. Chronic abdominal pain and persistent opioid use after bariatric surgery. Scand J Pain 2020;20(2):239–51.
57. King WC, Chen JY, Courcoulas AP, et al. Alcohol and other substance use after bariatric surgery: prospective evidence from a U.S. multicenter cohort study. Surg Obes Relat Dis 2017;13(8):1392–402.
58. Sarwer DB, Allison KC, Wadden TA, et al. Psychopathology, disordered eating, and impulsivity as predictors of outcomes of bariatric surgery. Surg Obes Relat Dis 2019;15(4):650–5.
59. Peña AS, Delko T, Couper R, et al. Laparoscopic adjustable gastric banding in Australian adolescents: should it be done? Obes Surg 2017;27(7):1667–73.
60. Utzinger LM, Gowey MA, Zeller M, et al. Loss of control eating and eating disorders in adolescents before bariatric surgery. Int J Eat Disord 2016;49(10): 947–52.
61. Goldschmidt AB, Khoury J, Jenkins TM, et al. Adolescent loss-of-control eating and weight loss maintenance after bariatric surgery. Pediatrics 2018;141(1): e20171659.
62. Garver WS, Newman SB, Gonzales-Pacheco DM, et al. The genetics of childhood obesity and interaction with dietary macronutrients. Genes Nutr 2013;8(3): 271–87.
63. Thaker VV. Genetic and epigenetic causes of obesity. Adolesc Med State Art Rev 2017;28(2):379–405.
64. Fullmer MA, Abrams SH, Hrovat K, et al. Nutritional strategy for adolescents undergoing bariatric surgery: report of a working group of the Nutrition Committee of NASPGHAN/NACHRI. J Pediatr Gastroenterol Nutr 2012;54(1):125–35.
65. Kaulfers A-MD, Bean JA, Inge TH, et al. Bone loss in adolescents after bariatric surgery. Pediatrics 2011;127(4):e956.
66. Flum DR, Belle SH, King WC, et al. Perioperative safety in the longitudinal assessment of bariatric surgery. N Engl J Med 2009;361(5):445–54.
67. Azam H, Shahrestani S, Phan K. Alcohol use disorders before and after bariatric surgery: a systematic review and meta-analysis. Ann Transl Med 2018; 6(8):148.
68. Salminen P, Helmiö M, Ovaska J, et al. Effect of laparoscopic sleeve gastrectomy vs laparoscopic Roux-en-Y gastric bypass on weight loss at 5 years among patients with morbid obesity: the SLEEVEPASS Randomized Clinical Trial. Jama 2018;319(3):241–54.
69. White B, Jamieson L, Clifford S, et al. Adolescent experiences of anti-obesity drugs. Clin Obes 2015;5(3):116–26.
70. Stanford FC, Alfaris N, Gomez G, et al. The utility of weight loss medications after bariatric surgery for weight regain or inadequate weight loss: a multi-center study. Surg Obes Relat Dis 2017;13(3):491–500.
71. Srivastava G, Fox CK, Kelly AS, et al. Clinical considerations regarding the use of obesity pharmacotherapy in adolescents with obesity. Obesity (Silver Spring) 2019;27(2):190–204.

72. Reiter-Purtill J, Ley S, Kidwell KM, et al. Change, predictors and correlates of weight- and health-related quality of life in adolescents 2-years following bariatric surgery. Int J Obes 2020;44(7):1467–78.
73. Schwimmer JB, Burwinkle TM, Varni JW. Health-related quality of life of severely obese children and adolescents. JAMA 2003;289(14):1813–9.
74. Sjöström L, Narbro K, Sjöström CD, et al. Effects of bariatric surgery on mortality in Swedish obese subjects. N Engl J Med 2007;357(8):741–52.
75. Perry CD, Hutter MM, Smith DB, et al. Survival and changes in comorbidities after bariatric surgery. Ann Surg 2008;247(1):21–7.

Revisional Bariatric Surgery

Katelin Mirkin, MD, Vamsi V. Alli, MD, Ann M. Rogers, MD*

KEYWORDS

- Bariatric • Revision • Reoperation • Complications • Weight loss surgery

KEY POINTS

- Revisional surgery is a growing subset of bariatric surgical procedures.
- These operations are generally more complex and more prone to complications than primary bariatric procedures.
- General principles exist for the evaluation of revisional patients.
- The approach to revision of different procedures will vary.

INTRODUCTION

Most of the bariatric procedures never require reoperation.[1] However, revisional procedures are a growing subset of bariatric operations, currently representing around 7% to 15% of the total number.[2–4] As primary bariatric volumes increase, inevitably so will the potential need for revisional surgeries. This increase has been demonstrated in multiple longitudinal studies in bariatric patients; notably, the long-term Swedish Obesity Study recently reported a 28% rate of revisional bariatric surgery in adults.[5] Similarly, a systematic review by Shoar and colleagues[6] reported rates of revisional bariatric surgery in up to 23.7% of adolescent patients.

Accepted nomenclature for various types of reoperative or revisional bariatric surgery include those that are "corrective" of primary bariatric operations in order to achieve their original desired function: a "conversion," in which one procedure is changed to another type, or "reversal," intended to restore normal or near-normal anatomy.[7] In this article, the authors use the words *reoperative* and *revisional* interchangeably.

INDICATIONS

Bariatric surgeons report that revisional surgery is primarily patient driven.[8] Potential indications for revision of a bariatric procedure include inadequate weight loss or postoperative weight regain; inadequate improvement or frank recurrence of a weight-related comorbidity such as type 2 diabetes; or complications related to the initial operation. Weight regain is the reported indication for more than half of revisional procedures.[8] Definitions of significant weight loss and weight regain vary, and it is now considered short

Minimally Invasive and Bariatric Surgery, Penn State Hershey Medical Center
* Corresponding author. 500 University Drive, H-149, Hershey, PA 17033.
E-mail address: arogers@pennstatehealth.psu.edu

Surg Clin N Am 101 (2021) 213–222
https://doi.org/10.1016/j.suc.2020.12.008
surgical.theclinics.com

sighted to classify the success or failure of a bariatric operation only in terms of weight. Nonetheless, one systematic review found that the most commonly used definition of "inadequate weight loss" after bariatric surgery was to lose less than 50% of excess weight.[9] The second most common definition cited in this review was less than 25% excess weight loss. One observational study of 300 bypass patients showed that, despite initial weight loss, 37% of patients regained 25% or more of their lost weight after a mean of 7 years,[10] so it is understandable that patients with such expectations might seek revision. Beyond weight regain, however, there exist innumerable other indications for revision, such as unrelenting gastroesophageal reflux disease (GERD), neuroglycopenia, refractory marginal ulcers and strictures, device and hardware complications, fistulae, intussusception, internal hernias, malnourishment, and pain.[5,8]

Clearly, nonoperative options exist for managing suboptimal weight loss, weight regain, and even comorbidity return, including adjunctive medications.[11] In addition, there is a variety of endoscopic and other surgical approaches designed to address weight and other complications after bariatric surgery; however, bariatric surgical revision is the focus of this article.

PREOPERATIVE EVALUATION

Before a revision is undertaken, multidisciplinary evaluation is appropriate. The patient's nutritional status should be assessed and any existing deficiencies should be repleted. Although protein deficiency is the most common macronutrient deficiency seen after bariatric surgery,[12] micronutrient abnormalities are not uncommon and should be corrected before major bariatric revisions. Behavioral and psychosocial assessment and intervention are also key at this juncture to determine if nonsurgical approaches would be helpful or preferable.

When surgical revision is, in fact, indicated, radiologic studies, such as an upper gastrointestinal series contrast study with admixed food or effervescent crystals, and diagnostic upper endoscopy are typically performed.[8,13] Three-dimensional computed tomographic reconstruction may also be helpful.[14] Review of prior operative reports is invaluable.

PREVALENCE AND DISTRIBUTION
Adjustable Gastric Band

At this time, adjustable gastric banding is the procedure that most commonly requires revision, with reported rates of 30% to 60%.[5,15] Hardware-related issues include tubing puncture, tubing disconnection, port diaphragm disruption, balloon rupture, port flip, and others. Some patients may undergo multiple procedures related to having had a band placed.[15] Conversions after band surgery are most often related to inadequate weight loss, often accompanied by dysphagia and maladaptive eating.[16] There is a substantial body of literature on conversion of band to bypass, band to sleeve, and even band to duodenal switch, with either 1 or 2 anastomoses.[17,18] There is a concomitant significant amount of literature addressing the controversy of whether such conversions are best performed in 1 or 2 stages.[19–21] What data exist seem to show that in whatever way such conversions are undertaken they can be performed safely, with a somewhat higher complication rate than that seen with a primary operation, but with similar weight loss and improvement of comorbidities.[22,23]

Nonadjustable Band/Gastroplasty

The nonadjustable gastric bands and stapled gastroplasties that were in use in variable geographic areas in the 1970s and 80s were most commonly revised by conversion to gastric bypass[24]; this is also true of the more widely employed vertical banded gastroplasty, described by Mason.[25] However, there is also literature on conversion of this latter procedure to sleeve gastrectomy (SG),[26] one-anastomosis gastric bypass (OAGB),[27] and duodenal switch (DS),[28,29] albeit with fairly high complication rates. Because the various stapled and banded gastroplasties are vanishing species, technical details regarding revision of such procedures are beyond the scope of this article.

Jejunoileal Bypass

Jejunoileal bypass, the first operation specifically designed for weight loss,[30] reported in the 1950s and subsequently abandoned for unacceptable malabsorptive complications and deaths, has been reversed, as well as converted to bypass and sleeve gastrectomy.[31–33] As the jejunoileal bypass operation was not standardized, the approach to revision of such a procedure should necessarily be individualized. Attention must be paid toward nutritional reeducation, preoperative correction of metabolic abnormalities, and often prerevisional enteral feeding of the defunctionalized limb in order to avoid complications related to bowel atrophy and size mismatch.

Roux-en-Y Gastric Bypass

Although the minority of gastric bypasses may require revision, globally, Roux-en-Y gastric bypass (RYGB) is by far the most commonly used revisional procedure performed after primary bariatric surgery of any type.[8] For revision after primary RYGB, pouch reduction is the most commonly performed revisional procedure,[8] and this has been reported as an endoscopic or a surgical procedure and may include concomitant gastrojejunostomy (GJ) revision. Although pouch or stomal reduction does not always successfully lead to further weight loss, it can be shown to arrest further weight gain, at least in the short term.[34] "Salvage" banding of the GJ has also been reported to enhance postbypass weight loss.[35]

Another potential cause of complications after RYGB is gastrogastric fistula, which may have developed over time or have been present since—but not immediately apparent at—the time of the index operation. When such a fistula becomes symptomatic, either as weight regain, pain, or marginal ulceration, it may be treated either endoscopically or by surgical division or resection. Surgical therapy may also include partial remnant resection, downsizing of the pouch, and revision of the GJ anastomosis, particularly if the fistula has led to marginal ulceration with or without stricture. The management of this challenging entity may be complex.[36]

A difficult clinical issue is weight and comorbidity regain seen in the setting of an anatomically intact gastric bypass. Because of the elevated risks related to preoperative bariatric surgery and the possibility of limited benefit, often this is reasonably treated as a dietary or behavioral issue. However, in some cases it may be addressed through surgical revision, including procedures to increase limb length (either biliopancreatic or proximal alimentary limb) as well as through conversion to DS.[37–39] The bariatric literature has demonstrated additional weight loss with such procedures, at the cost of an elevated complication rate (**Table 1**).

Vertical Sleeve Gastrectomy

Now that SG is the most common operation for severe obesity in the world,[40] there naturally will be concomitant need for its revision. There exist multiple reports on resleeving and sleeve plication for weight regain and/or GERD based on fundal dilation, as well as seromyotomy or stricturoplasty for midbody stricture.[41,42] However, there is a far more extensive body of literature on the conversion of sleeve

Table 1
Comparison of primary and revisional Roux-en-Y gastric bypass outcomes

	Primary RYGB (%)	Revisional RYGB (%)
Leak	2.1	3.0
Hemorrhage	1.2	0–4.6
SSI	0.8–1	1–6.5
Stricture	0.2–0.4	0.9–1.8
Ulcer	0.4–2.0	0.9–2.6
Perforation	0.4	0–1.2
Hernia	1.2	7.6
Mortality	0.4	0
Total morbidity rate	6.5	10.3

Abbreviation: SSI, surgical site infection.

Data from Dardamanis D, Navez J, Coubeau L, et al. A retrospective comparative study of primary versus revisional Roux-en-Y gastric bypass: long-term results. *Obes Surg.*2018;28(8):2457-2464; and Axer S, Szabo E, Agerskov S, et al. Predictive factors of complications in revisional gastric bypass surgery: results from the Scandinavian Obesity Surgery Registry. Surg Obes Relat Dis.2019;15(12):2094-100.

to bypass, either to RYGB or to OAGB, or the addition of the DS or single-anastomosis duodenoileostomy (SADI) procedure for additional weight loss or comorbidity resolution[43–45] **(Table 2)**.

Biliopancreatic Diversion, with or Without Duodenal Switch

Although at this time these procedures account for less than 1% of all bariatric procedures performed globally,[3] there is reason to believe that the somewhat simpler SADI or loop version of the DS procedure may come to be used more frequently with time. It is anticipated that revisions including lengthening of the common channel or reversals of these procedures will become increasingly necessary, likely related to malabsorptive issues.[46,47]

OUTCOMES

Revisional RYGB is associated with decreased weight loss compared with primary RYGB.[48–50] However, revisional surgery can offer improvement in comorbid conditions, such as in the use of type 2 diabetes medications and overall glucose control.[51] As expected with any reoperative procedure, revisional bariatric surgery seems to be associated with greater morbidity. In a study of the Scandinavian Obesity Registry, revisional surgery was associated with a higher incidence of complications both intraoperatively and postoperatively, and an open approach to revisional procedures was an independent risk factor for intraoperative complications. Interestingly, indication for revision and type of primary operation were not predictive of complications.[52] Relative to primary bariatric procedures, revisional surgeries are associated with longer operative times, increased length of stay, more frequent conversions to open surgery, higher readmission rates, and higher rates of unplanned admissions to the intensive care unit (ICU).[49,53] In an analysis of the MBSAQIP data registry of patients who underwent SG, the incidence of complications requiring reoperation within 30 days was twice as high in patients undergoing revisional surgery, but there was no difference

Table 2
Conversional complications

Conversion from	Complication Rate	Complication Categories
Roux-en-Y gastric bypass	7%–44% overall 7.3% reoperation 24% readmit	4.3%–33% stricture 2.7%–22% leak 2.1%–34.5% SSI 4.3% ulcer 1.5%–2.3% hemorrhage 21% incisional hernia
Adjustable gastric band	3.7%–32% overall (16.5% RYGB, 7.7%–32% SG, 4.8%–62% for BPD-DS) 2.3%–6.5% reoperation (7.8% RYGB, 2.0% SG) Intraoperative 14.4%–19.7%	1.7%–13.3% stricture 0.3%–6.89% (1.7%–2.3% RYGB, 2.2%–33%SG) leak 0.9%–20.8% SSI 4.3% ulcer 1.2%–20% hemorrhage 8% incisional hernia
One-anastomosis gastric bypass	5%–35.2% overall	5.88%–7.7% leak 5% SSI 2.38%–17.65% hemorrhage 3.8% stenosis
Sleeve gastrectomy	6.7%–27.8%	2.78% hemorrhage 2.78% obstruction

Abbreviations: BPD-DS, biliopancreatic diversion with duodenal switch; SSI, surgical site infection.
Data from Refs.[7,22,43,52,59–65]

in length of stay or 30-day mortality.[53] The evaluation and management of complications after revisional bariatric surgery is similar to that after primary cases. Because the rate of complications may be higher, however, it is important to maintain a high index of suspicion.

APPROACH

As revisional surgery becomes more widespread, minimally invasive approaches are becoming increasingly commonplace. In the Scandinavian Obesity Registry study, the rate of open procedures decreased from 70.8% in 2007 to 8.5% in 2016.[52] The same registry reports, however, that revisional bariatric surgery carries a significantly higher rate of conversion to open surgery when started laparoscopically. There are growing numbers of reports in the literature on the benefits and risks of the robotic approach to revisional bariatric surgery. An MBSAQIP database study of patients undergoing revisional surgery, matching 1144 robotic and 1144 laparoscopic patients, reported that the former were associated with longer operative times, higher rates of ICU admission, more leaks, and more bleeding, but that both approaches were overall safe.[54] The definitive determination on the safety, cost, and applicability of robotics to revisional bariatric surgery is in evolution. Nonetheless, multiple smaller studies of revisional cases done through minimally invasive techniques report equivalent outcomes and low morbidity rates.[55,56]

INTERNATIONAL OPERATIONS AND EMERGING PROCEDURES

With the increase in bariatric surgery worldwide, along with greater ease of travel and international surgical options approved by US insurers,[57] bariatric surgeons in the United States can be expected to encounter revisional candidates who had their index operation elsewhere. However, innovative procedures are also developed and propagated in the United States, and all accredited bariatric programs will need the flexibility to manage patients with unusual or unfamiliar primary procedures or devices. One of the larger case series (n = 16) of patients undergoing conversion from OAGB to RYGB, indeed from a US bariatric program, reported a mean length of stay of 5.5 days, a rate of conversion to open surgery of 25%, and an overall (major and minor) complication rate of 37.5%.[58] These rates are significantly higher than what is reported in the primary RYGB literature and illustrate the difficulties that can be encountered in such less-common procedures.

DISCUSSION

Revisional bariatric surgery is on the increase in the United States and globally. It is important to point out that insurance policies and determinations that rule out bariatric revisions are outdated and discriminatory and are not driven by evidence. Obesity is understood to be a chronic and recurring disease as many others but one that responds favorably to surgical interventions. Just as most other medical and surgical therapies sometimes need alterations, additional approaches, or adjunctive therapies, so will bariatric surgery.

SUMMARY

Bariatric procedures are commonly performed, and there is reason to believe that reoperative surgery will be a growing part of most bariatric surgeons' practice. Revisional surgery can have a higher reported rate of morbidity, mortality, and inadequate weight loss, along with a lower rate of comorbidity resolution. Nonetheless, it can be safely performed, with excellent outcomes and improved quality of life for patients.[7]

CLINICS CARE POINTS

- Revisional surgery is a growing subset of bariatric surgical procedures.
- These operations are generally more complex and more prone to complications than primary bariatric procedures.
- General principles exist for the evaluation of revisional patients.
- The approach to surgical revision of different procedures will vary.

DISCLOSURE

The authors have nothing to disclose.

REFERENCES

1. Sudan R, Nguyen NT, Hutter MM, et al. Morbidity, mortality, and weight loss outcomes after reoperative bariatric surgery in the USA. J Gastrointest Surg 2015; 19:171–9.
2. Angrisani L, Santonicola A, Iovino P, et al. IFSO worldwide survey 2016: primary, endoluminal, and revisional procedures. Obes Surg 2018;28(12):3783–94.
3. Ponce J, DeMaria EJ, Nguyen NT, et al. American society for metabolic and bariatric surgery estimation of bariatric surgery procedures in 2015 and surgeon workforce in the United States. Surg Obes Relat Dis 2016;12(9):1637–9.

4. English WJ, DeMaria EJ, Hutter MM, et al. American society for metabolic and bariatric surgery 2018 estimate of metabolic and bariatric procedures performed in the United States. Surg Obes Relat Dis 2020;16(4):457–63.
5. Hjorth S, Näslund I, Andersson-Assarsson JC, et al. Reoperations after bariatric surgery in 26 years of follow-up of the swedish obese subjects study. JAMA Surg 2019;154(4):319–26.
6. Shoar S, Mahmoudzadeh H, Naderan M, et al. Long-term outcome of bariatric surgery in morbidly obese adolescents: a systematic review and meta-analysis of 950 patients with a minimum of 3 years follow-up. Obes Surg 2017;27(12): 3110–7.
7. Brethauer SA, Kothari S, Sudan R, et al. Systematic review of reoperative bariatric surgery: American society for metabolic and bariatric surgery revision task force. Surg Obes Relat Dis 2014;10:952–72.
8. Mahawar KK, Nimeri A, Adamo M, et al. Practices concerning revisional bariatric surgery: a survey of 460 Surgeons. Obes Surg 2018;28(9):2650–60.
9. Mann JP, Jakes AD, Hayden JD, et al. Systematic review of definitions of failure in revisional bariatric surgery. Obes Surg 2015;25(3):571–4.
10. Cooper TC, Simmons EB, Webb K, et al. Trends in weight regain following Roux-en-Y gastric bypass (RYGB) bariatric surgery. Obes Surg 2015;25(8):1474–81.
11. Alli V, Rogers AM. Role of the obesity medicine physician. The SAGES manual of bariatric surgery, 2nd edition. Eds. Kevin Reavis, Allison Barrett, Matthew Kroh. 2017.
12. Mohapatra S, Gangadharan K, Pitchumoni CS, et al. Malnutrition in obesity before and after bariatric surgery. Dis Mon 2020;66:100866;1–25.
13. Qiu J, Lundberg PW, Javier Birriel T, et al. Revisional bariatric surgery for weight regain and refractory complications in a single MBSAQIP accredited center: what are we dealing with? Obes Surg 2018;28(9):2789–95.
14. Latif MA, Fouda N, Omran E, et al. Role of imaging in assessment and detection of complications after bariatric surgery. Egypt J Radiol Nucl Med 2020; 51(41):1–9.
15. Ibrahim AM, Thumma JR, Dimick JB. Reoperation and Medicare expenditures after laparoscopic gastric band surgery. JAMA Surg 2017;152(9):835–42.
16. Tran TT, Pauli E, Lyn-Sue JR, et al. Revisional weight loss surgery after failed laparoscopic gastric banding: an institutional experience. Surg Endosc 2013;27(11): 4087–93.
17. Zhou R, Poirier J, Torquati A, et al. Short-term outcomes of conversion of failed gastric banding to laparoscopic sleeve gastrectomy or Roux-en-Y gastric bypass: a meta-analysis. Obes Surg 2019;29(2):420–5.
18. De Csepel J, Quinn T, Pomp A, et al. Conversion to a laparoscopic biliopancreatic diversion with a duodenal switch for failed laparoscopic adjustable silicone gastric banding. J Laparoendosc Adv Surg Tech A 2002;12(4):237–40.
19. Spaniolas K, Bates AT, Docimo S, et al. Single stage conversion from adjustable gastric banding to sleeve gastrectomy or Roux-en-Y gastric bypass: an analysis of 4875 patients. Surg Obes Relat Dis 2017;13:1880–6.
20. Debergh I, Defoort B, De Visschere M, et al. A one-step conversion from gastric banding to laparoscopic Roux-en-Y gastric bypass is as safe as a two-step conversion: a comparative analysis of 885 patients. Acta Chir Belg 2016;116(5): 271–7.
21. Obeid NR, Schwack BF, Kurian MS, et al. Single-stage versus 2-stage sleeve gastrectomy as a conversion after failed adjustable gastric banding: 30-day outcomes. Surg Endosc 2014;28:3186–92.

22. Coblijn UK, Verveld CJ, van Wagensveld BA, et al. Laparoscopic Roux-en-Y gastric bypass or laparoscopic sleeve gastrectomy as a revisional procedure after adjustable gastric band - a systematic review. Obes Surg 2013;23:1899–914.

23. Topart P, Becouarn G, Ritz P. Biliopancreatic diversion with duodenal switch or gastric bypass for failed gastric banding: retrospective study from two institutions with preliminary results. Surg Obes Relat Dis 2007;3:512–5.

24. Jones KB. Revisional bariatric surgery - safe and effective. Obes Surg 2001;11: 183–9.

25. Mason EE. Vertical banded gastroplasty for obesity. Arch Surg 1982;117(5): 701–6.

26. Salama TMS, Sabry K. Redo surgery after failed open VBG: laparoscopic mini-gastric bypass versus laparoscopic Roux en Y gastric bypass - which is better? Minim Invasive Surg 2016. https://doi.org/10.1155/2016/8737519.

27. Benlice C, Antoine HJ, Schauer PR. Laparoscopic conversion of a vertical banded gastroplasty to a sleeve gastrectomy in a morbidly obese patient with a complicated medical history. Obes Surg 2018;12:4095.

28. Greenbaum DF, Wasser SH, Riley T, et al. Duodenal switch with omentopexy and feeding jejunostomy - a safe and effective revisional operation for failed previous weight loss surgery. Surg Obes Relat Dis 2011;7:213–8.

29. Jain-Spangler K, Portenier D, Torquati A, et al. Conversion of vertical banded gastroplasty to stand-alone sleeve gastrectomy or biliopancreatic diversion with duodenal switch. J Gastrointest Surg 2013;17(4):805–8.

30. Buchwald H. The evolution of metabolic/bariatric surgery. Obes Surg 2014;24(8): 1126–35.

31. Dallal RM, Akhondzadeh M. Minimally invasive management of complications from jejunoileal bypass. Surg Obes Relat Dis 2006;2:226–7.

32. Tapper D, Hunt TK, Allen RC, et al. Conversion of jejunoileal bypass to gastric bypass to maintain weight loss. Surg Gynecol Obstet 1978;147(3):353–7.

33. Patel SM, Escalante-Tattersfield T, Szomstein S, et al. Sleeve gastrectomy after a jejunoileal bypass reversal: case report and review of the literature. Bariatric Times 2008.

34. Thompson CC, Chand B, Chen YK, et al. Endoscopic suturing for transoral outlet reduction increases weight loss after Roux-en-Y gastric bypass surgery. Gastroenterology 2013;145:129–37.

35. Irani K, Youn HA, Ren-Fielding CJ, et al. Midterm results for gastric banding as salvage procedure for patients with weight loss failure after Roux-en-Y gastric bypass. Surg Obes Relat Dis 2011;7:219–24.

36. Campos J, Galvao Neto M, Martins J, et al. Endoscopic, conservative, and surgical treatment of the gastrogastric fistula: the efficacy of a stepwise approach and its long-term results. Bariatr Surg Pract Patient Care 2015;10(2):62–7.

37. Buchwald H, Oien DM. Revision Roux-en-Y gastric bypass to biliopancreatic long-limb gastric bypass for inadequate weight response: case series and analysis. Obes Surg 2017;27(9):2293–302.

38. Caruana JA, Monte SV, Jacobs DM, et al. Distal small bowel bypass for weight regain after gastric bypass: safety and efficacy threshold occurs at <70% bypass. Surg Obes Relat Dis 2015;11(6):1248–55.

39. Parikh M, Pomp A, Gagner M. Laparoscopic conversion of failed gastric bypass to duodenal switch: technical considerations and preliminary outcomes. Surg Obes Relat Dis 2007;3(6):611–8.

40. Welbourn R, Hollyman M, Kinsman R, et al. Bariatric surgery worldwide: baseline demographic description and one-year outcomes from the Fourth IFSO Global Registry Report 2018. Obes Surg 2019;29(3):782–95.
41. Dapri G, Cadiere GB, Himpens J. Laparoscopic seromyotomy for long stenosis after sleeve gastrectomy with or without duodenal switch. Obes Surg 2009;19: 495–9.
42. Sudan R, Kasotakis G, Betof A, et al. Sleeve gastrectomy strictures: technique for robotic-assisted strictureplasty. Video case report. Surg Obes Relat Dis 2010;6: 434–6.
43. Iannelli A, Debs T, Martini F, et al. Laparoscopic conversion of sleeve gastrectomy to Roux-en-Y gastric bypass: indications and preliminary results. Surg Obes Relat Dis 2016;12:1533–8.
44. Moon RC, Fuentes AS, Teixeira AF, et al. Conversions after sleeve gastrectomy for weight regain: to a single and double anastomosis duodenal switch and gastric bypass at a single institution. Obes Surg 2019;29:48–53.
45. Greco F. Conversion of vertical sleeve gastrectomy to a functional single-anastomosis gastric bypass: technique and preliminary results using a non-adjustable ring instead of stapled division. Obes Surg 2017;27:896–901.
46. Hamoui N, Chock B, Anthone G, et al. Revision of the duodenal switch: indications, technique, and outcomes. J Am Coll Surg 2007;204(4):603–8.
47. Mitzman B, Cottam D, Goripathi R, et al. Stomach intestinal pylorus sparing (SIPS) surgery for morbid obesity: retrospective analyses of our preliminary experience. Obes Surg 2016;26:2098–104.
48. Pędziwiatr M, Małczak P, Wierdak M, et al. Revisional gastric bypass is inferior to primary gastric bypass in terms of short- and long-term outcomes-systematic review and meta-analysis. Obes Surg 2018;28(7):2083–91.
49. Dardamanis D, Navez J, Coubeau L, et al. A retrospective comparative study of primary versus revisional Roux-en-Y gastric bypass: long-term results. Obes Surg 2018;28(8):2457–64.
50. Mora Oliver I, Cassinello Fernández N, Alfonso Ballester R, et al. Revisional bariatric surgery due to failure of the initial technique: 25 years of experience in a specialized Unit of obesity surgery in spain. Cir Esp 2019;97(10):568–74.
51. Aleassa EM, Hassan M, Hayes K, et al. Effect of revisional bariatric surgery on type 2 diabetes mellitus. Surg Endosc 2019;33(8):2642–8.
52. Axer S, Szabo E, Agerskov S, et al. Predictive factors of complications in revisional gastric bypass surgery: results from the scandinavian obesity surgery registry. Surg Obes Relat Dis 2019;15(12):2094–100.
53. El Chaar M, Stoltzfus J, Melitics M, et al. 30-Day outcomes of revisional bariatric stapling procedures: first report based on MBSAQIP data registry. Obes Surg 2018;28(8):2233–40.
54. Acevedo E, Mazzei M, Zhao H, et al. Outcomes in conventional laparoscopic versus robotic-assisted revisional bariatric surgery: a retrospective, case-controlled study of the MBSAQIP database. Surg Endosc 2020;34(4):1573–84.
55. Gray KD, Moore MD, Elmously A, et al. Perioperative outcomes of laparoscopic and robotic revisional bariatric surgery in a complex patient population. Obes Surg 2018;28(7):1852–9.
56. Rebecchi F, Ugliono E, Allaix ME, et al. Robotic Roux-en-Y gastric bypass as a revisional bariatric procedure: a single-center prospective cohort study. Obes Surg 2020;30(1):11–7.
57. Available at: https://wwwnc.cdc.gov/travel/page/medical-tourism. Accessed January 12, 2021.

58. Landreneau JP, Barajas-Gamboa JS, Strong AT, et al. Conversion of one-anastomosis gastric bypass to Roux-en-Y gastric bypass: short-term results from a tertiary referral center. Surg Obes Relat Dis 2019;15:1896–902.
59. Noel P, Nedelcu M, Nocca D, et al. Revised sleeve gastrectomy: another option for weight loss failure after sleeve gastrectomy. Surg Endosc 2014;28(4): 1096–102.
60. Berende CA, de Zoete JP, Smulders JF, et al. Laparoscopic sleeve gastrectomy feasible for bariatric revision surgery. Obes Surg 2012;22(2):330–4.
61. Khrucharoen U, Juo YY, Chen Y, et al. Indications, operative techniques, and outcomes for revisional operation following mini-gastric bypass-one anastomosis gastric bypass: a systematic review. Obes Surg 2020;30(4):1564–73.
62. Tran DD, Nwokeabia ID, Purnell S, et al. Revision of Roux-en-Y gastric bypass for weight regain: a systematic review of techniques and outcomes. Obes Surg 2016;26(7):1627–34.
63. Elnahas A, Graybiel K, Farrokhyar F, et al. Revisional surgery after failed laparoscopic adjustable gastric banding: a systematic review. Surg Endosc 2013;27(3): 740–5.
64. Sharples AJ, Charalampakis V, Daskalakis M, et al. Systematic review and meta-analysis of outcomes after revisional bariatric surgery following a failed adjustable gastric band. Obes Surg 2017;27(10):2522–36.
65. Dang JT, Switzer NJ, Wu J, et al. Gastric band removal in revisional bariatric surgery, one-step versus two-step: a systematic review and meta-analysis. Obes Surg 2016;26(4):866–73.

Physiologic Mechanisms of Weight Loss Following Metabolic/Bariatric Surgery

James N. Luo, MD[a], Ali Tavakkoli, MD[b],*

KEYWORDS

- Bariatric surgery • Microbiome • Metabolism • Insulin resistance • Diabetes
- Bariatric physiology

KEY POINTS

- Bariatric/metabolic surgery currently is the most effective treatment modality for morbid obesity and its metabolic comorbidities.
- The mechanism of bariatric surgery is a complex physiologic dialogue involving the endocrine, immune, nervous, and digestive systems.
- The bariatric microbiome represents an evolving frontier in metabolic research with major therapeutic implications.

INTRODUCTION

The origin of bariatric surgery largely is rooted in empiricism. The early search for their mechanisms similarly was guided by anatomic understandings alone. Bariatric operations initially were viewed as restrictive, malabsorptive, or a combination of both. As the strong antidiabetic effects of surgery have been documented in multiple randomized studies, it has become clear that underlying mechanisms of surgery are more complex. This complex biology has yet to be elucidate fully, although significant progress has been made. No single theory has emerged as the dominate unifying mechanism. It is plausible, if not likely, that multiple mechanisms are responsible for postoperative weight and metabolic changes, with some degree of overlap.

A key clinical observation with respect to postbariatric metabolic improvements has been that many patients leave the hospital after their index operation with significant improvement in their diabetes but prior to any significant weight loss. This has led to

Conflict of Interest: The authors have no relevant commercial or financial conflicts of interest to disclose.
a Department of Surgery, Brigham and Women's Hospital, Harvard Medical School, 20 Shattuck Street, Thorn 1503, Boston, MA 02115, USA; b Division of General and GI Surgery, Laboratory for Surgical and Metabolic Research, Department of Surgery, Brigham and Women's Hospital, Harvard Medical School, 75 Francis Street, Boston, MA 02115, USA
* Corresponding author.
E-mail address: atavakkoli@bwh.harvard.edu
Twitter: @JamesNLuo (J.N.L.); @BWHSurgMetab (A.T.)

the concept of weight-independent metabolic benefits of bariatric surgery. Among the possible explanations, studies have shown an early rise in hepatic insulin sensitivity.[1] Within 1 week following Roux-en-Y gastric bypass (RYGB), homeostatic model assessment of insulin resistance (HOMA-IR), which is a measure of hepatic glucose resistance, decreases by as much as 50%, with significant improvement in hepatic insulin sensitivity and decreased basal glucose production.[2,3] As hepatocyte and muscle adiposity decreases after surgery, this early effect is followed by an increase in peripheral insulin sensitivity, which then contributes to long-term glycemic control and diabetes improvement.[1] Understanding the mechanisms behind these early changes in glucose homeostasis catalyzed intense ongoing efforts to elucidate postbariatric physiology. This article presents the most well-studied mechanisms and omits potential mechanisms that have not yet amassed a sufficient body of evidence (**Fig. 1**).

HORMONAL EFFECTS OF BARIATRIC SURGERY

Bariatric surgery has been shown to affect several of the key obesity-related hormones. These hormonal changes were some of the earliest physiologic changes studied after bariatric surgery and were thought to be the driving mechanism. Further research, however, has revealed a more complex picture. GLP-1 and ghrelin have emerged as among the most important and well-studied bariatric hormones. Although there are many hormonal changes noted following bariatric surgery, it has been difficult to discern which changes are the drivers, and which are the consequences, of postbariatric physiology (**Table 1**).

Ghrelin

Ghrelin is a gastrointestinal (GI) peptide hormone with orexigenic properties. Secreted primarily by fundus of the stomach, it is an endogenous ligand of the growth hormone secretagogue receptor 1a.[4,5] Ghrelin has several key functions; chief among them is the transmission of hunger signal to the central nervous system.[4] In addition to

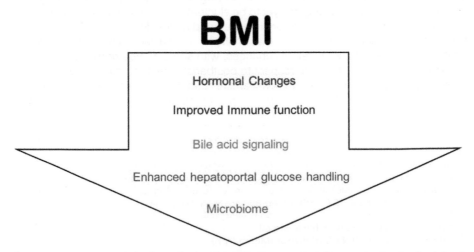

Fig. 1. An overview of the hypothesized mechanisms underlying postbariatric physiology. Available evidence suggests that the overall physio-metabolic transformation following bariatric. surgery likely reflects the cumulative effects of all of these mechanisms.

Table 1
Commonly studied hormones in bariatric physiology

Hormone	Primary Action	Role in Obesity/ Diabetes	Postbariatric Changes
Ghrelin	Hunger transmission	↑ Hunger/appetite ↑ Insulin sensitivity ↑ Lipogenesis	↓ In short-term and ↑ in long-term following RYGB ↓ Following SG
Leptin	Hunger suppression	↓ Hunger ↑ Energy expenditure	↓ Both RYGB and SG
GLP-1	Incretin effect	↑ Glucose-dependent insulin secretion ↓ Glucagon secretion	↑ Both RYGB and SG
Adiponectin	Target tissue dependent	Anti-inflammation ↑ Insulin sensitivity	↑ Both RYGB and SG
Secretin	Pancreatic secretion	Brown adipose tissue activation	↑ RYGB (limited human data)
Oxyntomodulin	Gastric acid modulation in oxyntic glands	↓ Appetite ↓ Food intake	↑ RYGB in response to oral glucose stimulation
Obestatin	Ghrelin antagonism	↓ Food intake ↓ Jejunal contraction ↓ Body weight	Remains inconclusive. Small human study suggests ↓ RYGB
Gastrin	Promotes gastric acid secretion	↑ Satiety	↓ RYGB ↑ SG
CCK	Promotes gallbladder contraction, pancreatic enzyme secretion	↑ Insulin secretion	↑ Both RYGB and SG (limited human data)

regulating hunger, it decreases insulin secretion, increases insulin sensitivity in the pancreas, increases lipogenesis, and augments gastric motility.[4] As the primary hunger hormone, it plays a major role in regulating caloric consumption. The effect of bariatric surgery on circulating ghrelin levels vary by the type of operation as well as the temporal distance from surgery. Following RYGB, ghrelin level is observed to decrease in the short term (<3 months) and increase in the long term.[6] Falling level of ghrelin has been observed as early as 1 day after RYGB and continues to fall for several weeks thereafter.[7,8] After this initial postoperative fall, ghrelin level begins to rise toward baseline and continues to do so when measured at 12 months.[8] Given these observations, many investigators have postulated that ghrelin likely plays a role in the short-term decrease in hunger following RYGB.[6]

A falling level of ghrelin is also observed following vertical sleeve gastrectomy (SG). At 1 month following SG, central nervous system changes associated with decreased circulating ghrelin were observed.[9] Unlike RYGB, however, the drop in ghrelin associated with SG appears to be durable. A randomized controlled trial of 69 patients reported by Kalinowski and colleagues[10] found that ghrelin level remains reduced at 12 months after SG. This sustained drop in ghrelin associated with SG likely is related to the surgical resection of the gastric fundus, where ghrelin is predominately secreted.

Leptin

Leptin is a circulating satiety factor, encoded by the *ob* gene, and secreted mostly by adipose tissue.[11] Leptin binds to its receptor, LRb, in the brain, resulting in hunger suppression and increased energy expenditure.[12] Mutation in the *ob* gene results in hyperphagia and severe early-onset obesity. Circulating leptin level is correlated with total body adipose tissue store and thus is elevated in obesity.[13] Following both RYGB and SG, fasting levels of leptin decrease significantly.[10] When measured at 12 months following bariatric surgery, lower leptin levels were correlated significantly with lower body mass index (BMI) and waist circumference.[14] This change in leptin level following bariatric surgery likely reflects diminished body fat rather than a driver of weight loss.

Glucagon-Like peptide

Glucagon-like peptide (GLP) 1 and GLP2 are coded by the proglucagon gene and are secreted, in equimolar quantities, by the intestinal enteroendocrine L cells.[15] At baseline, they are secreted continuously at low rates, and their secretion is stimulated after food intake with levels rising sharply within minutes of food consumption.[16] Although they are tandemly linked, GLP-1 and GLP-2 have quite diverging functions. GLP-1 has been one of the best studied hormones following weight loss surgery and has emerged as a key player in postbariatric physiology. GLP-1 is an incretin hormone, whose functions include glucose-dependent insulin secretion as well as inhibition of glucagon secretion, food intake, and gastric emptying.[16] Following RYGB, both total and active postprandial GLP-1 levels are increased significantly.[17,18] A similar postprandial increase is observed following SG.[19,20] The postprandial increase in GLP-1 following bariatric surgery is not seen in patients with comparable weight loss via caloric restriction or physical exercise.[21] This postsurgical increase in GLP-1 likely accounts, at least in part, for the rapid glycemic improvement observed in both RYGB and SG. Several studies have found, however, that GLP-1 antagonism has only a minimal impact on the antidiabetic effects of RYGB.[22] These observations suggest the postoperative increase in GLP-1 is unlikely to be the sole, or even perhaps the predominant, factor in the antidiabetic effects of bariatric surgery. Despite these questions regarding the importance of GLP-1 in postsurgical physiology, the therapeutic role of GLP-1 in weight and diabetes control remains undisputed with several Food and Drug Administration–approved medications (eg, liraglutide and dulaglutide) for both diabetes and weight management. Although such GLP-1 analogs replicate the dual effects of bariatric surgery, their magnetite is much more modest.

GLP-1's twin, GLP-2, has intestinotrophic and proabsorptive properties, and pharmacologic agonists of GLP-2 receptor have been used to treat short gut syndrome.[23] It has been much less well studies after bariatric surgery. Some studies have suggested that endogenous GLP-2 may possess a protective property against glucose intolerance, but its precise role in postbariatric surgery physiology remains uncertain.[24]

Adiponectin

Adiponectin is the most abundant peptide adipokine (cytokines secreted by adipocytes) with signaling targets in the liver, vascular endothelium, adipose tissues, and skeletal muscle.[25] Its signaling consequence include anti-inflammation and enhanced insulin sensitivity.[26] In general, adipose tissue adiponectin levels are decreased in obese patients, although there is variability in this trend depending on insulin sensitivity status. It has been shown that adiponectin expression in visceral fat is higher in obese patients who are insulin sensitive compared with those who are insulin resistance.[26,27] Adiponectin level increases following bariatric surgery, and this has been observed for both RYGB and SG.[28,29] It remains uncertain, however, as to whether this restoration is a driver of the metabolic benefit of surgery or a consequence of surgery and weight loss.

Secretin

Secretin is a 27–amino acid peptide hormone produced by S cells in the duodenum. It is stimulated by low luminal pH, and in turn stimulates pancreatic enzyme production, decreases stomach acid secretion, promotes insulin release, and decreases gastric motility.[23] Recently, secretin was found to be a nonadrenergic activator of brown adipose tissue in mice, capable of altering the expression of melanocortinergic peptides of hypothalamus.[30] This novel endocrine gut–brown fat–brain axis likely plays a role in regulating satiety.[30] In a small human study of 1 week and 3 months following RYGB, postprandial secretin more than doubled after surgery.[31] Although these novel observations are intriguing, more human studies are required to place the role of secretin in its proper physiologic context.

Oxyntomodulin

Oxyntomodulin is a 37-amino acid hormone produced by L cells in the gut via posttranslational modification of the proglucagon hormone. Its name derives from its inhibitory effect of the oxyntic glands of the stomach. In both rodents and humans, oxyntomodulin has been shown to inhibit appetite and food intake.[32] Following RYGB, oxyntomodulin level increases in response to oral glucose stimulation.[33] A comparable rise in oxyntomodulin is not seen following diet-induced weight loss.[33] When assessed at 18 months after RYGB, oxyntomodulin level has been found to be associated with favorable changes in eating behavior and is independently predictive of successful weight loss.[34]

Other Hormones

Several additional hormonal changes have also been linked to postbariatric physiology, although existing evidence varies on their potential contribution to weight loss or glycemic improvement. Cholecystokinin (CCK), in addition to promoting gallbladder contraction and aiding in digestion, has been shown to promote insulin secretion.[35] In general, CCK levels appears to increase after bariatric surgery, but this has not correlated well with weight loss or glycemic improvement.[36,37] Gastrin level also appears to change following bariatric surgery. Increased gastrin level has been observed following SG whereas the opposite has been observed following RYGB.[7,8,38] These changes likely reflect their respective anatomic changes. Lastly, obestatin is an antagonistic hormone of ghrelin that suppresses food intake and decreases body weight.[39] Some groups have reported a decrease in obestatin following bariatric surgery.[40] All these findings further highlight the complexity of postbariatric surgical hormonal changes and perhaps lead us to question the mechanistic importance of these changes.

POSTSURGICAL CHANGES IN INTESTINAL AND PORTAL PHYSIOLOGY AND FUNCTION

Given that surgery leads to significant anatomic changes in the GI tract, it is not surprising that several studies have highlighted changes in intestinal physiology that may contribute to the antidiabetic changes after surgery. This was acknowledged by the

Second Diabetes Surgery Summit in 2016, which concluded that the GI tract constitutes a clinically and biologically meaningful target for the management of refractory type 2 diabetes mellitus.[41] Some of the these hormonal changes are in fact a direct result of these changes in GI anatomy. There also are, however, documented changes in intestinal metabolism itself, which may have mechanistic benefits and significance.

Changes in Intestinal Glucose Absorption and Utilization

Although overall malabsorption does not play a major role in outcomes of most common bariatric operations,[42] an important change in post-RYGB intestinal physiology is a decrease in proximal intestinal absorptive capacity, which may in turn account for greater glucose delivery into the distal small bowel and be one of the drivers of enhanced GLP-1 secretion after RYGB.[43]

Several groups, including the authors', have shown that after RYGB, there also is an increase in intestinal glucose utilization.[44] The small bowel at rest requires energy for its multiple functions, and, after surgery, there is a shift toward glucose use as reflected in PET scans of both rodent and human subjects. Saeidi and colleagues[45] have reported in rodent models that following RYGB, there is a reprograming of the Roux limb, resulting in increased glucose uptake and utilization. Furthermore, this increased glucose utilization help support the increased energic needs of the Roux limb after RYGB. In this sense, the small intestine acts as a major destination for glucose disposal. Although it is tempting to consider this increase in glucose utilization as the direct driver of the antidiabetic effects of surgery, it is unlikely that this change alone is sufficient to drive the multiple benefits of surgery. The authors believe that these changes, including the increase in intestinal glucose utilization, lead to a lowering of portal glucose levels, which, in turn, alters hepatic insulin sensitivity and likely drives the early weight-independent metabolic benefits of bariatric operations.

Changes in Portal Vein Milieu and Portal Glucose Levels

Decades-old studies have shown that glucose infusion into the portal vein resulted in up-regulation of hepatic glucose uptake machinery that was not observed with systemic infusion.[46] These studies have highlighted the importance of portal vein in glucose sensing and hepatic glucose regulation and led to multiple studies investigating the precise elements of this hepatoportal glucose sensing apparatus. Current data suggest that portal glucose is sensed by neurons expressing sodium glucose transporter 3 (SLGT3), which in turn activates the region of the brain controlling food intake, thus leading to centrally driven decrease in caloric intake.[47] Additionally, portal glucose sensing has been shown to directly trigger glucose-lowering effects. In rodents, stimulation of the portal sensor SLGT3 results in lowering of systemic glucose.[48] Moreover, this portal-mediated glucose-lowering effect was more pronounced in diabetic rodents, suggesting that this effect might be up-regulated in diabetes.

Overall, it appears that the intestine and the portal glucose-regulatory machinery play a critical role in maintaining glucose homeostasis and affecting postbariatric glycemic improvement. The portal vein—being the central conduit linking the intestines with the liver—serves as the physiologic canary in the coal mine of the gut-liver glycemic axis. Changes in the intestines following bariatric surgery is reflected in the portal milieu, which in turn influences hepatic glucose metabolism. In this regard, the authors believe the exquisite changes in portal glycemic and hormonal environments are key relays in facilitating postbariatric metabolic changes. Because of these vital roles, the portal glucose pathway represents a potential antidiabetic therapeutic target.

IMPROVED IMMUNE SYSTEM FUNCTION

The immune system's role in obesity, insulin resistance, and bariatric surgery is an actively expanding frontier of research with profound therapeutic implications. Ongoing research no doubt will continue to expand, and perhaps revise, these understandings. From an immune perspective, obesity is viewed as a state of chronic low-grade sterile inflammation, characterized by modest increases in systemic markers of inflammation without overt clinical symptoms.[49] This chronic state of inflammation is believed to play an active role in many of the metabolic derangements seen in morbid obesity, including insulin resistance.[50] Much of this is orchestrated by adipose tissue itself, which is not a mere storage of fat but rather a complex microenvironment (**Fig. 2**). In addition to adipocytes, there is a biologically active vascular-stromal component of adipose tissue, composed of macrophages, fibroblasts, and endothelial cells.[51] Besides adipokines, such as leptin and adiponectin, adipose tissue secrete myriad immune cytokines, including interleukin (IL)-1, IL-6, tumor necrosis factor (TNF)-α, and interferon (INF)-γ, among others.[52]

Both adipocytes and stromal cells in white adipose tissue contribute to systemic inflammation and metabolic dysfunction.[53] TNF-α and INF-γ both have been linked to insulin resistance via differing pathways.[54,55] Increased IL-1 and IL-6 are associated with increased HOMA-IR.[56] Excessive lipid accumulation results in adipocyte expansion beyond its effective diffusion capacity, resulting in cellular hypoxia and cell death, leading to the ensuing inflammatory response.[57,58] Over-capacitated adipocytes also increase circulating free fatty acids, which in and of themselves are cytotoxic.

In concert with innate immunity, adaptive immunity is also prominently involved in obesity-related inflammation. White adipose tissue from obese patients show increased CD4+ and CD8+ T-lymphocytes.[55] Increased activated lymphocytes have been linked to insulin resistance. T-lymphocytes from obese patients tend to exhibit the proinflammatory type 1 helper T cell (T_H1) phenotype, and the abundance of T_H1 cells has been found to correlate positively with the degree of insulin resistance.[59] Furthermore, there are 2 types of macrophages typically found in white adipose tissue: M1 and M2. M1 macrophages secrete a proinflammatory cytokine profile and are attracted to necrotic adipocytes.[60] M2 macrophages secrete an anti-inflammatory cytokine profile and are the resident macrophages in adipose tissue.[60] The relative

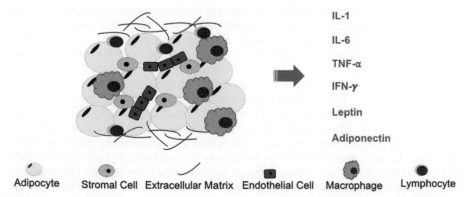

Fig. 2. Simplified schematic of adipose tissue. Lipid-laden adipocytes, endothelial cells, stromal cells, macrophages, and lymphocytes, among others, form a complex immunologically and hormonally active network. In addition to adipokines, adipose tissue produces several key inflammatory cytokines.

proportion of M1 and M2 plays an important role in mediating inflammation and insulin resistance in morbid obesity.

In general, bariatric surgery is associated with decreased circulating markers of inflammation, including C-reactive protein.[61,62] Bariatric surgery also reduces the abundance of white adipose tissue, which is itself a major source of inflammation.[61] Bariatric surgery does not affect the number of adipocytes but results in the reduction of its lipid content. Moreover, it has been observed that in obesity, insulin's ability to suppress lipolysis is attenuated, which results in leakage of free fatty acid. Following bariatric surgery, there is improved response to insulin and catecholamine signaling and reduced free fatty acid leakage.[63] There also is significant change to the immune cellular profile in response to bariatric surgery.[64] Two important changes include reduction of helper T cell T_H1 lymphocytes with decrease in T_H1:type 2 helper T cell (T_H2) ratio, and increase in the proportion of M2 macrophage.[61] In addition to circulating immune improvement, bariatric surgery improved local intestinal immunity. Following both RYGB and SG, there is a reduction in proinflammatory cytokines IL-17, IL-23, and INF-γ in the jejunum, which correlated with weight loss and glucose-triggered insulin response.[62] Overall, these postbariatric changes are associated with amelioration of excessive inflammation and restoration of metabolic health.

BARIATRIC SURGERY AND BILE ACIDS

Bile acids (BAs) are biologic detergents that are essential for the absorption of fat-soluble nutrients. Although this is their primary claim to fame, BAs' full physiologic function extends far beyond lipid digestion. They play key roles in signal transduction and inflammation.[65] Cholesterol 7-Alpha-hydroxylase (CYP7A1) is the rate-limiting enzyme in BA synthesis. As part of their enterohepatic circulation, nearly all BAs are resorbed in the small intestine. What escapes enter the colon and are biotransformed by the gut microbiota via a variety of organic chemical reactions (eg, deconjugation, dehydrogenation, dihydroxylation, and epimerization) and ultimately are returned to the liver or excreted in the feces.[66]

Research thus far have identified 2 main signaling cascades, through which BAs participate in glucose and metabolic homeostasis. First, the farnesoid X receptor (FXR). FXR is part of the nuclear receptor superfamily, found primarily in the liver, kidney, and intestine. BAs are endogenous ligands of FXR. One consequence of BA activation of FXR is suppression of CYP7A1, the rate-limiting enzyme in BA synthesis.[67] In addition to this regulatory feedback inhibition, FXR activation also down-regulates gluconeogenesis, up-regulates glycolysis and glycogen synthesis, and increases glucose tolerance and insulin sensitivity.[68] FXR−/− mice exhibit both impaired glucose tolerance and diminished insulin sensitivity.[69]

The second BA pathway involves the G-protein–coupled BA receptor 1 (GPBAR1), also known as TGR5. TGR5 is found in the small intestine, stomach, and liver, among other organs. TGR5 activation results in myriad physiologic responses, including cellular growth and differentiation via AKT and PIP3 as well as anti-inflammation via down-regulation of nuclear factor κB.[70] TGR5 also exert several key metabolic functions. First, BA activation of TGR5 results in dose-dependent GLP-1 secretion.[71] Second, activating TGR5 on adipose tissue macrophages decreases LPS-induced inflammatory cytokines and protect against insulin resistance.[72] Third, TGR5 activation has been shown to increase energy expenditure in brown adipose tissue and to prevent obesity and insulin resistance.[73]

Both FXR and TGR5 have been implicated in the metabolic consequences of bariatric surgery. It has long been known that bariatric surgery is associated with global changes in the BA pool, including increased circulating BA following both RYGB and SG.[74,75] These changes have been linked to improved glucose homeostasis. Much of the recent work on the role of BAs in bariatric physiology has focused on SG. Ryan and colleagues[76] reported significantly attenuated weight loss and glucose improvement in FXR knockout mice following SG. This finding implied that FXR signaling plays a key role in bariatric physiology and is necessary to achieve to the full weight and glycemic benefits of SG. Although further mechanistic studies is required to fully understand this effect, especially given the potential confounding properties of FXR knockout mice compared with wild-type mice.[77] Similarly, expression of TGR5 has been found to increase significantly after SG with enhanced signaling in the ileum and brown adipose tissue.[78] Furthermore, it appears that intact TGR5 signaling is necessary for the full weight and glycemic effects of SG.[78] Recently, the authors' group has shown that following SG in mice, there is an increase in sulfated BA level, which in turn activates TGR5, resulting in increased GLP-1 and improved glucose tolerance.[79]

BARIATRIC MICROBIOME: NEXT FRONTIER

In recent years, the importance of the gut microbiome in metabolic health and GI surgery has emerged to the forefront.[80,81] Obesity is associated with microbiome dysbiosis, characterized by decrease in both species diversity and richness as well as an increase in the ratio of Firmicute to Bacteroidetes.[82] Although the microbiota is always influenced by the peculiar conditions of the subject being studied, some general trends in the microbiome in response to bariatric surgery have emerged. These include some degree of restoration in diversity and richness,[83] increases in Bacteroidetes, and decreases in Firmicutes.[84] A more diverse core microbiome following RYGB has been associated with more successful weight loss.[85] Moreover, there is a bloom in *Akkermansia*.[86] *Akkermansia muciniphila* is associated with an overall healthier clinical profile.[87] Some microbiome changes, such as enriched Enterobacteriaceae and Fusobacteriaceae, may have implications beyond, or independent of, weight loss, because both have been linked to colorectal cancer pathogenesis.[88,89]

As knowledge and appreciation for the role of the microbiome in obesity grow, novel therapeutic approaches are being considered. Fecal microbiota transplant has been introduced successfully in gut-derived infectious diseases, such as fulminant *Clostridium difficile* colitis, but its consideration in obesity remains in its infancy. Liou and colleagues[90] reported in 2013 that fecal microbiota transplant from post-RYGB mice into germ-free nonoperated mice resulted in weight loss and decreased fat mass. Pilot human studies investigating transplanting microbiota from lean donors to obese patients with metabolic syndrome have resulted in increased insulin sensitivity,[91] although these benefits have thus far appeared transient, lasting less than 18 months.[92] In the first human randomized controlled trial of 22 obese and metabolically healthy patients, Allegretti and colleagues[93] showed microbiota transplanted from lean donors resulted in a shift in the obese recipients' microbiome profile toward that of their donors, but no significant difference in BMI at 12 weeks was observed. These findings suggest that the microbiome likely have an important role in obesity, metabolic health, and bariatric physiology, but they also highlight the complexity of the host-microbial dialogue and emphasize the importance of further understanding before the full therapeutic potential of the microbiome can be harnessed in combating obesity and metabolic disequilibrium.

SUMMARY

The battle against rising morbid obesity is joined. The field of bariatric surgery has evolved from experimental procedures for a challenging problem to a sophisticated multidisciplinary modality rooted in biology and physiology. Over the past 2 decades, the elegant mechanisms behind these operations have been gradually unveiled. Much has been learned, but much more learning remains. The increasing scientific understanding of bariatric physiology has allowed for the advent of more noninvasive treatments for obesity and metabolic syndrome. Ultimately, the aim should be to deliver the therapeutic efficacy of bariatric surgery without its attendant risk. In this ongoing effort, the words of Sir Winston Churchill are an apropos reminder : "This is not the end. It is not even the beginning of the end. But it is, perhaps, the end of the beginning."

CLINICS CARE POINTS

- Bariatric/metabolic surgery currently is the most effective treatment modality for morbid obesity and its metabolic comorbidities.

- The mechanism of bariatric surgery is a complex physiologic dialogue involving the endocrine, immune, nervous, and digestive systems.

- There are numerous hormonal changes following bariatric surgery, but many likely are results of the surgery rather than drivers of postsurgical physiology.

- Postsurgical changes in intestinal glucose absorption and portal milieu likely play key roles in postsurgical diabetes improvement.

- Obesity is a state of chronic low-grade inflammation. Bariatric surgery has been shown to reverse many proinflammatory changes associated with obesity and diabetes.

- The bariatric microbiome represents an evolving frontier in metabolic research with major therapeutic implications.

REFERENCES

1. He B, Chen L, Yu C, et al. Roux-en-Y gastric bypass increases hepatic and peripheral insulin sensitivity in rats with type 2 diabetes mellitus. Surg Obes Relat Dis 2014;10(3):485–93.
2. Jørgensen NB, Jacobsen SH, Dirksen C, et al. Acute and long-term effects of Roux-en-Y gastric bypass on glucose metabolism in subjects with Type 2 diabetes and normal glucose tolerance. Am J Physiol - Endocrinol Metab 2012; 303(1):122–31.
3. Bojsen-Møller KN, Dirksen C, Jørgensen NB, et al. Early enhancements of hepatic and later of peripheral insulin sensitivity combined with increased postprandial insulin secretion contribute to improved glycemic control after Roux-en-Y gastric bypass. Diabetes 2014;63(5):1725–37.
4. Müller TD, Nogueiras R, Andermann ML, et al. Ghrelin. Mol Metab 2015;4(6): 437–60.
5. Kojima M, Kangawa K. Ghrelin: Structure and function. Physiol Rev 2005;85(2): 495–522.
6. Xu HC, Pang YC, Chen JW, et al. Systematic review and meta-analysis of the change in ghrelin levels after Roux-en-Y Gastric Bypass. Obes Surg 2019; 29(4):1343–51.

7. Jacobsen SH, Olesen SC, Dirksen C, et al. Changes in gastrointestinal hormone responses, insulin sensitivity, and beta-cell function within 2 weeks after gastric bypass in non-diabetic subjects. Obes Surg 2012;22(7):1084–96.

8. Sundbom M, Holdstock C, Engström BE, et al. Early changes in ghrelin following Roux-en-Y gastric bypass: Influence of vagal nerve functionality? Obes Surg 2007;17(3):304–10.

9. Zhang Y, Ji G, Li G, et al. Ghrelin reductions following bariatric surgery were associated with decreased resting state activity in the hippocampus. Int J Obes 2019;43(4):842–51.

10. Kalinowski P, Paluszkiewicz R, Wróblewski T, et al. Ghrelin, leptin, and glycemic control after sleeve gastrectomy versus Roux-en-Y gastric bypass—results of a randomized clinical trial. Surg Obes Relat Dis 2017;13(2):181–8.

11. Ahima RS, Flier JS. LEPTIN. Annu Rev Physiol 2000;62:413–50.

12. Myers MG, Cowley MA, Münzberg H. Mechanisms of Leptin Action and Leptin Resistance. Annu Rev Physiol 2008;70(1):537–56.

13. Hamilton B, Paglia D, Kwan A, et al. Increased obese mRNA expression in omental fat cells from massively obese humans. Nat Med 1995;1(9):953–6.

14. Terra X, Auguet T, Guiu-Jurado E, et al. Long-term changes in leptin, chemerin and ghrelin levels following different bariatric surgery procedures: Roux-en-Y gastric bypass and sleeve gastrectomy. Obes Surg 2013;23(11):1790–8.

15. Drucker DJ. Mechanisms of Action and Therapeutic Application of Glucagon-like Peptide-1. Cell Metab 2018;27(4):740–56.

16. Drucker DJ, Habener JF, Holst JJ. Discovery, characterization, and clinical development of the glucagon-like peptides. J Clin Invest 2017;127(12):4217–27.

17. Hutch CR, Sandoval D. The role of GLP-1 in the metabolic success of bariatric surgery. Endocrinology 2017;158(12):4139–51.

18. Laferrère B, Heshka S, Wang K, et al. Incretin levels and effect are markedly enhanced 1 month after Roux-en-Y gastric bypass surgery in obese patients with type 2 diabetes. Diabetes Care 2007;30(7):1709–16.

19. Nannipieri M, Baldi S, Mari A, et al. Roux-en-Y gastric bypass and sleeve gastrectomy: Mechanisms of diabetes remission and role of gut hormones. J Clin Endocrinol Metab 2013;98(11):4391–9.

20. McCarty TR, Jirapinyo P, Thompson CC. Effect of sleeve gastrectomy on ghrelin, GLP-1, PYY, and GIP Gut hormones: a systematic review and meta-analysis. Ann Surg 2020;272(1):72–80.

21. Laferrère B, Teixeira J, McGinty J, et al. Effect of weight loss by gastric bypass surgery versus hypocaloric diet on glucose and incretin levels in patients with type 2 diabetes. J Clin Endocrinol Metab 2008;93(7):2479–85.

22. Jiménez A, Casamitjana R, Viaplana-Masclans J, et al. GLP-1 action and glucose tolerance in subjects with remission of type 2 diabetes after gastric bypass surgery. Diabetes Care 2013;36(7):2062–9.

23. Meek CL, Lewis HB, Reimann F, et al. The effect of bariatric surgery on gastrointestinal and pancreatic peptide hormones. Peptides 2016;77:28–37.

24. Baldassano S, Rappa F, Amato A, et al. GLP-2 as beneficial factor in the glucose homeostasis in mice fed a high fat diet. J Cell Physiol 2015;230(12):3029–36.

25. Achari AE, Jain SK. Adiponectin, a therapeutic target for obesity, diabetes, and endothelial dysfunction. Int J Mol Sci 2017;18(6):1321.

26. Sams VG, Blackledge C, Wijayatunga N, et al. Effect of bariatric surgery on systemic and adipose tissue inflammation. Surg Endosc 2016;30(8):3499–504.

27. Sirbu AE, Buburuzan L, Kevorkian S, et al. Adiponectin expression in visceral adiposity is an important determinant of insulin resistance in morbid obesity. Endokrynol Pol 2018;69(3):252–8.
28. Kelly AS, Ryder JR, Marlatt KL, et al. Changes in inflammation, oxidative stress and adipokines following bariatric surgery among adolescents with severe obesity. Int J Obes 2016;40(2):275–80.
29. Gómez-Martin JM, Balsa JA, Aracil E, et al. Circulating adiponectin increases in obese women after sleeve gastrectomy or gastric bypass driving beneficial metabolic changes but with no relationship with carotid intima-media thickness. Clin Nutr 2018;37(6):2102–6.
30. Schnabl K, Li Y, Klingenspor M. The gut hormone secretin triggers a gut–brown fat–brain axis in the control of food intake. Exp Physiol 2020;105(8):1206–13.
31. Modvig IM, Andersen DB, Grunddal KV, et al. Secretin release after Roux-en-Y gastric bypass reveals a population of glucose-sensitive S cells in distal small intestine. Int J Obes 2020;44(9):1859–71.
32. Cohen MA, Ellis SM, Le Roux CW, et al. Oxyntomodulin suppresses appetite and reduces food intake in humans. J Clin Endocrinol Metab 2003;88(10):4696–701.
33. Laferrère B, Swerdlow N, Bawa B, et al. Rise of oxyntomodulin in response to oral glucose after gastric bypass surgery in patients with type 2 diabetes. J Clin Endocrinol Metab 2010;95(8):4072–6.
34. Nielsen MS, Ritz C, Wewer Albrechtsen NJ, et al. Oxyntomodulin and glicentin may predict the effect of bariatric surgery on food preferences and weight loss. J Clin Endocrinol Metab 2020;105(4):dgaa061.
35. Pathak V, Flatt PR, Irwin N. Cholecystokinin (CCK) and related adjunct peptide therapies for the treatment of obesity and type 2 diabetes. Peptides 2018;100: 229–35.
36. Peterli R, Steinert RE, Woelnerhanssen B, et al. Metabolic and hormonal changes after laparoscopic Roux-en-Y gastric bypass and sleeve gastrectomy: A randomized, prospective trial. Obes Surg 2012;22(5):740–8.
37. Dirksen C, Jørgensen NB, Bojsen-Møller KN, et al. Gut hormones, early dumping and resting energy expenditure in patients with good and poor weight loss response after Roux-en-Y gastric bypass. Int J Obes 2013;37(11):1452–9.
38. Grong E, Græslie H, Munkvold B, et al. Gastrin secretion after bariatric surgery—response to a protein-rich mixed meal following Roux-En-Y gastric bypass and sleeve gastrectomy: a pilot study in normoglycemic women. Obes Surg 2016; 26(7):1448–56.
39. Zhang JV, Ren PG, Avsian-Kretchmer O, et al. Medicine: Obestatin, a peptide encoded by the ghrelin gene, opposes ghrelin's effects on food intake. Science (80-) 2005;310(5750):996–9.
40. Dogan U, Ellidag HY, Aslaner A, et al. The impact of laparoscopic sleeve gastrectomy on plasma obestatin and ghrelin levels. Eur Rev Med Pharmacol Sci 2016; 20(10):2113–22.
41. Rubino F, Nathan DM, Eckel RH, et al. Metabolic surgery in the treatment algorithm for type 2 diabetes: A joint statement by international diabetes organizations. Diabetes Care 2016;39(6):861–77.
42. Odstrcil EA, Martinez JG, Santa Ana CA, et al. The contribution of malabsorption to the reduction in net energy absorption after long-limb Roux-en-Y gastric bypass. Am J Clin Nutr 2010;92(4):704–13.
43. Pal A, Rhoads DB, Tavakkoli A. Foregut exclusion disrupts intestinal glucose sensing and alters portal nutrient and hormonal milieu. Diabetes 2015;64(6): 1941–50.

44. Pal A, Rhoads DB, Tavakkoli A. Portal milieu and the interplay of multiple antidiabetic effects after gastric bypass surgery. Am J Physiol Gastrointest Liver Physiol 2019;316(5):G668–78.
45. Saeidi N, Meoli L, Nestoridi E, et al. Reprogramming of intestinal glucose metabolism and glycemic control in rats after gastric bypass. Science 2013; 341(6144):406–10.
46. Adkins BA, Myers SR, Hendrick GK, et al. Importance of the route of intravenous glucose delivery to hepatic glucose balance in the conscious dog. J Clin Invest 1987;79(2):557–65.
47. Mithieux G. Metabolic effects of portal vein sensing. Diabetes Obes Metab 2014; 16:56–60.
48. Pal A, Rhoads DB, Tavakkoli A. Effect of portal glucose sensing on systemic glucose levels in SD and ZDF Rats. PLoS One 2016;11(11):e0165592.
49. Medzhitov R. Origin and physiological roles of inflammation. Nature 2008; 454(7203):428–35.
50. Heilbronn L, Campbell L. Adipose tissue macrophages, low grade inflammation and insulin resistance in human obesity. Curr Pharm Des 2008;14(12):1225–30.
51. Hajer GR, Van Haeften TW, Visseren FLJ. Adipose tissue dysfunction in obesity, diabetes, and vascular diseases. Eur Heart J 2008;29(24):2959–71.
52. Wang Z, Nakayama T. Inflammation, a link between obesity and cardiovascular disease. Mediators Inflamm 2010;2010:17.
53. Fantuzzi G. Adiponectin and inflammation: Consensus and controversy. J Allergy Clin Immunol 2008;121(2):326–30.
54. Hotamisligil GS, Shargill NS, Spiegelman BM. Adipose expression of tumor necrosis factor-α: Direct role in obesity-linked insulin resistance. Science 1993; 259(5091):87–91.
55. Duffaut C, Zakaroff-Girard A, Bourlier V, et al. Interplay between human adipocytes and T lymphocytes in obesity: CCL20 as an adipochemokine and T lymphocytes as lipogenic modulators. Arterioscler Thromb Vasc Biol 2009;29(10): 1608–14.
56. Charles BA, Doumatey A, Huang H, et al. The roles of IL-6, IL-10, and IL-1RA in obesity and insulin resistance in African-Americans. J Clin Endocrinol Metab 2011;96(12):E2018–22.
57. O'Rourke RW. Inflammation in obesity-related diseases. Surgery 2009;145(3): 255–9.
58. Mosser DM, Edwards JP. Exploring the full spectrum of macrophage activation. Nat Rev Immunol 2008;8(12):958–69.
59. Viardot A, Heilbronn LK, Samocha-Bonet D, et al. Obesity is associated with activated and insulin resistant immune cells. Diabetes Metab Res Rev 2012;28(5): 447–54.
60. Rull A, Camps J, Alonso-Villaverde C, et al. Insulin resistance, inflammation, and obesity: Role of monocyte chemoattractant protein-1 (orCCL2) in the regulation of metabolism. Mediators Inflamm 2010;2010:11.
61. Villarreal-Calderón JR, Cuéllar RX, Ramos-González MR, et al. Interplay between the adaptive immune system and insulin resistance in weight loss induced by bariatric surgery. Oxid Med Cell Longev 2019;2019:3940739.
62. Subramaniam R, Aliakbarian H, Bhutta HY, et al. Sleeve Gastrectomy and Roux-en-Y gastric bypass attenuate pro-inflammatory small intestinal cytokine signatures. Obes Surg 2019;29:3824–32.
63. Frikke-Schmidt H, O'Rourke RW, Lumeng CN, et al. Does bariatric surgery improve adipose tissue function? Obes Rev 2016;17(9):795–809.

64. Zhang H, Wang Y, Zhang J, et al. Bariatric surgery reduces visceral adipose inflammation and improves endothelial function in type 2 diabetic mice. Arterioscler Thromb Vasc Biol 2011;31(9):2063–9.
65. Chiang JYL. Bile acids: Regulation of synthesis. J Lipid Res 2009;50(10): 1955–66.
66. Hofmann AF. Chemistry and enterohepatic circulation of bile acids. Hepatology 1984;4(2 S):4S–14S.
67. Goodwin B, Jones SA, Price RR, et al. A regulatory cascade of the nuclear receptors FXR, SHP-1, and LRH-1 represses bile acid biosynthesis. Mol Cell 2000;6(3): 517–26.
68. Albaugh VL, Banan B, Ajouz H, et al. Bile acids and bariatric surgery. Mol Aspects Med 2017;56:75–89.
69. Ma K, Saha PK, Chan L, et al. Farnesoid X receptor is essential for normal glucose homeostasis. J Clin Invest 2006;116(4):1102–9.
70. Guo C, Chen WD, Wang YD. TGR5, not only a metabolic regulator. Front Physiol 2016;7:646.
71. Katsuma S, Hirasawa A, Tsujimoto G. Bile acids promote glucagon-like peptide-1 secretion through TGR5 in a murine enteroendocrine cell line STC-1. Biochem Biophys Res Commun 2005;329(1):386–90.
72. Perino A, Pols TWH, Nomura M, et al. TGR5 reduces macrophage migration through mTOR-induced C/EBPβ differential translation. J Clin Invest 2014; 124(12):5424–36.
73. Chen X, Lou G, Meng Z, et al. TGR5: a novel target for weight maintenance and glucose metabolism. Exp Diabetes Res 2011;2011:853501.
74. McGavigan AK, Garibay D, Henseler ZM, et al. TGR5 contributes to glucoregulatory improvements after vertical sleeve gastrectomy in mice. Gut 2017;66(2): 226–34.
75. Patti ME, Houten SM, Bianco AC, et al. Serum bile acids are higher in humans with prior gastric bypass: Potential contribution to improved glucose and lipid metabolism. Obesity 2009;17(9):1671–7.
76. Ryan K, Tremaroli V, Clemmensen C, et al. FXR affects weight loss in SG - nature.pdf. Nature 2014;509(7499):183–8.
77. Tian J, Huang S, Sun S, et al. Bile acid signaling and bariatric surgery. Liver Res 2017;1(4):208–13.
78. Ding L, Sousa KM, Jin L, et al. Vertical sleeve gastrectomy activates GPBAR-1/ TGR5 to sustain weight loss, improve fatty liver, and remit insulin resistance in mice. Hepatology 2016;64(3):760–73.
79. Chaudhari SN, Harris DA, Aliakbarian H, et al. Bariatric surgery reveals a gut-restricted TGR5 agonist with anti-diabetic effects. Nat Chem Biol 2020; 17(1):20–9.
80. Shogan BD, Belogortseva N, Luong PM, et al. Collagen degradation and MMP9 activation by Enterococcus faecalis contribute to intestinal anastomotic leak. Sci Transl Med 2015;7(286):286ra68.
81. Alverdy JC, Luo JN. The influence of host stress on the mechanism of infection: Lost microbiomes, emergent pathobiomes, and the role of interkingdom signaling. Front Microbiol 2017;8:322.
82. Ley RE, Bäckhed F, Turnbaugh P, et al. Obesity alters gut microbial ecology. Proc Natl Acad Sci U S A 2005;102(31):11070–5.
83. Davies NK, O'Sullivan JM, Plank LD, et al. Altered gut microbiome after bariatric surgery and its association with metabolic benefits: A systematic review. Surg Obes Relat Dis 2019;15(4):656–65.

84. Luijten JCHBM, Vugts G, Nieuwenhuijzen GAP, et al. The importance of the microbiome in bariatric surgery: a systematic review. Obes Surg 2019;29(7):2338–49.
85. Gutiérrez-Repiso C, Moreno-Indias I, Hollanda A de, et al. Gut microbiota specific signatures are related to the successful rate of bariatric surgery. Am J Transl Res 2019;11(2):942–52.
86. Peat CM, Kleiman SC, Bulik CM, et al. The intestinal microbiome in bariatric surgery patients. Eur Eat Disord Rev 2015;23(6):496–503.
87. Dao MC, Belda E, Prifti E, et al. Akkermansia muciniphila abundance is lower in severe obesity, but its increased level after bariatric surgery is not associated with metabolic health improvement. Am J Physiol - Endocrinol Metab 2019; 317(3):E446–59.
88. Garrett WS. The gut microbiota and colon cancer. Science 2019;364(6446): 1133–5.
89. Arthur JC, Perez-Chanona E, Mühlbauer M, et al. Intestinal inflammation targets cancer-inducing activity of the microbiota. Science 2012;338(6103):120–3.
90. Liou AP, Paziuk M, Luevano J-M, et al. Conserved shifts in the gut microbiota due to gastric bypass reduce host weight and adiposity. Sci Transl Med 2013;5(178): 178–219.
91. Vrieze A, Van Nood E, Holleman F, et al. Transfer of intestinal microbiota from lean donors increases insulin sensitivity in individuals with metabolic syndrome. Gastroenterology 2012;143(4):913–6.e7.
92. Kootte RS, Levin E, Stroes ESG, et al. Clinical and translational report improvement of insulin sensitivity after lean donor feces in metabolic syndrome is driven by baseline intestinal microbiota composition cell metabolism clinical and translational report improvement of insulin sensitivity. Cell Metab 2017;26:611–9.
93. Allegretti JR, Kassam Z, Mullish BH, et al. Effects of fecal microbiota transplantation with oral capsules in obese patients. Clin Gastroenterol Hepatol 2020;18(4): 855–63.e2.

Obesity, Cancer, and Risk Reduction with Bariatric Surgery

Peter R.A. Malik, MSc(c), BHSc[a,b],
Aristithes G. Doumouras, MD, MPH[a], Roshan S. Malhan, BHSc[a],
Yung Lee, MD[a], Vanessa Boudreau, MD, MSc[a,b],
Karen Barlow, HonsBSc[a], Marta Karpinski, MSc, BHSc[b],
Mehran Anvari, MBBS, PhD, FRCSC, FACS[a,*]

KEYWORDS

- Bariatric surgery • Cancer risk • Risk reduction • Obesity • Cancer survivorship

KEY POINTS

- Obesity has revealed strong links to cancer of the esophagus, stomach, colon, rectum, liver, gallbladder, pancreas, breast, uterus, ovary, kidney, and thyroid.
- The evidence for surgical weight loss in the prevention of cancers is highest for hormone-related cancers, which show both biologic plausibility and strong associations in observational research.
- Other obesity-related cancers (eg, colorectal, pancreatic) show more variable evidence, whereas no associations have been seen between surgical weight loss and nonobesity-related cancers.
- Bariatric surgery is tolerable in patients with cancer and has been shown to improve quality of life; however, further research is required to determine the impact on cancer prognosis.

INTRODUCTION

Increasing Incidences of Noncommunicable Diseases in North America and Across the Globe

The incidence rates of noncommunicable diseases (NCDs), such as obesity, are increasing in North America and throughout the world.[1,2] Between 2008[1] and 2013,[2] the prevalence of obesity in high-income North America has increased from 29.2% to 30.6% in men, and from 30% to 32.5% in women. Between 1980 and

[a] Department of Surgery and Centre for Minimal Access Surgery, St. Joseph's Healthcare, 50 Charlton Avenue East, Rm T2141 Hamilton, Ontario L8N 4A6, Canada; [b] Department of Health Research Methods, Evidence & Impact, Faculty of Health Sciences, McMaster University Medical Centre, 1280 Main Street West, 2C Area, Hamilton, Ontario L8S 4K1, Canada
* Corresponding author.
E-mail address: anvari@mcmaster.ca

Surg Clin N Am 101 (2021) 239–254
https://doi.org/10.1016/j.suc.2020.12.003
0039-6109/21/© 2020 Elsevier Inc. All rights reserved.

surgical.theclinics.com

2008, the average body mass index (BMI) for men and women in high-income regions of North America increased by 1.1 and 1.2 kg/m^2 per decade, respectively.[1] This trend has also been observed globally, where the average BMI has increased by approximately 0.45 kg/m^2 per decade, from 1980 to 2008.[2] Consequently, the increasing prevalence of obesity, and associated comorbidities, coincides with the average BMI increases observed globally.[1,2] As the impact of communicable diseases decreases, the prevention of NCDs has been prioritized as a significant public health goal,[3–5] particularly in developing and low-income countries,[6] where most of the NCD burden lies.

In addition to obesity, cancer is an NCD associated with one of the highest rates of patient morbidity and mortality, and costs to health care systems worldwide.[6–8] As of 2018, the greatest incident cancers in men were malignancies of the lungs, prostate, colon/rectum, stomach, and liver.[9] Cancers with the highest incidence in women include malignancies of the breast, colon/rectum, lung, cervix uteri, and thyroid.[9] It is estimated that cancer accounts for 169.3 million years of healthy life lost annually,[10] with an incidence rate projected to increase from 12.7 million cases in 2008 to 22.2 million cases by 2030.[10,11] This dramatic increase has been attributed to increased risk factors, such as global mean age, consumption of tobacco and alcohol, nutritional habits, and inadequate levels of physical activity.[12] Because of the modifiable nature of drug and alcohol use, nutrition, and physical activity, these risk factors have been the main target for NCD prevention.

Connection Between Obesity and Cancer Incidence

Substantial evidence suggests obesity is a risk factor for the development of several cancer types.[13,14] There is compelling evidence demonstrating a link between increased BMI and increased incidence of cancers of the esophagus, stomach, colon, rectum, liver, gallbladder, pancreas, breast, uterus, ovary, kidney, and thyroid.[13] Evidence supporting a similar association in cancers of the brain, spinal cord, testis, lungs, and skin is inconclusive.[13] Studies examining the mechanism of this BMI-related modulation of cancer risk have focused on the role of sex hormones, insulin, insulin-like growth factors, and adipokines.[9,13,15] Increased adiposity is thought to lead to disruptions in the cellular signaling pathways involving these biomolecules, ultimately resulting in increased proliferation and decreased apoptosis of cancer cells.[9,13,15] Notably, evidence suggests that weight loss can also influence these pathways, lending further support to the hypothesis that body weight plays a role in moderating cancer risk.[9]

Hormone-Related Cancers

Hormone-related cancers, such as prostate, endometrial, and breast cancer, have been positively associated with obesity. A meta-analysis of 23 studies found that an increase of 5 kg/m^2 in BMI corresponded to an 8% increase in advanced prostate cancer risk in a dose-dependent manner.[16] Another meta-analysis examining breast cancer found adult weight gain (relative risk [RR] 1.07; 95% confidence interval [CI], 1.05–1.09) and greater body adiposity (RR 1.11; 95% CI, 1.08–1.14) increased the risk of breast cancer in postmenopausal women.[17] This relation was only true for hormone receptor-positive cancers, but not for those that were hormone receptor-negative.[17] Studies pooling the results of endometrial cancer cohorts have found that BMI is positively associated with estrogen-dependent (odds ratio [OR] 1.20 per 2 kg/m^2 increase; 95% CI, 1.19–1.21) and independent cancers (OR 1.12 per 2 kg/m^2 increase; 95% CI, 1.09–1.14).[18] Therefore, the current data support a strong association between obesity and hormone-related cancers.

Nonhormone Obesity-Related Cancers

Colorectal, esophageal, and pancreatic cancer incidence rates have been strongly correlated with obesity. The results of several meta-analyses have demonstrated a significant positive association between BMI and incidence of colorectal cancer.[19–22] A dose-response relationship has been identified between colorectal cancer risk and increased BMI.[22] Similarly, a study on esophageal adenocarcinoma found a 16% increase in cancer risk for every 1 kg/m^2 increase in BMI.[23] A meta-analysis seeking to understand the relationship between pancreatic cancer and obesity also found statistically significant dose-response relationships, with and without adjusting for known risk factors (adjusted RR 1.19; 95% CI, 1.10–1.29).[24] These dose-response associations provide supporting evidence for a relationship between obesity and colorectal, esophageal, and pancreatic cancers. Chronic inflammation and hormonal imbalances resulting from increased BMI may be involved in the observed increase in cancer risk, although the exact mechanisms underlying this relationship remain unclear and warrant further investigation.

Obesity and Cancer Survival

Obesity may also influence the extent of disease-free survivorship following successful cancer treatment. Evidence examining several types of cancer suggests recurrence is more likely among obese patients.[25–28] A potential underlying mechanism for this phenomenon relates to the fact that tumor cells are able to induce the conversion of typical adipocytes into cancer-associated adipocytes, which in turn aids in tumor progression.[29]

Furthermore, cancer-related mortality has been linked to obesity in a dose-dependent manner.[30] Higher risk of mortality for any cancer type was shown for men and women with baseline obesity (hazard ratio [HR] 1.23; 95% CI, 1.01–1.50) and in women with chronic obesity over a 25-year period (HR 2.16; 95% CI, 1.47–3.18). Among men and women who experienced a short-term annual decrease in BMI of 0.50 kg/m^2 per year, risk of mortality from any cancer type decreased (HR 0.73; 95% CI, 0.55–0.97). Therefore, the management of obesity may be an effective strategy for improving cancer survivorship.

Obesity and Complications Related to Cancer Treatment

Obesity's impact on cancer is not limited to increased incidence, but also appears to play a role in disease course once cancer has developed. Numerous studies have linked obesity to an increased risk of mortality and recurrence following a cancer diagnosis.[31–33] In addition, length of hospital stay[34,35] and operative time,[36] which significantly impact hospital costs, have also been linked to increased BMI. Higher BMI has been associated with surgical complications and increased mortality.[30,37–43] Elevated BMI has been used as a predictor of conversion to an open procedure in several studies on different types of cancer.[37–39] Specific surgical complications, such as lymphedema in patients with breast cancer, are more common among those with increased BMI.[40–42]

Obesity also appears to influence adjuvant and neoadjuvant administration of chemotherapy and radiotherapy. Those classified as overweight and obese are at an increased likelihood to receive intentionally decreased doses of chemotherapy, despite a lack of consensus regarding whether reduced dosing is recommended, or whether it prevents increased risk of toxicity.[44,45] Insufficient locoregional control as a result of reduced dosing poses a threat of cancer recurrence and may hinder remission of incident cancers. Furthermore, there is some evidence suggesting an increased risk of complications following radiotherapy in obese patients, indicating that obesity may hinder multiple stages of the cancer treatment pathway.[46] Overall, there is mounting evidence that obesity has a detrimental effect on those undergoing cancer treatments, which can undoubtedly affect survivorship and quality of life. This finding alludes to a potential protective effect of weight loss on cancer progression.[47]

DISCUSSION

Although the role of excessive body weight in elevating cancer risk has been well established in the medical literature,[13] the role of surgical weight loss in the development of cancer and cancer-related outcomes is less clearly defined. In 2014, the *American Society of Clinical Oncology Position Statement on Obesity and Cancer* made several recommendations for reducing cancer risk. Among the recommendations outlined, weight management was suggested only to those with a current cancer diagnosis, falling short of recommending intentional weight loss as a prophylactic measure for reducing cancer risk.[48] In 2016, the International Agency for Research on Cancer cited insufficient evidence to endorse intentional weight loss as a means to reduce one's risk of developing cancer, despite identifying 13 cancers as obesity-related diseases.[13]

Bariatric surgery has proven efficacious for treating obesity and for helping to resolve obesity-associated complications, such as type 2 diabetes, sleep apnea, cardiovascular disease, dyslipidemia, and hypertension.[49,50] As a result, many investigators have turned to bariatric surgery for a durable and effective measure for intentional weight loss. Bariatric surgery has thus become the clinical tool of choice for studying the effects of reducing adiposity on subsequent cancer risk. Although investigations into a proposed link have become more frequent in recent years, the viability of bariatric surgery as a cancer prevention strategy, and the mechanism by which it may mitigate cancer risk, remains poorly understood and continues to be an area of active research.

The current research base evaluating cancer outcomes following intentional weight loss requires a nuanced appraisal. Randomized controlled trials (RCTs) are unlikely to be conducted in this area because of the financial costs, large sample size requirements, and extended time horizons necessary to examine the relationship between long-term, sustained weight loss, and the detection of incident cancer. Indeed, studies published to date are primarily observational in nature, supported by a combination of biomarker mechanistic studies to further investigate the biologic plausibility of this relationship. Methodological issues, such as bias arising from potential prognostic imbalances owing to the nonrandom sampling strategies used in observational research,[14,51] make it challenging to draw sound inferences and conclusions about the nature of this relationship.[52]

Furthermore, results of many studies are often in conflict with one another, suggesting that intentional weight loss via bariatric surgery may demonstrate variable effects. Currently available data suggest that bariatric surgery confers a stronger benefit in reducing overall cancer risk in women compared with men[53]; however, further research is needed to provide more reliable evidence for the role of sex as an effect modifier in this relationship. Another prominent point of discordance comes from the examination of colorectal cancer risk following bariatric surgery.[54] Observational cohorts have reported a paradoxic increase[55,56] or decrease[57,58] in colorectal cancer risk depending on the bariatric population under study. Interpretation of the range of plausible results has generated the prevailing theory of differential effects of bariatric surgery, depending on the anatomic site of the cancer. Additional confounders may be contributory, such as the surgical approach adopted (Roux-en-Y gastric bypass [RYGB] versus laparoscopic sleeve gastrectomy versus biliopancreatic diversion with duodenal switch) and detection bias as a result of short follow-up durations or undetected neoplasms at the time of index surgery. Factors such as the degree of gut microbiota alterations leading to intestinal dysbiosis–driven carcinogenesis, metabolic dysfunction, liver steatosis, and circulating estrogen levels are likely to modulate the purported benefits of bariatric surgery in the context of cancer risk reduction.[59]

Discussed later are the most salient findings as they pertain to cancer risk following bariatric surgery, including cancer incidence and mortality, and the possible mechanisms involved.

Bariatric Surgery and the Prevention of Hormone-Related Cancers

In hormone-related cancers, Schauer and colleagues[58] reported statistically significant decreases in postmenopausal breast cancer (HR 0.58; 95% CI, 0.44–0.77), endometrial cancer (HR 0.50; 95% CI, 0.37–0.67), and pancreatic cancer (HR 0.46; 95% CI, 0.22–0.97) among those who had undergone bariatric surgery compared with matched nonsurgical controls. Mackenzie and colleagues[56] matched 8794 patients undergoing bariatric surgery to nonsurgical controls and found a similar and consistent decrease in risk for all hormone-related cancers (OR 0.23; 95% CI, 0.18–0.30), corresponding to a 5-fold reduction in the incidence of hormone-related cancers following bariatric surgery, with RYGB patients receiving the largest benefit (OR 0.16; 95% CI, 0.11–0.24). Bariatric surgery was also associated with incidence rates of individual cancers, including cancers of the breast (OR 0.25; 95% CI, 0.19–0.33), endometrium (OR 0.21; 95% CI, 0.13–0.35), and prostate (OR 0.37; 95% CI, 0.17–0.76).[56] Wiggins and colleagues[60] similarly found a statistically significant reduction in breast cancer risk and bariatric surgery (pooled OR 0.50; 95% CI, 0.25–0.99), but not for endometrial (pooled OR 0.47; 95% CI, 0.08–2.65) or prostate cancers (pooled OR 0.82; 95% CI, 0.39–1.73).

The Swedish Obese Subjects study,[53] a large cohort of 1420 women undergoing bariatric surgery and 1447 matched controls, revealed an association between bariatric surgery and reduced risk of hormone-related cancers in women (HR 0.71; 95% CI, 0.59–0.85), particularly for endometrial cancer (HR 0.56; 95% CI, 0.35–0.89). A similar effect has been demonstrated for breast cancer in both premenopausal (HR 0.72; 95% CI, 0.54–0.94) and postmenopausal women (HR 0.55; 95% CI, 0.42–0.72).[61] It is hypothesized that the risk of breast and endometrial cancer may be mitigated via bariatric surgery because of a decrease in circulating estrogen levels, and an increase in sex hormone–binding globulin, which diminishes the oncogenic impulse.[62]

Bariatric Surgery and the Prevention of Nonhormone Obesity-Related Cancers

Beginning in 2008,[63,64] initial evidence derived from prospective cohort studies of bariatric patients matched to nonbariatric controls demonstrated a reduction in cancer incidence following surgery. However, because of the limited sample size and event frequency, conclusions about site-specific associations could not be drawn. More recently, evidence from large cohorts mounted enough data to interpolate site-specific associations.[53,56,58,65] Interestingly, cohort studies have shown that weight loss is not a necessary cause for cancer risk reduction.[64,66] Although investigators cite lack of statistical power,[64] it has been argued that this finding suggests mechanisms are independent of obesity resolution and can be partially attributable to improvements in obesity-related comorbidity.

Data pooled across population-based cohort studies show bariatric surgery leads to a benefit in cancer risk reduction,[56,58,60] especially for obesity-related cancers. Wiggins and colleagues[60] found a significant decrease in overall cancer risk following bariatric surgery (pooled OR 0.72; 95% CI 0.59–0.87), a result that has been reproduced by Schauer and colleagues[58] (HR 0.67; 95% CI 0.60–0.74). For obesity-related cancers, both meta-analyses found a significant reduction in cancer incidences following bariatric procedures (Wiggins and colleagues, pooled OR 0.55; 95% CI, 0.31–0.96; Schauer and colleagues, HR 0.59; 95% CI, 0.51–0.69). For colorectal cancers, Wiggins and colleagues were unable to find a significant reduction (pooled OR 1.39; 95% CI, 0.96–2.02), whereas Schauer and colleagues were able to make a statistically significant determination (HR 0.59; 95% CI, 0.36–0.97). Similarly, Wiggins and colleagues found esophageal cancers (pooled OR 0.79; 95% CI, 0.43–1.44) were not significantly associated with bariatric surgery. Schauer and colleagues noted significantly more cases of esophageal cancer in the control group when compared with the bariatric population but were unable to generate a HR. Schauer and colleagues analyzed additional cancer types individually and found a significant reduction in pancreatic cancer (HR 0.46; 95% CI, 0.22–0.97), whereas cancers of the liver, gallbladder, rectum, and thyroid were statistically insignificant, but had a HR of less than one.

Bariatric Surgery and Evidence for Increased Risk with Non-Hormone Obesity-Related Cancers

It is suspected that the primary mechanism by which bariatric surgery protects against cancer promotion is through a reduction of obesity-related risk factors; however, this prediction is not always borne out empirically. In select instances, bariatric surgery has been shown to increase risk of esophageal,[67–69] gastric,[70,71] and colorectal cancer.[72] Cohort studies have shown that esophageal cancer risk may not decrease following bariatric surgery[73] and may in fact be increased. Similarly, cancer of the remnant stomach following RYGB has similarly been reported.[74,75] The single anastomosis duodeno-ileal (SADI) bypass procedure has recently been endorsed by the International Federation for the Surgery of Obesity and Metabolic Disorders[76] (IFSO), in part, because of its demonstrated clinical feasibility in comparison to more complex bariatric procedures.[77] However, case reports have linked SADI with the development of gastroesophageal cancer,[78,79] although the novelty of this procedure necessitates adequately powered RCTs to further explore a causal link.[80]

Conflicting evidence exists on whether bariatric surgery reduces the risk of colorectal cancer development. A recent systematic review and meta-analysis reported a 35% reduction in risk for those who had undergone bariatric surgery compared with nonsurgical controls.[81] However, whether bariatric surgery increases or decreases colorectal cancer risk is widely debated in the literature. Many cohort studies have reported increased colorectal cancer risk[82,83] and polyp formation[84] after bariatric surgery. This finding is in conflict with other evidence pointing toward reduced colorectal cancer risks.[85] Interestingly, Mackenzie and colleagues[56] found that RYGB, but not gastric banding or LSG (lateral sleeve gastrectomy), was associated with an increased risk of colorectal cancer (OR 2.63; 95% CI, 1.17–5.95). Studies of colorectal cancer biomarkers have also provided mixed mechanistic support. Kant and colleagues[86,87] found that biomarkers for colorectal cancer risk do not increase at 6 months following sleeve gastrectomy, whereas the opposite was found in patients who underwent gastric bypass. Lower levels of inflammation biomarkers and improved glucose regulation were observed following RYGB in another study.[88]

A possible explanation for these findings relates to the contributions of comorbidities, such as gastroesophageal reflux disease[89,90] (GERD), *Helicobacter pylori* infections,[91] and dysregulation of insulin and IGF-1 secretions. Of note, these ailments are more prevalent in the obese surgical population.[92,93] Whether bariatric surgery itself leads to the worsening of symptoms, such as GERD and gastric-emptying disturbances, has been a topic of debate in the surgical literature.[94] In addition, most malignancies reported following bariatric surgery are derived from case reports and case series; thus, the relationship between specific bariatric surgical procedures and new cancer onset requires further discernment. Nevertheless, it is important to note that such a relationship has neither been exclusively confirmed or denied in the literature.[95]

Bariatric Surgery and Cancer Survivorship

The existing literature examining the impact of previous bariatric surgery on cancer prognosis has produced conflicting results. There is a lack of meta-analyzed data on bariatric surgery's effect on cancer prognosis or survivorship, with most published reviews on this topic being narrative in nature. A cost-effectiveness study of bariatric surgery in patients with early-stage, low-risk endometrial cancer[96] determined that weight-loss surgery was a viable therapeutic option given the improved quality of life following the procedure. In a population-based cohort study of patients with colorectal cancer,[82] it was determined that the mortality of patients with rectal cancer and a history of weight-loss surgery was 3-fold compared with that in patients without prior bariatric surgery (disease-specific HR 3.70; 95% CI, 2.00–6.90). A propensity matched analysis by Hussan and colleagues[97] seems to contradict this finding and instead indicates that prior bariatric surgery resulted in fewer colorectal cancer surgery complications, and a lower total hospital cost. The discordant results of these studies may be attributable to differences in study design, with the study by Hussan and colleagues using database information to perform their propensity matched analysis. Similarly, Tao and colleagues[82] used a large patient registry to retrospectively analyze the risk of cancer incidence. Given the methodological flaws associated with these study designs, including limitations of a retrospective analysis, it is unsurprising that such inconsistencies exist. As it stands, the relationship between cancer prognosis and bariatric surgery is poorly understood and requires additional high-quality research.

Nonsurgical Weight Loss and Cancer Risk Reduction

Studies that investigate the effects of lifestyle modification interventions (caloric restriction or dieting) on cancer risk reduction carry methodological limitations, such as recall bias and issues with determining temporality. Long follow-up periods are a prerequisite for any investigation into weight loss and associated cancer risk. Therefore, factors that lead to high rates of attrition, as well as volatility in weight-loss estimates over extended durations, significantly compromise the validity of these studies.

In line with the poor internal validity of these studies, and their risk of bias, the results of systematic reviews examining various lifestyle interventions on cancer risk are mixed. An analysis and appraisal of systematic reviews on gastrointestinal cancers determined that there are limited data to support significant cancer risk reduction following nonsurgical weight-loss strategies.[98] Alternatively, a systematic review found that endometrial cancer risk following self-reported intentional weight loss ranged from estimates of (HR 0.61; 95% CI, 0.40–0.92) to (RR 0.96; 95% CI, 0.61–1.52).

FUTURE DIRECTIONS
Future Research

The use of bariatric surgery for cancer prevention and treatment will be restricted to a limited subset of patients in clinic. Future research in this area will likely focus on identifying the prognostic factors that can be used to deliver precise care to those patients that would most benefit from bariatric surgery. In fact, preliminary work in this area has already begun in an effort to better serve patients desiring weight loss[99]; however, research into optimizing the use of bariatric surgery in the context of cancer prevention and treatment is still lacking.

Based on the systematic literature search used to inform this article, several future research areas have been identified, including research to determine the types of cancer that are most affected by weight-loss surgery, and the effect of different bariatric procedures on cancer mitigation and proliferation. Furthermore, a clearer understanding of the safety profile, and contraindications for the use of bariatric surgery for cancer risk reduction will be required before clinical guidelines can be established.

In addition, studies aimed at understanding the effect of bariatric surgery on cancer prognosis are currently lacking. The literature supports a connection between obesity and worsening chemotherapy or radiotherapy usage and outcomes.[25,44,45] Despite this, research examining whether bariatric surgery can reverse or mitigate these treatment challenges could not be found. Upcoming research should seek to determine if bariatric surgery can mitigate the impact elevated BMI has on cancer treatment utilization and resulting complications.

A Search of the Clinical Trial Database

A search of ClinicalTrials.gov yields a plethora of upcoming studies examining the potential utility of bariatric surgery in cancer treatment and prophylaxis. Several upcoming studies examining breast cancer seek to characterize the impact of bariatric surgery on cancer incidence[100,101] and recurrence.[102] Additional trials examining the utility of bariatric surgery as an adjunct to typical endometrial cancer treatment have been proposed.[102,103] Another upcoming trial seeks to examine the effect of bariatric surgery on gut health as a potential indication of future colorectal cancer.[104] Taken together, future research into the utility of bariatric surgery investigates breast and endometrial cancer.

Barriers to Addressing the Gaps in Research

Several issues will limit the applicability and quality of future research in this area. First, there is a lack of existing and planned RCTs, meaning much of the evidence for the relationship between bariatric surgery and cancer risk is based on nonrandomized cohorts. Observational study designs are more susceptible to selection bias, thus limiting the quality of evidence generated. Second, given that cancer outcomes can occur several years following an intervention, future studies will require long-term follow-up periods, making such studies expensive and time-consuming. The associated financial and resource burden makes these studies challenging to conduct. In addition, the screening procedures typically used by these studies likely introduce lead time bias, which may skew the study results. Unless these methodological limitations are addressed by future researchers, the upcoming research in this field is likely to be limited, and of low methodological quality.

APPLICATION

Multiple physician stakeholder groups have published statements regarding the current use of bariatric surgery as it pertains to intentional weight loss for cancer risk reduction. The IFSO position statement discussing the indications for bariatric surgery includes the following statement: "Weight loss, induced or not by surgery, reduces the risks of gastrointestinal, genitourinary, reproductive, and hematopoietic malignancies."[105] Although not an explicit endorsement of cancer risk reduction as an indication for bariatric surgery, this does support a consensus agreement that obesity surgery provides a protective effect.

The American Society for Metabolic and Bariatric Surgery has recently released a similar position statement discussing the relationship between obesity and cancer.[106] They conclude that "Obesity increases the risk for development of many types of cancer, and successful treatment of obesity by various methods, including bariatric surgery, can mitigate this risk."[106] The statement emphasizes the importance of cancer screening for patients with obesity; however, it does not explicitly suggest the use of bariatric surgery for cancer prevention or treatment.[106] Furthermore, the position statement makes clear that additional research is needed, and concrete clinical practice guidelines are yet to be established.[106]

The utility of bariatric surgery in resolving obesity-related disorders, other than cancer, is an area of current exploration.[107] Existing precedent shows the potential utility of metabolic surgery for the treatment of nonalcoholic fatty liver disease.[108] In addition, bariatric procedures have been used as an initial step for patients with early-stage gastric lesions who require rapid weight loss before a curative procedure.[109] Given the increasing obesity rates observed globally, bariatric surgery will play a larger role in disease management, especially as higher BMIs become perceived as the new normal.[110] Endoscopic screening will need to be implemented to identify risk factors for those who will benefit from bariatric surgery. This large-scale surveillance will provide the added benefit of early detection of cancerous lesions.[111]

SUMMARY

Obesity and cancer are NCDs that have grown in prevalence for several decades. A plethora of cancer varieties has been linked to obesity in a dose-dependent manner. Obesity may also impact the management and curative potential in patients with cancer. Elevated BMI has been shown to lead to marked increases in complications following cancer surgery and may negatively impact cancer prognosis.

Bariatric surgery has proven to be an effective and durable weight-loss treatment for obesity and obesity-related comorbidities. Several articles have suggested a potential protective effect of weight-loss interventions on cancer incidence, prognosis, and mortality. Currently, evidence suggests bariatric surgery improves the risk of overall cancer development. Site-specific associations have been found for some obesity-related cancers, and hormone-related cancers, such as endometrial cancer. To elucidate the relationship between bariatric surgery and cancer prognosis more clearly, additional research will be required; however, there is consensus that obesity results in greater operative costs, and higher complication rates. Studies on lifestyle modification are prone to methodological flaws, which explains their conflicting findings.

Case reports and case series have indicated a potential increase in the likelihood of some cancers after bariatric surgery, particularly in the remnant stomach. The validity of these claims is in conflict within the literature, and information stratified by surgical approach is lacking. Several upcoming clinical trials focus on bariatric surgery utility for breast and endometrial cancers. These studies will need to overcome a variety of issues associated with measuring the longitudinal development of cancer. Future research will seek to determine the conditions under which patients benefit the most from bariatric surgery's effect on cancer incidence. Stakeholders agree that cancer is linked to obesity, and that bariatric surgery can provide some benefit in improving cancer outcomes, although current guidelines and position statements fall short of recommending bariatric surgery to patients based on demonstrated protective effects. However, there is evidence of bariatric procedures being used for other obesity-related diseases, giving precedent for the expanded use of these surgeries.

CLINICS CARE POINTS

- Associations between bariatric surgery and cancer risk reductions are strongest for hormone-related cancers.
- Indications for bariatric surgery in the context of cancer risk management will likely rely on factors such as the type of cancer, bariatric surgery technique, and patient comorbidity profiles.
- Cancer risk reduction should play a small role in clinical decision making when considering the broad benefits of bariatric surgery.
- Weight loss of any type should be suggested by clinicians to patients as a preventative measure to reduce their risk of developing cancer and improve cancer prognosis.

DISCLOSURE

The authors have nothing to disclose.

REFERENCES

1. Finucane MM, Stevens GA, Cowan MJ, et al. National, regional, and global trends in body-mass index since 1980: systematic analysis of health examination surveys and epidemiological studies with 960 country-years and 9.1 million participants. Lancet 2011;377(9765):557–67.
2. Ng M, Fleming T, Robinson M, et al. Global, regional, and national prevalence of overweight and obesity in children and adults during 1980-2013: a systematic analysis for the Global Burden of Disease Study 2013. Lancet 2014; 384(9945):766–81.
3. Kluge HHP, Wickramasinghe K, Rippin HL, et al. Prevention and control of non-communicable diseases in the COVID-19 response. Lancet 2020;395(10238): 1678–80.
4. World Health Organization. WHO tools to prevent and control noncommunicable diseases 2014. Available at: https://www.who.int/nmh/ncd-tools/en/. Accessed April 19, 2020.
5. Word Health Organization. Preventing noncommunicable diseases. Available at: https://www.who.int/activities/preventing-noncommunicable-diseases. Accessed April 19, 2020.
6. Schmidt C. The fight against non-communicable disease in emerging economies. Nature 2018;562(7727):S65–7.
7. Habib SH, Saha S. Burden of non-communicable disease: global overview. Diabetes Metab Syndr Clin Res Rev 2010;4(1):41–7.
8. Pan American Health Organization, World Health Organization. Noncommunicable disease prevention and control. Available at: https://www.paho.org/salud-en-las-americas-2017/?p=1391. Accessed April 19, 2020.
9. Bray F, Ferlay J, Soerjomataram I, et al. Global cancer statistics 2018: GLOBOCAN estimates of incidence and mortality worldwide for 36 cancers in 185 countries. CA Cancer J Clin 2018;68(6):394–424.

10. Soerjomataram I, Lortet-Tieulent J, Parkin DM, et al. Global burden of cancer in 2008: a systematic analysis of disability-adjusted life-years in 12 world regions. Lancet 2012;380(9856):1840–50.

11. Bray F, Jemal A, Grey N, et al. Global cancer transitions according to the Human Development Index (2008-2030): a population-based study. Lancet Oncol 2012; 13(8):790–801.

12. Ferlay J, Shin HR, Bray F, et al. Estimates of worldwide burden of cancer in 2008: GLOBOCAN 2008. Int J Cancer 2010;127(12):2893–917.

13. Lauby-Secretan B, Scoccianti C, Loomis D, et al. Body fatness and cancer–viewpoint of the IARC Working Group. N Engl J Med 2016;375(8):794–8.

14. Basen-Engquist K, Chang M. Obesity and cancer risk: recent review and evidence. Curr Oncol Rep 2011;13(1):71–6.

15. Calle EE, Kaaks R. Overweight, obesity and cancer: epidemiological evidence and proposed mechanisms. Nat Rev Cancer 2004;4(8):579–91.

16. Continuous Update Project Report: diet, nutrition, physical activity, and prostate cancer. 2014. Available at: www.wcrf.org/sites/default/files/Prostate-Cancer-2014-Report.pdf. Accessed April 19, 2020.

17. Chan DSM, Abar L, Cariolou M, et al. World Cancer Research Fund International: Continuous Update Project-systematic literature review and meta-analysis of observational cohort studies on physical activity, sedentary behavior, adiposity, and weight change and breast cancer risk. Cancer Causes Control 2019;30(11):1183–200.

18. Setiawan VW, Yang HP, Pike MC, et al. Type I and II endometrial cancers: have they different risk factors? J Clin Oncol 2013;31(20):2607–18.

19. Ben Q, An W, Jiang Y, et al. Body mass index increases risk for colorectal adenomas based on meta-analysis. Gastroenterology 2012;142(4):762–72.

20. Hong S, Cai Q, Chen D, et al. Abdominal obesity and the risk of colorectal adenoma: a meta-analysis of observational studies. Eur J Cancer Prev 2012;21(6): 523–31.

21. Lee YJ, Myung SK, Cho B, et al. Adiposity and the risk of colorectal adenomatous polyps: a meta-analysis. Cancer Causes Control 2011;22(7):1021–35.

22. Okabayashi K, Ashrafian H, Hasegawa H, et al. Body mass index category as a risk factor for colorectal adenomas: a systematic review and meta-analysis. Am J Gastroenterol 2012;107(8):1175–85 [quiz: 1186].

23. Thrift AP, Shaheen NJ, Gammon MD, et al. Obesity and risk of esophageal adenocarcinoma and Barrett's esophagus: a Mendelian randomization study. J Natl Cancer Inst 2014;106(11):dju252.

24. Berrington de Gonzalez A, Sweetland S, Spencer E. A meta-analysis of obesity and the risk of pancreatic cancer. Br J Cancer 2003;89(3):519–23.

25. Lee K, Kruper L, Dieli-Conwright CM, et al. The impact of obesity on breast cancer diagnosis and treatment. Curr Oncol Rep 2019;21(5):41.

26. Fleming JB, Gonzalez RJ, Petzel MQ, et al. Influence of obesity on cancer-related outcomes after pancreatectomy to treat pancreatic adenocarcinoma. Arch Surg 2009;144(3):216–21.

27. Meyerhardt JA, Catalano PJ, Haller DG, et al. Influence of body mass index on outcomes and treatment-related toxicity in patients with colon carcinoma. Cancer 2003;98(3):484–95.

28. Dignam JJ, Polite BN, Yothers G, et al. Body mass index and outcomes in patients who receive adjuvant chemotherapy for colon cancer. J Natl Cancer Inst 2006;98(22):1647–54.

29. Park J, Morley TS, Kim M, et al. Obesity and cancer–mechanisms underlying tumour progression and recurrence. Nat Rev Endocrinol 2014;10(8):455–65.
30. Taghizadeh N, Boezen HM, Schouten JP, et al. BMI and lifetime changes in BMI and cancer mortality risk. PLoS One 2015;10(4):e0125261.
31. Xing P, Li JG, Jin F, et al. Prognostic significance of body mass index in breast cancer patients with hormone receptor-positive tumours after curative surgery. Clin Invest Med 2013;36(6):E297–305.
32. Liu LN, Lin YC, Miaskowski C, et al. Association between changes in body fat and disease progression after breast cancer surgery is moderated by menopausal status. BMC Cancer 2017;17(1):863.
33. McCall NS, Simone BA, Mehta M, et al. Onco-metabolism: defining the prognostic significance of obesity and diabetes in women with brain metastases from breast cancer. Breast Cancer Res Treat 2018;172(1):221–30.
34. Hendifar A, Osipov A, Khanuja J, et al. Influence of body mass index and albumin on perioperative morbidity and clinical outcomes in resected pancreatic adenocarcinoma. PLoS One 2016;11(3):e0152172.
35. Chen K, Pan Y, Zhai ST, et al. Laparoscopic gastrectomy in obese gastric cancer patients: a comparative study with non-obese patients and evaluation of difference in laparoscopic methods. BMC Gastroenterol 2017;17(1):78.
36. Chen H, Sui W. Influence of obesity on short- and long-term outcomes after laparoscopic distal gastrectomy for gastric cancer. J BUON 2017;22(2):417–23.
37. Rottoli M, Bona S, Rosati R, et al. Laparoscopic rectal resection for cancer: effects of conversion on short-term outcome and survival. Ann Surg Oncol 2009;16(5):1279–86.
38. Tekkis PP, Senagore AJ, Delaney CP. Conversion rates in laparoscopic colorectal surgery: a predictive model with, 1253 patients. Surg Endosc 2005;19(1):47–54.
39. Kunisaki C, Makino H, Takagawa R, et al. Predictive factors for surgical complications of laparoscopy-assisted distal gastrectomy for gastric cancer. Surg Endosc 2009;23(9):2085–93.
40. Ridner SH, Dietrich MS, Stewart BR, et al. Body mass index and breast cancer treatment-related lymphedema. Support Care Cancer 2011;19(6):853–7.
41. Vignes S, Porcher R, Champagne A, et al. Predictive factors of response to intensive decongestive physiotherapy in upper limb lymphedema after breast cancer treatment: a cohort study. Breast Cancer Res Treat 2006;98(1):1–6.
42. Jammallo LS, Miller CL, Singer M, et al. Impact of body mass index and weight fluctuation on lymphedema risk in patients treated for breast cancer. Breast Cancer Res Treat 2013;142(1):59–67.
43. Calle EE, Rodriguez C, Walker-Thurmond K, et al. Overweight, obesity, and mortality from cancer in a prospectively studied cohort of U.S. adults. N Engl J Med 2003;348(17):1625–38.
44. Griggs JJ, Sorbero ME, Lyman GH. Undertreatment of obese women receiving breast cancer chemotherapy. Arch Intern Med 2005;165(11):1267–73.
45. Wolin KY, Carson K, Colditz GA. Obesity and cancer. Oncologist 2010;15(6):556–65.
46. Wang LS, Murphy CT, Ruth K, et al. Impact of obesity on outcomes after definitive dose-escalated intensity-modulated radiotherapy for localized prostate cancer. Cancer 2015;121(17):3010–7.
47. Zhang S, Ikramuddin S, Beckwith HC, et al. The impact of bariatric surgery on breast cancer recurrence: case series and review of literature. Obes Surg 2020;30(2):780–5.

48. Ligibel JA, Alfano CM, Courneya KS, et al. American Society of Clinical Oncology position statement on obesity and cancer. J Clin Oncol 2014; 32(31):3568–74.

49. Jarolimova J, Tagoni J, Stern TA. Obesity: its epidemiology, comorbidities, and management. Prim Care Companion CNS Disord 2013;15(5).

50. Pontiroli AE, Ceriani V, Sarro G, et al. Incidence of diabetes mellitus, cardiovascular diseases, and cancer in patients undergoing malabsorptive surgery (biliopancreatic diversion and biliointestinal bypass) vs medical treatment. Obes Surg 2019;29(3):935–42.

51. Mctiernan A. Obesity and cancer: the risks, science, and potential management strategies. Oncology 2005;19(7):871–81 [discussion: 881–2, 885–6].

52. Sterne JA, Hernan MA, Reeves BC, et al. ROBINS-I: a tool for assessing risk of bias in non-randomised studies of interventions. BMJ 2016;355:i4919.

53. Anveden A, Taube M, Peltonen M, et al. Long-term incidence of female-specific cancer after bariatric surgery or usual care in the Swedish Obese Subjects Study. Gynecol Oncol 2017;145(2):224–9.

54. Davidson LE, Adams TD. Does bariatric surgery increase or reduce colorectal cancer risk-is the jury still out? JAMA Surg 2020;11:11.

55. Aravani A, Downing A, Thomas JD, et al. Obesity surgery and risk of colorectal and other obesity-related cancers: an English population-based cohort study. Cancer Epidemiol 2018;53:99–104.

56. Mackenzie H, Markar SR, Askari A, et al. Obesity surgery and risk of cancer. Br J Surg 2018;105(12):1650–7.

57. Bailly L, Fabre R, Pradier C, et al. Colorectal cancer risk following bariatric surgery in a nationwide study of French individuals with obesity. JAMA Surg 2020; 155(5):395–402.

58. Schauer DP, Feigelson HS, Koebnick C, et al. Bariatric surgery and the risk of cancer in a large multisite cohort. Ann Surg 2019;269(1):95–101.

59. Sinclair P, Brennan DJ, le Roux CW. Gut adaptation after metabolic surgery and its influences on the brain, liver and cancer. Nat Rev Gastroenterol Hepatol 2018;15(10):606–24.

60. Wiggins T, Antonowicz SS, Markar SR. Cancer risk following bariatric surgery-systematic review and meta-analysis of national population-based cohort studies. Obes Surg 2019;29(3):1031–9.

61. Feigelson HS, Caan B, Weinmann S, et al. Bariatric surgery is associated with reduced risk of breast cancer in both premenopausal and postmenopausal women. Ann Surg 2020;272(6):1053–9.

62. Byers T, Sedjo RL. Does intentional weight loss reduce cancer risk? Diabetes Obes Metab 2011;13(12):1063–72.

63. Christou NV, Lieberman M, Sampalis F, et al. Bariatric surgery reduces cancer risk in morbidly obese patients. Surg Obes Relat Dis 2008;4(6):691–5.

64. Sjostrom L, Gummesson A, Sjostrom CD, et al. Effects of bariatric surgery on cancer incidence in obese patients in Sweden (Swedish Obese Subjects Study): a prospective, controlled intervention trial. Lancet Oncol 2009;10(7): 653–62.

65. Ostlund MP, Lu Y, Lagergren J. Risk of obesity-related cancer after obesity surgery in a population-based cohort study. Ann Surg 2010;252(6):972–6.

66. Schauer DP, Feigelson HS, Koebnick C, et al. Association between weight loss and the risk of cancer after bariatric surgery. Obesity (Silver Spring) 2017; 25(Suppl 2):S52–7.

67. Melstrom LG, Bentrem DJ, Salvino MJ, et al. Adenocarcinoma of the gastro-esophageal junction after bariatric surgery. Am J Surg 2008;196(1):135–8.

68. Burton PR, Ooi GJ, Laurie C, et al. Diagnosis and management of oesophageal cancer in bariatric surgical patients. J Gastrointest Surg 2016;20(10):1683–91.

69. Allen JW, Leeman MF, Richardson JD. Esophageal carcinoma following bariatric procedures. JSLS 2004;8(4):372–5.

70. Orlando G, Pilone V, Vitiello A, et al. Gastric cancer following bariatric surgery: a review. Surg Laparosc Endosc Percutan Tech 2014;24(5):400–5.

71. Fleetwood VA, Petersen L, Millikan KW. Gastric adenocarcinoma presenting after revisional Roux-en-Y gastric bypass. Am Surg 2016;82(8):e186–7.

72. Derogar M, Hull MA, Kant P, et al. Increased risk of colorectal cancer after obesity surgery. Ann Surg 2013;258(6):983–8.

73. Maret-Ouda J, Tao W, Mattsson F, et al. Esophageal adenocarcinoma after obesity surgery in a population-based cohort study. Surg Obes Relat Dis 2017;13(1):28–34.

74. Escalona A, Guzman S, Ibanez L, et al. Gastric cancer after Roux-en-Y gastric bypass. Obes Surg 2005;15(3):423–7.

75. Wu CC, Lee WJ, Ser KH, et al. Gastric cancer after mini-gastric bypass surgery: a case report and literature review. Asian J Endosc Surg 2013;6(4):303–6.

76. Brown WA, Ooi G, Higa K, et al. SADI-S/OADS IF-ATFRTLO. Single anastomosis duodenal-ileal bypass with sleeve gastrectomy/one anastomosis duodenal switch (SADI-S/OADS) IFSO position statement. Obes Surg 2018;28(5):1207–16.

77. Lee Y, Ellenbogen Y, Doumouras AG, et al. Single- or double-anastomosis duodenal switch versus Roux-en-Y gastric bypass as a revisional procedure for sleeve gastrectomy: a systematic review and meta-analysis. Surg Obes Relat Dis 2019;15(4):556–66.

78. Aggarwal S, Bhambri A, Singla V, et al. Adenocarcinoma of oesophagus involving gastro-oesophageal junction following mini-gastric bypass/one anastomosis gastric bypass. J Minim Access Surg 2019;16(2):175–8.

79. Guirat A, Addossari HM. One anastomosis gastric bypass and risk of cancer. Obes Surg 2018;28(5):1441–4.

80. Bruzzi M, Chevallier JM, Czernichow S. One-anastomosis gastric bypass: why biliary reflux remains controversial? Obes Surg 2017;27(2):545–7.

81. Almazeedi S, El-Abd R, Al-Khamis A, et al. Role of bariatric surgery in reducing the risk of colorectal cancer: a meta-analysis. Br J Surg 2020;107(4):348–54.

82. Tao W, Konings P, Hull MA, et al. Colorectal cancer prognosis following obesity surgery in a population-based cohort study. Obes Surg 2017;27(5):1233–9.

83. Tao W, Artama M, von Euler-Chelpin M, et al. Colon and rectal cancer risk after bariatric surgery in a multicountry Nordic cohort study. Int J Cancer 2020;147(3):728–35.

84. Hussan H, Drosdak A, Le Roux M, et al. The long-term impact of Roux-en-Y gastric bypass on colorectal polyp formation and relation to weight loss outcomes. Obes Surg 2020;30(2):407–15.

85. Kedrin D, Gandhi SC, Wolf M, et al. Bariatric surgery prior to index screening colonoscopy is associated with a decreased rate of colorectal adenomas in obese individuals. Clin Transl Gastroenterol 2017;8(2):e73.

86. Kant P, Perry SL, Dexter SP, et al. Mucosal biomarkers of colorectal cancer risk do not increase at 6 months following sleeve gastrectomy, unlike gastric bypass. Obesity (Silver Spring) 2014;22(1):202–10.

87. Kant P, Sainsbury A, Reed KR, et al. Rectal epithelial cell mitosis and expression of macrophage migration inhibitory factor are increased 3 years after Roux-en-Y gastric bypass (RYGB) for morbid obesity: implications for long-term neoplastic risk following RYGB. Gut 2011;60(7):893–901.

88. Afshar S, Malcomson F, Kelly SB, et al. Biomarkers of colorectal cancer risk decrease 6 months after Roux-en-Y gastric bypass surgery. Obes Surg 2018; 28(4):945–54.

89. Acosta A, Streett S, Kroh MD, et al. White Paper AGA: POWER - practice guide on obesity and weight management, education, and resources. Clin Gastroenterol Hepatol 2017;15(5):631–49.e10.

90. Alexandre L, Long E, Beales IL. Pathophysiological mechanisms linking obesity and esophageal adenocarcinoma. World J Gastrointest Pathophysiol 2014;5(4): 534–49.

91. Dantas AC, Santo MA, de Cleva R, et al. Influence of obesity and bariatric surgery on gastric cancer. Cancer Biol Med 2016;13(2):269–76.

92. Ulrich CM, Himbert C, Holowatyj AN, et al. Energy balance and gastrointestinal cancer: risk, interventions, outcomes and mechanisms. Nat Rev Gastroenterol Hepatol 2018;15(11):683–98.

93. Kant P, Hull MA. Excess body weight and obesity–the link with gastrointestinal and hepatobiliary cancer. Nat Rev Gastroenterol Hepatol 2011;8(4):224–38.

94. Lieverse RJ, Jansen JB, Masclee AA, et al. Gastrointestinal disturbances with obesity. Scand J Gastroenterol Suppl 1993;200:53–8.

95. Musella M, Berardi G, Bocchetti A, et al. Esophagogastric neoplasms following bariatric surgery: an updated systematic review. Obes Surg 2019;29(8):2660–9.

96. Neff R, Havrilesky LJ, Chino J, et al. Bariatric surgery as a means to decrease mortality in women with type I endometrial cancer - an intriguing option in a population at risk for dying of complications of metabolic syndrome. Gynecol Oncol 2015;138(3):597–602.

97. Hussan H, Stanich PP, Gray DM 2nd, et al. Prior bariatric surgery is linked to improved colorectal cancer surgery outcomes and costs: a propensity-matched analysis. Obes Surg 2017;27(4):1047–55.

98. Coe PO, O'Reilly DA, Renehan AG. Excess adiposity and gastrointestinal cancer. Br J Surg 2014;101(12):1518–31 [discussion: 1531].

99. Severin R, Sabbahi A, Mahmoud AM, et al. Precision medicine in weight loss and healthy living. Prog Cardiovasc Dis 2019;62(1):15–20.

100. The Cleveland Clinic. Effects of bariatric surgery on breast density improvement and impact on breast cancer risk in severe obese patients. 2020. Available at: https://ClinicalTrials.gov/show/NCT04170335. Accessed April 19, 2020.

101. Tarah B, Indiana University. Pilot study of the effect of weight loss on breast tissue and blood biomarkers in women at increased risk for breast cancer. 2020. Available at: https://ClinicalTrials.gov/show/NCT02681120. Accessed April 19, 2020.

102. Toronto University Health Network. Bariatric surgery for fertility-sparing treatment of atypical hyperplasia and grade 1 cancer of the endometrium. 2013. Available at: https://ClinicalTrials.gov/show/NCT04008563. Accessed April 19, 2020.

103. Brigham Women's Hospital, Dana-Farber Cancer Institute. Laparoscopic hysterectomy and weight loss surgery in obese patients with endometrial carcinoma/intraepithelial neoplasia. 2022. Available at: https://ClinicalTrials.gov/show/NCT04278183. Accessed April 19, 2020.

104. Leuven KU. Impact of bariatric surgery on the gut environment. 2021. Available at: https://ClinicalTrials.gov/show/NCT04345328. Accessed April 19, 2020.
105. De Luca M, Angrisani L, Himpens J, et al. Indications for surgery for obesity and weight-related diseases: position statements from the International Federation for the Surgery of Obesity and Metabolic Disorders (IFSO). Obes Surg 2016; 26(8):1659–96.
106. Ghiassi S, El Chaar M, Aleassa EM, et al. ASMBS position statement on the relationship between obesity and cancer, and the role of bariatric surgery: risk, timing of treatment, effects on disease biology, and qualification for surgery. Surg Obes Relat Dis 2020;16(6):713–24.
107. Selby LV, Ejaz A, Brethauer SA, et al. Fatty liver disease and primary liver cancer: disease mechanisms, emerging therapies and the role of bariatric surgery. Expert Opin Investig Drugs 2020;29(2):107–10.
108. Lee Y, Doumouras AG, Yu J, et al. Complete resolution of nonalcoholic fatty liver disease after bariatric surgery: a systematic review and meta-analysis. Clin Gastroenterol Hepatol 2019;17(6):1040–60.e11.
109. Gianos M, Abdemur A, Szomstein S, et al. Laparoscopic sleeve gastrectomy as a step approach for morbidly obese patients with early stage malignancies requiring rapid weight loss for a final curative procedure. Obes Surg 2013; 23(9):1370–4.
110. Henretta MS, Copeland AR, Kelley SL, et al. Perceptions of obesity and cancer risk in female bariatric surgery candidates: highlighting the need for physician action for unsuspectingly obese and high risk patients. Gynecol Oncol 2014; 133(1):73–7.
111. Gagne DJ, Papasavas PK, Maalouf M, et al. Obesity surgery and malignancy: our experience after 1500 cases. Surg Obes Relat Dis 2009;5(2):160–4.

Diabetes Risk Reduction and Metabolic Surgery

John D. Scott, MD[a],*, Sean C. O'Connor, MD[b]

KEYWORDS

- Metabolic surgery • Type 2 diabetes mellitus • Roux-en-Y gastric bypass
- Vertical sleeve gastrectomy • Duodenal switch
- Single-anastomosis duodeno-ileal bypass

KEY POINTS

- Type 2 diabetes mellitus (T2D) is an insidious, chronic medical condition that has a low rate of remission when treated with medication and lifestyle changes alone.
- The incidence of T2D diabetes continues to rise and have a negative impact on the economic well-being of the American health care system.
- Metabolic surgery has been shown to be effective in treating T2D and has afforded patients the best opportunity for remission.
- There are several surgical procedures, including the Roux-en-Y gastric bypass, the vertical sleeve gastrectomy, and the biliopancreatic diversion, that have been shown to be effective in patients with T2D.
- Metabolic surgery is highly underutilized, and increasing access to surgical care may help decrease expenditure on T2D related disease and complications.

INTRODUCTION

Type 2 diabetes mellitus (T2D) remains among the most common chronic medical conditions in the United States. The National Diabetes Statistics Report, published by the Centers for Disease Control and Prevention (CDC), reports that 10.2% of Americans (34.2 million) carried a diagnosis of T2D in 2018, an increase from 7% in 2002.[1] The disease remains underdiagnosed, however, with another 2.8% of Americans (7.3 million) meeting the laboratory criteria for T2D, without a formal diagnosis. Older adults ages greater than 65 have had the sharpest increase in disease burden from 2000 to 2017 (15.8% to 19.1% prevalence, respectively); however, all age groups, including children 10 years old to 19 years old, have experienced significant increases over the past 2 decades.

[a] Department of Surgery, Division of Minimal Access and Bariatric Surgery, Prisma Health, 905 Verdae Boulevard Suite 202, Greenville, SC 29607, USA; [b] Department of Surgery, Division of Minimal Access and Bariatric Surgery, Prisma Health, 701 Grove Road, Greenville, SC 29601, USA
* Corresponding author.
E-mail address: John.Scott@prismahealth.org

Surg Clin N Am 101 (2021) 255–267
https://doi.org/10.1016/j.suc.2020.12.004
0039-6109/21/© 2020 Elsevier Inc. All rights reserved.

surgical.theclinics.com

The demographics of diabetic patients have remained consistent, with elderly patients age greater than 65, male patients, and Native Americans carrying the greatest burden of disease. The racial distribution of disease in descending order is Native Americans (14.7%), Hispanic (12.5%), blacks (11.7%), non-Hispanic Asians (9.2%), and non-Hispanic whites (7.5%). Hispanics and blacks have been found to have a 2-fold to 3-fold risk of developing T2D during the course of their life compared with their white counterparts (**Fig. 1**). Although central obesity and the development of subsequent metabolic syndrome is associated with insulin resistance (IR) in the general population, the relationship clearly is stronger in some ethnic groups over others. For example, after controlling for obesity, behavioral factors and body fat distribution, blacks continue to have higher IR compared with whites, whereas the difference in IR between Hispanics and whites appears associated with obesity and fat distribution.[2] The black population, therefore, is particularly vulnerable to developing T2D in spite of lower rates of metabolic syndrome and similar environmental exposures.[3]

Although the prevalence of T2D has been increasing nationwide, the burden of disease always has remained highest across the Southern states. Arkansas and Alabama became the first 2 states to have greater than 9% of the population diagnosed in 2001. By 2015, the entire Southeast and Southwestern regions reported greater than 9% prevalence as well as Indiana, Ohio, Pennsylvania, and Michigan.[4] The reason for this trend is multifactorial; however, Southern states tend to have higher populations of nonwhite ethnicities, who are particularly at risk for the disease. In addition, lower socioeconomic class places patients at higher risk for developing the disease, independent of access to medical care. Disparities continue to exist in countries with nationalized health care systems meant to improve access to care, with lower education and income level independent risk factors for the development of T2D.[5,6]

The economic impact of T2D both on individuals and the health care system at large is substantial and is increasing steadily. Between the years of 2012 and 2017, the total direct treatment costs of all diabetics in the United States increased by 21%, from $188 billion to $237 billion. Indirect costs also increased by 19%, resulting in a total

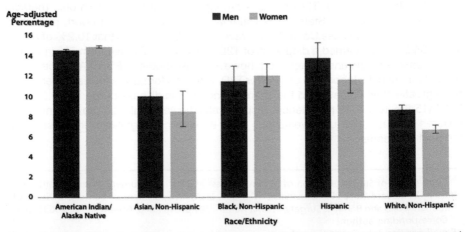

Fig. 1. Trends in age-adjusted prevalence of diagnosed diabetes, undiagnosed diabetes, and total diabetes among adults aged 18 years or older, United States, 1999 to 2016. (*From* Centers for Disease Control. National Diabetes Statistics Report 2020. Estimates of Diabetes and Its Burden in the United States.; 2020.)

of $327 billion expense to the US health care system, making up 9.3% of total health care spending.[7] The increase in the prevalence of disease is partially to blame; however, novel, more-expensive treatment strategies also play a role. The annual costs per person due to diabetes management increased from $8417 to $9601 in the same time frame.[1] Management of T2D is becoming more burdensome financially both on individual patients and health care system at large; therefore, the pursuit of a durable cure has intensified.

COMORBIDITIES ASSOCIATED WITH TYPE 2 DIABETES MELLITUS

The most common and feared comorbidities associated with T2D are atherosclerosis, nephropathy, and retinopathy. All of these are the direct result of the damage chronic hyperglycemia has on the vasculature throughout the body through multiple pathways. The atherosclerotic lesions found in diabetic patients are identical to those in nondiabetic patients and share a similar pathogenesis. A chronic hyperglycemic state causes an overproduction of adenosine triphosphate through the electron transport chain, of which superoxide is a by-product. This oxidative stress signals macrophage recruitment to the intimal lining and the subsequent retention of low-density lipoprotein in foam cells. In addition to recruiting inflammatory mediators to the intimal lining, reactive oxygen species within the plaque core causes apoptosis of macrophages, destabilizing the plaque structure as well as breaking down the fibrous cap.[8] The result is a higher risk of plaque rupture and thrombotic events in diabetics compared with nondiabetics with a similar atherosclerotic burden.[9]

Furthermore, microvascular effects of hyperglycemia are due primarily to vascular permeability, which leads to the high rates of nephropathy and retinopathy seen in diabetics. The initial finding in diabetic nephropathy is albuminuria, due to increased renal perfusion and degradation of the glomerular basement membrane. Oxidative stress combined with alterations to endothelial membrane surface proteins, called advanced glycosylation end-product, signals apoptosis of podocytes that maintain the endothelial lining. In addition, proinflammatory signals cause glomerulosclerosis, which exacerbates the glomerular basement membrane permeability. The result is a complete breakdown of plasma filtration through the glomeruli, leading to an intrinsic nephropathy.[10] The CDC reports that diabetes is the leading cause of end-stage renal disease, accounting for 38% of cases, followed by hypertension (26%) and glomerulonephritis (16%).[11]

A similar pathway leads to macular edema, angiogenesis, and vitreous hemorrhage that cause retinopathy in these patients. The same oxidative stress and advanced glycosylation end-product production causes apoptosis of pericytes that line the retinal capillaries. This leads to increased permeability of the vascular walls and ultimately macular edema. Retinal ischemia ensues as a result of apoptosis, and the retina reacts by up-regulating vascular growth factors, such as vascular endothelial growth factor and erythropoietin. This leads to microvascular overgrowth and hemorrhage within the retina, ultimately exacerbating vision loss.[8,10]

PHYSIOLOGIC EFFECTS OF METABOLIC SURGERY ON TYPE 2 DIABETES MELLITUS

The effect of bariatric surgery on the neurohormonal axis of energy metabolism recently has gained increased attention. Anatomic alterations change nutrient presentation to the gut, thereby altering the up-regulation and down-regulation of a variety of intestinal hormones and modulators, each of which has paracrine and endocrine effects on glucose metabolism, energy storage, and appetite.[12] Glucagon-like peptide 1 (GLP-1) is 30–amino acid peptide produced in the L cells of the distal small bowel.

GLP-1 is described as an incretin, a metabolic hormone that can stimulate a decrease in blood sugar levels. GLP-1 does this by directly increasing the release of insulin and inhibiting the release of glucagon.[13] Certain bariatric surgical procedures increase the delivery of nutrients and food particles to the distal small bowel and L cells, leading to their stimulation and release of GLP-1. It is the profound hypersecretion of GLP-1 after bariatric surgery that seems to have the most effect on postoperative plasma glucose levels. Other gut hormones, especially peptide YY (PYY), glucose-dependent insulino-tropic polypeptide, and oxyntomodulin, also are potential agents that work in a complicated, poorly understood concert to maintain energy homeostasis.[14] These hormone levels also are affected by bariatric procedures and are targets for pharma-cologic intervention in an effort to replicate the success of the GLP-1 pathway alter-ations commonly used today in medical practice.

Because of the effects of bariatric surgical procedures on the function of this neurohormonal axis of energy metabolism, a more clinically appropriate and relevant term for this class of procedures is metabolic surgery rather than bariatric surgery, which implies only weight loss benefits. As the concept of metabolic surgery is pro-moted to primary care physicians and patients, the positive effects of the surgery on T2D are highlighted and the weight-reduction effects become secondary. This termi-nology may decrease the inherent bias against weight loss surgery and patients who suffer from obesity.

PATIENT EVALUATION

Metabolic surgery provides superior glucose control and remission of T2D compared with medical management alone.[15] Not all diabetic patients respond equally, however, with T2D remission rates ranging widely from 30% to 80%, when patients are followed further than 5 years after their operation.[16] The durability of glycemic control is dependent on β-cell function at the time of surgery. As diabetes progresses over time, β-cell are required to maintain hyperinsulinemia in the face of persistent hyperglycemia and peripheral IR. This metabolic stress combined with the systemic inflammatory state ultimately causes damage and death to the islet cells of the pancreas, commonly referred to as *burnout*. The severity of disease is measured by the residual secretory function of the pancreas that ultimately declines if hypergly-cemia goes unchecked.

In mild disease, residual β-cell are able to provide sustained insulin production over time after surgery, whereas severe diabetics suffer shorter remission of disease due to the lack of islet cell reserves.[17] Older age, longer duration of disease, higher hemoglo-bin A_{1c} (HbA_{1c}), use of more than 2 diabetes medications, and insulin requirement prior to surgery can act as surrogate markers for islet cell function and all have been associated with worse glycemic control after 5 years after surgery.[18] This infor-mation can be used clinically to predict patient outcomes when discussing the risks and benefits of metabolic surgical options. Patients with severe disease may choose a lower risk surgical option if the chances of remission are similar between vertical sleeve gastrectomy, gastric bypass, or duodenal switch (DS) (**Fig. 2**).

Aminian and colleagues created and externally validated an individualized scoring system based on a patient's severity of disease to aid in the decision between vertical sleeve gastrectomy (VSG) and Roux-en-Y gastric bypass (RYGB).[17] The individualized metabolic surgery (IMS) score is based on preoperative diabetes medications, preop-erative insulin use, duration of diabetes, and glycemic control defined as HbA_{1c} greater than 7%. They performed a retrospective review of 659 patients who had at least 5 years of follow-up after either VSG or RYGB, assigning a point system to the

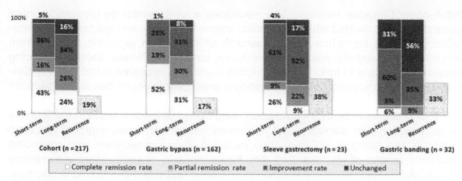

Fig. 2. Short-term and long-term diabetes remission and recurrence rates according to procedure type. (*From* Brethauer SA, Aminian A, Romero-Talamás H, et al. Can diabetes be surgically cured? Long-term metabolic effects of bariatric surgery in obese patients with type 2 diabetes mellitus. *Ann Surg.* 2013;258(4):628-637; with permission.)

each of these characteristics based on their impact on long-term remission (defined as HbA$_{1c}$ <7% without medications). In patients with severe disease (>95 IMS score), they found no difference in glycemic control between VSG or RYGB, with long-term remission rates approximately only 12%. VSG is recommended in these patients because the risk of RYGB does not result in more reward. In patients with moderate disease (25–95 IMS score), however, RYGB resulted in 35% improvement in T2D remission (60% vs 25%; P = .0001), prompting the investigators to recommend RYGB for patients who fall in this category as the higher-risk procedure results in significant rewards. Patients with mild disease (<25 IMS score) saw the highest rates of disease remission with only marginal differences between VSG and RYGB. Because RYGB resulted in a significant reduction in the number of diabetes medications over SG, however, the investigators suggest RYGB to for these patients as well. These data were used to create a user-friendly calculator that can be utilized in the office to aid in the discussion of the risks and potential benefits of surgical options.[19]

One criticism of the widespread distribution and use of the IMS is the lack of data for other alternative surgical options, such as the one-anastomosis gastric bypass (OAGB), the DS, and a modification of the DS: the single-anastomosis duodeno-ileal bypass with VSG (SADI-S). The physiologic effects of the DS and its variants are discussed later. The OAGB initially was described by Rutledge and colleagues,[20] in 1997, as the mini–gastric bypass and has gained wide acceptance in the international community. In the era of high-utilization of the gastric sleeve as an alternative to the RYGB and the DS, the OAGB has not yet achieved widespread adoption in the United States. Recent studies have demonstrated positive physiologic effects of the OAGB and its modifications on T2D.[21] As additional studies reveal the relative strengths of all operations to place T2D into remission, the procedure selection algorithm for surgeons and patients will become more robust and accurate.

SURGICAL OPTIONS
Roux-en-Y Gastric Bypass

The RYGB has become the mainstay of metabolic surgery since the publication in 1995 of the landmark article by Pories and colleagues,[22] delightfully entitled, "Who Would Have Thought It? An Operation Proves To Be the Most Effective Therapy for

Adult-onset Diabetes Mellitus." The mechanisms of its effect on glycemic control generally can be divided into 2 categories: calorie restriction and gut hormone stimulation.[23] Calorie restriction has a cascade of effects on glycemic control, from reducing postprandial glycemic load, reducing lipotoxicity through lipolysis, reducing hepatic steatosis, and free radical reduction leading to improved β-cell survival. Calorie restriction is accomplished by creating a small gastric pouch that restricts caloric intake as well as proximal small bowel bypass that causes malabsorption of calories. The proximal enteric bypass also causes rapid transit of food particles to the terminal ileum, which in turn stimulates gut hormones. These hormones augment glycemic control by regulating insulin production, reducing glucagon secretion, and enhancing peripheral uptake of glucose; and they have anorexic properties that also reduce caloric intake. This powerful combination of caloric restriction and hormone augmentation has allowed the RYGB to stand the test of time as the standard metabolic surgical intervention.[19]

The antidiabetic effects are showcased by the acute improvements in glycemic control postoperatively, even prior to any weight loss. Within the first 6 days of surgery, patients experience improvements in their postprandial blood glucose levels and may eliminate the need for diabetic medications altogether.[24] Wallenius and colleagues[25] studied fasting blood glucose, insulin, GLP-1 levels, and IR at 2 days, 3 weeks, and 12 months in diabetic patients undergoing RYGB and SG. They found significant reductions in fasting blood glucose at 3 weeks, with decreased insulin levels (**Fig. 3**) and IR as soon as 2 days following surgery, which continued to improve over the 12-month extent of the study.[25]

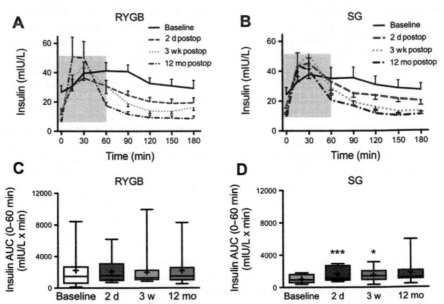

Fig. 3. Within-group plasma insulin levels 0 minutes to 180 minutes after a modified 30-g oral glucose tolerance test at baseline, 2 days, 3 weeks, and 12 months after ([A] and [C]) LRYGB or ([B] and [D]) LVSG after Roux-en-Y gastric bypass, RYGB (see panels A and B) or after vertical sleeve gastrectomt, VSG (panels C and D). AUC, area under the curve. (*From* Wallenius V, Dirinck E, Fändriks L, Maleckas A, le Roux CW, Thorell A. Glycemic Control after Sleeve Gastrectomy and Roux-En-Y Gastric Bypass in Obese Subjects with Type 2 Diabetes Mellitus. Obes Surg. 2018;28(6):1461-1472; with permission.)

The durability of glycemic control has been corroborated by the 5-year follow-up of the STAMPEDE (Surgical Treatment and Medications Potentially Eradicate Diabetes Efficiently) trial, which randomized patients to intensive medical management, RYGB, or SG.[13] Ultimately, patients in the surgical arm achieved the highest rates of remission (HbA$_{1c}$ <6.5% without medications): 30.6% after RYGB, 23.4% after VSG, and 0 patients in the medical therapy group. After 5 years, patients requiring insulin in the RYGB arm dropped by 35%, and 45% of patients required no diabetic medications at all. This study was performed on all patients regardless of severity of diabetes, even though it now is understood that remission rates vary depending on an individual patient's severity of disease.[14] Even so, the ability to achieve immediate glycemic control along with durable diabetes remission has established the RYGB as the gold standard metabolic procedure since the 1990s.

Vertical Sleeve Gastrectomy

The concept of the VSG was born from the restrictive portion of the DS and later used as a stand-alone operation.[26] Until recently, its effects on T2D were thought to be limited to calorie restriction and weight loss with very little effect on the gut hormone axis. In spite of the lack of intestinal bypass, however, GLP-1 and PYY levels have been found to increase perioperatively to levels that rival the RYGB.[27] The small gastric reservoir results in rapid transit of food particles into the small bowel, stimulating the intestinal enteroendocrine axis in a way similar to bypass procedures. Wallenius and colleagues found that GLP-1 levels increased similarly 2 days postoperatively; however, patients who underwent RYGB maintained higher levels at 3 weeks and 12 months.[25] Ultimately, they found that both early glycemic control and late glycemic control were similar between VSG and RYGB in spite of less weight loss. Although GLP-1 may play a role in early glycemic control, there clearly are other non–weight-dependent pathways that contribute to the durable euglycemic effect of SG.

This theory has been supported by the 5-year follow-up of the STAMPEDE trial, which showed no significant difference in HbA$_{1c}$ between VSG and RYGB. Diabetic remission rates (HbA$_{1c}$ <6.5% without medication) were better in the surgical arm with no significant difference between the 2 procedures (23.4% vs 30.6%; $P = .043$).[13] These findings have been corroborated in a large metanalysis by Guraya and Strate,[28] who also noted that 5-year remission rates were lower after SG; however, this difference did not reach statistical significance ($P = .07$). Clearly the metabolic effects of VSG are potent but largely have been overshadowed by the gastric bypass through the early years of bariatric surgery. When attempting to predict successful remission for an individual patient, the choice between these 2 procedures is less important than patient severity of disease preoperatively. A thorough assessment of a patient's goals and risk tolerance can be assessed using the Web-based Metabolic and Bariatric Surgery Accreditation and Quality Improvement Program risk/benefit calculator, which can empower patient and surgeon to make an informed decision.[29]

Biliopancreatic Diversion with Duodenal Switch

The mechanisms of glycemic control from biliopancreatic diversion (BPD) with DS are identical to RYGB; however, they are augmented by the technique. A much longer portion of jejunum is excluded by creating a 150-cm Roux limb and a 100-cm common channel (**Fig. 4**). Restriction is achieved by performing a VSG first, and dumping symptoms are mitigated by locating the Roux anastomosis to the postpyloric duodenum. This anatomic arrangement results in a decreased absorptive capacity for nutrients and a more rapid transit of food particles to the terminal ileum, thereby stimulating

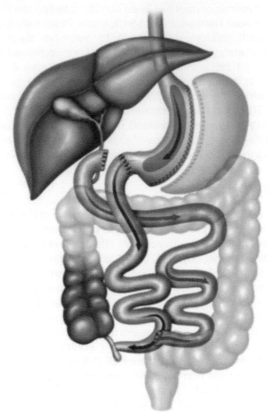

Fig. 4. BPD-DS. (*From* Biertho L, Lebel S, Marceau S, Hould FS, Julien F, Biron S. Biliopancreatic Diversion with Duodenal Switch: Surgical Technique and Perioperative Care. *Surg Clin North Am*. 2016;96(4):815-826; with permission.)

distal ileal hormone release (PYY and GLP-1). Studies of superobese patients (BMI >50 kg/m^2) have shown increased weight loss and glycemic control compared with RYGB; however, this comes at the expense of more potential adverse outcomes, such as gastroesophageal reflux disease (GERD), vitamin deficiencies, and diarrhea.[30] Mingrone and colleagues performed an RCT where they showed a 63% T2D remission rate on 5-year follow-up after BPD-DS compared with 37% in the RYGB group.[15] Compared with RYGB for weight loss and antidiabetic effects, BPD-DS is more effective; however, it also is the more technically challenging operation and can be associated with higher complication rates. As robotic surgery is changing current paradigms, the DS and its variants are becoming more feasible. The DS should be utilized, however, in patients who are able to realize the maximum rewards while being able to tolerate potential longer term nutritional complications.

Diabetes remission is but one of the many goals a patient may have when pursuing metabolic surgery, and these must all be considered when tailoring the correct procedure to a patient. A review of the Bariatric Outcomes Longitudinal Database showed that BPD-DS resulted in an average greater weight loss and improved resolution of diabetes mellitus and hypertension but was inferior to RYGB in resolution of GERD symptoms and associated with a greater number of nutritional complications.[31] The ideal candidate should have mild-severity to moderate-severity T2D, minimal preoperative GERD, BMI greater than 50kg/m^2 and desire for substantial weight loss, and proved dietary compliance, because nutritional supplementation is required for life.

Single-Anastomosis Duodeno-ileal Bypass with Vertical Sleeve Gastrectomy

In the past 5 years, interest has grown in the SADI-S as an alternative to the DS.[32] The procedure involves creation of a VSG and division of the proximal duodenum as performed in the DS; however, a section of ileum 250 cm to 300 cm from the ileocolonic valve is brought up as a loop anastomosis to the duodenum (**Fig. 5**). The theoretic advantages include a technically simpler operation to perform with only 1 anastomosis, less potential internal hernia, and improved vitamin absorption because food is exposed to bile and pancreatic fluid through the entire length of the efferent limb. Current comparative studies have confirmed shorter operative times with equivalent weight loss; however, the rate of postoperative vitamin deficiencies remained unchanged between the 2 procedures.[33]

One of the largest studies by Sánchez-Pernaute and colleagues[34] followed the glycemic control of 97 patients after SADI-S. They found that 5 years after SADI-S, between 70% and 84% of their population were off all diabetic medication and maintaining HbA$_{1c}$ less than 6. Successful long-term remission was more likely in non–insulin-dependent versus insulin-dependent diabetics (75% vs 38.4%, respectively) and in patients who had a shorter duration of disease prior to surgery. Like

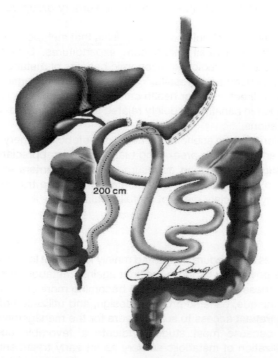

Fig. 5. SADI-S. (*From* Wu A, Tian J, Cao L, Gong F, Wu A, Dong G. Single-anastomosis duodeno-ileal bypass with sleeve gastrectomy (SADI-S) as a revisional surgery. *Surg Obes Relat Dis.* 2018;14(11):1686-1690; with permission.)

DS, the SADI-S appears to be an excellent procedure for superobese, diabetic patients; however, it is technically simpler and has some potential advantages. Concerns about afferent loop syndrome and gastroesophageal reflux remain, and long term, comparative studies are needed to identify the procedures best clinical application.

ECONOMIC IMPLICATIONS OF METABOLIC SURGERY FOR TYPE 2 DIABETES MELLITUS

As discussed previously, T2D is an insidious, chronic medical condition that is associated with a host of medical comorbidities, including microvascular complications (retinopathy, nephropathy, and neuropathy) as well as macrovascular disease states (myocardial infarctions, strokes, and amputations). Intense medical treatment of T2D has not demonstrated widespread effectiveness in halting the progression of the disease, and the cost of associated medical and surgical comorbidity continues to add to the financial burden on health care systems. Metabolic surgery halts the advancement of the disease process and, in 1 study, surgery was associated with a 65% decrease in microvascular and macrovascular complications related to T2D.[35] The Swedish Obesity Subjects Study (SOS), known for its extreme long-term follow-up, demonstrated a decrease in the cumulative incidence of microvascular and macrovascular complications with a mean follow-up of 17.6 years.[36] O'Brien and colleagues[37] also reported a significantly lower risk for the development of neuropathy, retinopathy, and nephropathy. In addition to decreases in the relative incidence of complications, hospitalizations, and surgeries associated with T2D, metabolic surgery has also shown a relative cost savings in medication usage. The SOS group also demonstrated decreased medication costs in the surgery group versus nonsurgical controls.[38]

In light of these savings, it should not be surprising that metabolic surgery affords an opportunity to decrease overall health care expenditures. Several studies have attempted to measure and predict the economic benefits of metabolic surgery in patients with T2D with encouraging results.[39–42] On a macroeconomic level, metabolic surgery may reduce direct costs for health care systems, but it may be more difficult to predict the economic benefits to society related to decreasing disability associated with T2D complications.

Despite the evidence of the economic benefits of metabolic surgery, it remains highly underutilized, perhaps due to preexisting bias and underappreciation of the metabolic effects of surgery.[43] As long as insurance policy barriers exist that prevent many patients from utilizing surgical treatments for T2D, the true economic benefit of metabolic surgery to society may not be fully realized.

SUMMARY

Since its inception as a procedure performed mainly for weight loss, metabolic surgery has evolved into a powerful weapon in the fight against metabolic disease. The physiologic impacts of these surgeries quickly are becoming more understood, leading to refinements in technique, bariatric program design, and utilization of pharmacologic adjuvant therapy. Patient access to surgical care for the management of T2D should be unrestricted, because most studies indicate a favorable cost/benefit ratio. Increasing the utilization of metabolic surgery as an early treatment option for T2D will slow the progression of the disease, decrease medical and surgical comorbidity, increase wellness and quality of life, and decrease overall health care expenditures over the lifetime of patients.

CLINICS CARE POINTS

- T2D incidence and prevalence are increasing in the United States.
- T2D is associated with microvascular comorbidity (nephropathy, neuropathy, and retinopathy) and macrovascular comorbidity (myocardial infarction, stroke, and limb ischemia).
- Metabolic surgery alters the levels of several key gut hormones that are responsible for maintaining energy metabolism.
- GLP-1 may play an important role in the remission of T2D after bariatric surgery.
- Metabolic surgery has variable effects on T2D, depending on the severity of disease and extend of comorbidity.
- The STAMPEDE trial demonstrated superiority of RYGB and VSG over medical management of T2D after 5 years.
- BPD may be more effective for the resolution of T2D compared with RYGB but may be associated with more potential complications.
- The SADI-S procedure is a modification of the BPD that has shown promise as a metabolic procedure.
- Several studies have indicated that metabolic surgery provides economic benefits compared with medical therapy for T2D.

DISCLOSURE

Authors have nothing to disclose.

REFERENCES

1. Centers for Disease Control and Prevention. National diabetes statistics report 2020: estimates of diabetes and its burden in the United States. Atlanta (GA). 2020.
2. Haffner SM, D'Agostino R, Saad MF, et al. Increased insulin resistance and insulin secretion in nondiabetic African-Americans and Hispanics compared with non-Hispanic whites: The insulin resistance atherosclerosis study. Diabetes 1996; 45(6):742–8.
3. Osei K, Gaillard T. Disparities in cardiovascular disease and type 2 diabetes risk factors in blacks and whites: dissecting racial paradox of metabolic syndrome. Front Endocrinol (Lausanne) 2017;8:204.
4. Centers for Disease Control. Diabetes data and statistics. 2019. Available at: https://www.cdc.gov/diabetes/data/. Accessed August 1, 2020.
5. Agardh E, Allebeck P, Hallqvist J, et al. Type 2 diabetes incidence and socio-economic position: a systematic review and meta-analysis. Int J Epidemiol 2011;40:804–18.
6. Wemrell M, Bennet L, Merlo J. Understanding the complexity of socioeconomic disparities in type 2 diabetes risk: a study of 4.3 million people in Sweden. What are the new findings? BMJ Open Diabetes Res Care 2019;7:749.
7. National Center for Health Statistics. Health of the United States -2018. Trend Tables; (2018). Available at: https://www.cdc.gov/nchs/hus/contents2018.htm# Table_042. Accessed April 9, 2020.
8. Brownlee M. Biochemistry and molecular cell biology of diabetic complications. Nature 2001;414(6865):813–20.

9. Wei M, Gaskill SP, Haffner SM, et al. Effects of diabetes and level of glycemia on all-cause and cardiovascular mortality: The San Antonio heart study. Diabetes Care 1998;21(7):1167–72.

10. Rask-Madsen C, King GL. Vascular complications of diabetes: mechanisms of injury and protective factors. Cell Metab 2013;17(1):20–33.

11. Centers for Disease Control. Chronic kidney disease in the United States. Atlanta (GA). 2019.

12. Dimitriadis GK, Randeva MS, Miras AD. Potential hormone mechanisms of bariatric surgery. Curr Obes Rep 2017;6(3):253–65.

13. Nauck MA, Meier JJ. The incretin effect in healthy individuals and those with type 2 diabetes: physiology, pathophysiology, and response to therapeutic interventions. Lancet Diabetes Endocrinol 2016;4(6):525–36.

14. Koliaki C, Liatis S, Dalamaga M, et al. The implication of gut hormones in the regulation of energy homeostasis and their role in the pathophysiology of obesity. Curr Obes Rep 2020. https://doi.org/10.1007/s13679-020-00396-9.

15. Mingrone G, Panunzi S, De Gaetano A, et al. Bariatric-metabolic surgery versus conventional medical treatment in obese patients with type 2 diabetes: 5 Year follow-up of an open-label, single-centre, randomised controlled trial. Lancet 2015;386(9997):964–73.

16. Schauer PR, Bhatt DL, Kirwan JP, et al. Bariatric surgery versus intensive medical therapy for diabetes - 5-year outcomes. N Engl J Med 2017;376(7):641–51.

17. Surgery AC, Aminian A, Brethauer SA, et al. Individualized metabolic surgery score: procedure selection based on diabetes severity. Ann Surg 2017; 266(August):2017.

18. Stacy Brethauer MA, Aminian A, Romero-Talamás H, et al. Can diabetes be surgically cured?: long-term metabolic effects of bariatric surgery in obese patients with type 2 diabetes. Ann Surg 2013. https://doi.org/10.1097/SLA. 0b013e3182a5034b.

19. Available at: https://riskcalc.org/Metabolic_Surgery_Score/. Accessed August 1, 2020.

20. Rutledge R, Kular K, Manchanda N. The mini-gastric bypass original technique. Int J Surg 2019;61:38–41.

21. Guenzi M, Arman G, Rau C, et al. Remission of type 2 diabetes after omega loop gastric bypass for morbid obesity. Surg Endosc 2015;29(9):2669–74.

22. Pories WJ, Swanson MS, MacDonald KG, et al. Who Would Have Thought It? An operation proves to Be the most effective therapy for adult-onset diabetes mellitus. Vol 222. Lippincott-Raven Publishers; 1995;222(3):339-50.

23. Nguyen NT, Blackstone RP, Morton JM, et al. The ASMBS textbook of bariatric surgery. Vol 1; Springer International Publishing, 2020. doi:10.1007/978-3-030-27021-6.

24. Gudbrandsen OA, Dankel SN, Skumsnes L, et al. Short-term effects of Vertical sleeve gastrectomy and Roux-en-Y gastric bypass on glucose homeostasis. Sci Rep 2019;9(1). https://doi.org/10.1038/s41598-019-51347-x.

25. Wallenius V, Dirinck E, Fändriks L, et al. Glycemic control after sleeve gastrectomy and roux-En-Y gastric bypass in obese subjects with type 2 diabetes mellitus. Obes Surg 2018;28(6):1461–72.

26. Hamoui N, Anthone GJ, Kaufman HS, et al. Sleeve gastrectomy in the high-risk patient. Obes Surg 2006;16(11):1445–9.

27. Peterli R, Wölnerhanssen B, Peters T, et al. Improvement in glucose metabolism after bariatric surgery: comparison of laparoscopic roux-en-Y gastric bypass and laparoscopic sleeve gastrectomy. Ann Surg 2009;250(2):234–41.

28. Guraya SY, Strate T. Surgical outcome of laparoscopic sleeve gastrectomy and Roux-en-Y gastric bypass for resolution of type 2 diabetes mellitus: a systematic review and meta-analysis. World J Gastroenterol 2020;26(8):865–76.
29. Available at: https://www.facs.org/quality-programs/mbsaqip/calculator. Accessed August 1, 2020.
30. Skogar ML, Sundbom M. Duodenal switch is superior to gastric bypass in patients with super obesity when evaluated with the bariatric analysis and reporting outcome system (BAROS). Obes Surg 2017;27(9):2308–16.
31. Sudan R, Jain-Spangler K. Tailoring bariatric surgery: sleeve gastrectomy, roux-en-Y gastric bypass and biliopancreatic diversion with duodenal switch. J Laparoendosc Adv Surg Tech A 2018;28(8):956–61.
32. Sánchez-Pernaute A, Herrera MA, Pérez-Aguirre ME, et al. Single anastomosis duodeno-ileal bypass with sleeve gastrectomy (SADI-S). One to three-year follow-up. Obes Surg 2010;20(12):1720–6.
33. Moon RC, Kirkpatrick V, Gaskins L, et al. Safety and effectiveness of single-versus double-anastomosis duodenal switch at a single institution. Surg Obes Relat Dis 2019;15(2):245–52.
34. Sánchez-Pernaute A, Rubio MÁ, Cabrerizo L, et al. Single-anastomosis duodenoileal bypass with sleeve gastrectomy (SADI-S) for obese diabetic patients. Surg Obes Relat Dis 2015;11(5):1092–8.
35. Johnson BL, Blackhurst DW, Latham BB, et al. Bariatric surgery is associated with a reduction in major macrovascular and microvascular complications in moderately to severely obese patients with type 2 diabetes mellitus. J Am Coll Surg 2013;216(4):545–58.
36. Sjöström L, Peltonen M, Jacobson P, et al. Association of bariatric surgery with long-term remission of type 2 diabetes and with microvascular and macrovascular complications. JAMA 2014;311(22):2297–304.
37. O'Brien R, Johnson E, Haneuse S, et al. Microvascular outcomes in patients with diabetes after bariatric surgery versus usual care: a matched cohort study. Ann Intern Med 2018;169(5):300–10.
38. Keating C, Neovius M, Sjöholm K, et al. Health-care costs over 15 years after bariatric surgery for patients with different baseline glucose status: results from the Swedish Obese Subjects study [published correction appears in Lancet Diabetes Endocrinol. 2015 Dec;3(12):e11]. Lancet Diabetes Endocrinol 2015; 3(11):855–65.
39. Wan B, Fang N, Guan W, et al. Cost-effectiveness of bariatric surgery versus medication therapy for obese patients with type 2 diabetes in china: a markov analysis. J Diabetes Res 2019;2019:1341963.
40. Makary MA, Clark JM, Shore AD, et al. Medication utilization and annual health care costs in patients with type 2 diabetes mellitus before and after bariatric surgery [published correction appears in Arch Surg. 2011 Jun;146(6):659. Clarke, Jeanne M [corrected to Clark, Jeanne M]]. Arch Surg 2010;145(8):726–31.
41. Borisenko O, Adam D, Funch-Jensen P, et al. Bariatric surgery can lead to net cost savings to health care systems: results from a comprehensive european decision analytic model. Obes Surg 2015;25(9):1559–68.
42. Warren JA, Ewing JA, Hale AL, et al. Cost-effectiveness of bariatric surgery: increasing the economic viability of the most effective treatment for type II diabetes mellitus. Am Surg 2015;81(8):807–11.
43. Gasoyan H, Tajeu G, Halpern MT, et al. Reasons for underutilization of bariatric surgery: the role of insurance benefit design. Surg Obes Relat Dis 2019;15(1): 146–51.

Cardiovascular Risk Reduction Following Metabolic and Bariatric Surgery

Vance L. Albaugh, MD, PhD[a], Tammy L. Kindel, MD, PhD[b],
Steven E. Nissen, MD[c], Ali Aminian, MD[d],*

KEYWORDS

- Diabetes • Obesity • Metabolic surgery • Cardiovascular risk • Bariatric surgery

KEY POINTS

- Cardiovascular disease (CVD) remains a significant burden to the health care systems globally and remains the leading cause of mortality worldwide.
- Although lifestyle, dietary, and pharmacologic interventions produce modest improvements in body weight and cardiovascular (CV) risk factors, no studies have demonstrated that nonsurgical weight loss is associated with improved CV morbidity or mortality.
- Only marked weight loss associated with metabolic surgery is likely to decrease CV and all-cause–related mortality in obese patients, reducing both macrovascular and microvascular complications.

INTRODUCTION

Cardiovascular disease (CVD) remains the greatest contributor to overall mortality among men and women in the United States and other developed countries.[1] The past 50 years have brought tremendous advances in CVD management and treatment. The increasing prevalence and incidence of obesity and diabetes, however, have partially eroded prior gains in CVD morbidity and mortality reduction.[2] This review discusses the current state of CVD risk assessment and reduction and presents an overview of recent trials that have taken aim at CVD. Emphasis is placed on metabolic or bariatric surgery (metabolic surgery) as an underutilized treatment with the potential for significant CV risk reduction and the potential mechanisms of these effects.

[a] Department of General Surgery, Bariatric and Metabolic Institute, Cleveland Clinic, Cleveland, OH, USA; [b] Department of Surgery, Medical College of Wisconsin, Milwaukee, WI, USA; [c] Department of Cardiovascular Medicine, Heart & Vascular Institute, Cleveland Clinic, Cleveland, OH, USA; [d] Department of General Surgery, Bariatric and Metabolic Institute, Cleveland Clinic, 9500 Euclid Avenue, M61, Cleveland, OH 44195, USA
* Corresponding author.
E-mail address: aminiaa@ccf.org

Surg Clin N Am 101 (2021) 269–294
https://doi.org/10.1016/j.suc.2020.12.012
0039-6109/21/© 2020 Elsevier Inc. All rights reserved.

surgical.theclinics.com

NATURE OF THE PROBLEM—CARDIOVASCULAR MORBIDITY AND MORTALITY

Improvement in life expectancy in the United States and other countries increased from the mid-twentieth century to the early 2000s. This improvement was in part driven by improved CVD treatment that included not only procedural interventions (eg, coronary artery bypass grafting and percutaneous coronary intervention for acute myocardial infarction [MI]) but also novel drug therapies for diseases associated with increased CV risk (eg, hypertension and hyperlipidemia). Age-specific mortality rates for coronary heart disease showed steep declines from the 1960s to the 1980s, with risk factor modification (eg, smoking cessation) and improved treatments for modifiable CVD risk factors (eg, hypertension and hyperlipidemia).

Despite these advances in treatment and prevention, improvements in mortality for coronary heart disease slowed in the 1990s. Unfortunately, the coronary heart disease mortality rate began to increase in the early 2000s.[3] Over the past decade, the rate of increase in life expectancy has slowed and begun to slightly decrease over the past several years.[4] This decrease in life expectancy partially is attributable to the rising prevalence of metabolic or organ system diseases, including obesity and diabetes.[4] Even though the gains in CVD morbidity and mortality reduction have not been entirely lost, this trend calls for critical reassessment and intervention.

Heart disease remains the leading cause of death in the United States[5,6] (**Fig. 1**). Of the 10 leading causes of death in the United States, obesity likely contributes directly and indirectly to each of these causes. Obesity is a chronic metabolic disease associated with many CV risk factors. Given the increasing epidemics of obesity and

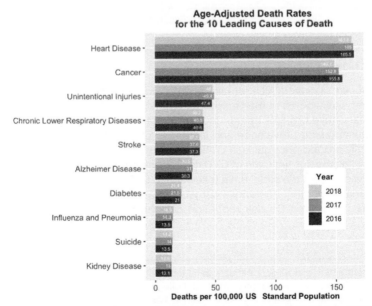

Fig. 1. Age-adjusted death rates for the leading causes of death in the United States in 2016 to 2018. The 10 leading causes of death accounted for 73.8% of all deaths in the United States in 2018. Causes of death are ranked according to number of deaths. Rankings for 2018 were the same as in 2017 and 2016. (*Data from* Murphy SL, Xu J, Kochanek KD, Arias E. Mortality in the United States, 2017. NCHS Data Brief. 2018;(328):1-8. And Xu J, Murphy SL, Kockanek KD, Arias E. Mortality in the United States, 2018. NCHS Data Brief. 2020;(355):1-8.)

diabetes and their effects on CV risk, treatment guidelines currently recommend consideration of metabolic surgery in selected patients for treatment of diabetes[7] and CV risk reduction.[8] Collectively, metabolic surgery is defined as procedures that influence metabolism by inducing weight loss and altering gastrointestinal physiology.

CARDIOVASCULAR RISK PREDICTION AND REDUCTION

Much of the progress regarding treatment of CVD over the past several decades[9] has come from an understanding of CVD pathophysiology and its associated risk factors. Well-designed, longitudinal, cohort studies (eg, the Framingham Heart Study) have identified important CVD risk factors and shaped current approaches to CVD risk reduction (Table 1). Most CVD risk factors are modifiable through lifestyle changes, including dietary habits, physical activity, and smoking cessation.[10,11] Others are modifiable through pharmacologic strategies, which have profoundly changed the treatment paradigms for hypertension,[12] hypercholesterolemia,[13] and diabetes.

In addition to the Framingham Study, other cohort studies (see Table 1) have helped define methods for calculation of primary CVD risk (eg, United Kingdom Prospective Diabetes Study [UKPDS] and European Systemic Coronary Risk Evaluation [SCORE] algorithm). These models are helpful for primary risk prediction and prevention. The progression and refinement of risk models readily can be seen, because previous variables have been removed (eg, left ventricular hypertrophy) and replaced with better documented variables to determine disease risk (ie, systolic blood pressure). Newer risk models use precise markers of glycemic control (ie, hemoglobin [Hgb]A_{1c}) instead of mere presence or absence of diabetes, and some include measures of obesity (eg, body mass index) for risk stratification, underscoring the importance of diabetes and obesity in predicting CVD risk.

High-quality evidence has demonstrated that diabetes confers a 2-fold or greater increase in risk of CVD morbidity and mortality.[14,15] This markedly increased risk makes identifying effective treatments of diabetes and obesity of high importance for targeting CV risk reduction. Several newer risk models have included assessment of lifetime risk and 1 (Individualized Diabetes Complications [IDC] Risk Score[16]) assesses the potential for reduction after treatment with metabolic surgery. The IDC risk score (see Table 1) uses predictive models and individual patient characteristics to give estimates for all-cause mortality as well as coronary artery disease (CAD), cerebrovascular attack (CVA), and diabetic nephropathy. The IDC risk score provides personalized 10-year risk predictions for individual patients with and without metabolic surgery. This individualized approach allows each patient and his/her physicians to see their potential risks and benefits of metabolic surgery compared with usual care.

RANDOMIZED TRIALS FOR OBESITY AND DIABETES EXAMINING CARDIOVASCULAR MORBIDITY AND MORTALITY

Medical or lifestyle therapies for obesity have not shown consistent benefits in randomized clinical trials (Table 2). Of these trials, the largest and longest randomized trial examining nonsurgical weight loss was the Look AHEAD: Action for Health in Diabetes study.[17] When Look AHEAD began recruiting, obesity was recognized as an important CVD risk factor, but few studies had explored interventions to decrease CVD risk by weight loss achieved through lifestyle interventions. Look AHEAD demonstrated that an intensive lifestyle intervention (eg, decreased caloric intake, increased physical activity) compared with usual care was associated with a modest but

Table 1
Representative models for cardiovascular risk assessment

Model	Year	Variables Included	Cardiovascular Disease Estimate	Notes
Framingham[117]	1976	Age, sex, obesity, smoking status, diabetes, HLD, HTN, EKG-LVH, inactivity	8-y risk of CHD onset	Only applicable to persons without previous CVD history
Framingham update[118,119]	1991, 1998	Age, sex, total cholesterol, HDL, SBP, smoking status, diabetes, EKG-LVH	10-y CHD onset	Only applicable to persons without previous CVD history
UKPDS Risk Engine	2001	Age, sex, race, smoking status, SBP, TC, HDL, HbA$_{1c}$ time since diabetes diagnosis	10-y risk of nonfatal/fatal CAD/CVA	Model specific to patients with diabetes
SCORE[120]	2003	Age, sex, TC, SBP, smoking status	10-y fatal CV event	Age used as measure of exposure time instead of simple risk
Reynolds Risk Score[121]	2007	Age, sex, smoking status, TC, HDL, hsCRP, HgbA$_{1c}$ (if diabetes), parental history of MI at <60 y old	10-y CVD risk	Model altered/optimized for women
QRISK1/QRISK2[122,123]	2007, 2008	Age, sex, ethnicity, body mass index, SBP, TC:HDL, Townsend score, smoking status, family history of (CAD <60 y, type 2 diabetes mellitus, treated HTN, rheumatoid arthritis, atrial fibrillation, chronic kidney disease)	10-y CVD risk	Predicts CVD onset (ie, CAD, CVA, TIA)
QRISK-Lifetime[124]	2010	Age, sex, ethnicity, body mass index, SBP, TC:HDL, Townsend score, smoking status, family history of (CAD <60 y, type 2 diabetes mellitus, treated HTN,	Lifetime risk of CVD	Model for early prediction and potential intervention

Model	Year	Variables	Risk estimate	Description
		rheumatoid arthritis, atrial fibrillation, chronic and/or kidney disease)		
Pooled cohort equation[125,126]	2017	Age, sex, race, TC, LDL, HDL, treatment with statin, SBP, HTN treatment, history of diabetes, smoking status, aspirin therapy	10-y risk of atherosclerotic CVD	Predicts CVD onset
LIFE-CVD[127]	2019	Age, sex, race, parental history of MI, BMI, non-HDL, SBP, smoking status, diabetes mellitus	10-y risks	Estimates 10-y absolute CVD risk reduction, lifetime risk reduction, and gain in CVD-free life expectancy
IDC risk score[16]	2020	Age, sex, race, BMI, smoking status, HTN, HLD, COPD, CHF, CHD, CVA, diabetic neuropathy, PAD, nephropathy, dialysis, SBP, DBP, HgbA₁c creatinine, triglycerides, insulin use, diabetes medications, lipid-lowering medications, antihypertensives, aspirin therapy, warfarin therapy	10-y risk for developing diabetes complications with and without metabolic surgery	Machine learning approach to estimate 10-y risk of all-cause mortality, CAD, CVA, and diabetic nephropathy

Abbreviations: BMI, body mass index; CHD, coronary heart disease; CHF, congestive heart failure; COPD, chronic obstructive pulmonary disease; DPB, diastolic blood pressure; EKG-LVH, electrocardiogram with evidence of left ventricular hypertrophy; HLD, hyperlipidemia; hsCRP, high-sensitivity C-reactive protein; HTN, hypertension; PAD, peripheral arterial disease; SBP, systolic blood pressure; TC, total cholesterol.
Data from Refs.[16,117–127]

Table 2
Notable nonsurgical trials examining morbidity and mortality in patients with obesity

Trial	Study Type	Patient Population	Primary Endpoint	Follow-up	Intervention(s)	Sample Size (Intervention vs Control)	Findings
Look AHEAD[17]	RCT	Overweight or obese patients with diabetes	CV morbidity and mortality	9.6 Years	Intensive lifestyle intervention vs standard diabetes treatment	2570 vs 2575	No difference in primary endpoint Terminated early due to futility
SCOUT trial[128]	RCT	Overweight or obese patients with CAD, diabetes, or CAD and diabetes	Composite (MI, CVA, resuscitation after cardiac arrest, CV mortality)	3.4 Years	Sibutramine vs placebo	4906 vs 4898	Increased risk (16%) of nonfatal MI, post hoc evaluation showed benefit of modest weight loss[129]
CAMELLIA-TIMI 61[130]	RCT	Overweight or obese patients with CAD or multiple CAD risk factors	Composite (MI, CVA, or CV mortality)	3.3 y	Lorcaserin vs placebo	5135 vs 5083	No difference in primary endpoint despite weight loss
The Light Study[131]	RCT	Overweight or obese patients with increased CV risk	Composite (MI, CVA, or CV mortality)	2.3 y	Naltrexone-bupropion vs placebo	4456 vs 4454	Terminated early, inconclusive

Abbreviations: IGT, impaired glucose tolerance; NGT, normal glucose tolerance; RCT, randomized clinical trial.
Data from Refs.[17,128,130,131]

significant decrease in total body weight (6% vs 3.5% at the end of the trial). This weight loss was accompanied by improved blood pressure, diabetes control (HgbA$_{1c}$), and cholesterol.[18] Despite the weight loss and beneficial improvements in biomarkers, however, the trial was stopped early due to futility (median follow-up, 9.6 years) and showed no difference in major CV events between the treatment groups. Disappointingly, the modest weight loss observed did not translate to any improvement in CV mortality. In post hoc analysis, those with significant weight loss (>10%) had a 20% lower risk of the primary outcome (composite of death from CV causes, nonfatal acute MI, nonfatal stroke, and angina admission) and 21% lower risk of secondary outcomes (primary outcomes as well as CVD-related interventions, congestive heart failure hospitalizations, peripheral vascular disease, and total mortality).[19] This highlights the importance of meaningful and substantial weight loss in obese individuals to produce a CVD benefit.

Aside from trials examining therapies for obesity and CVD outcomes, several trials focused on diabetes management have shaped current practice but failed to show any benefits on macrovascular outcomes (cardiovascular [CV] morbidity and mortality). The Diabetes Control and Complications Trial demonstrated that intensive glucose control slowed progression of microvascular complications (eg, retinopathy and nephropathy) in patients with type 1 diabetes mellitus.[20] The UKPDS[21] extended these findings and confirmed the safety of intensive glucose control in type 2 diabetes mellitus,[22] although CV risk reduction was observed only with extended (>10 years) treatment.[23] Additional follow-up studies have examined intensive glycemic control to improved CV morbidity and mortality, but these trials (eg, Action to Control Cardiovascular Risk in Diabetes [ACCORD],[24] Action in Diabetes and Vascular Disease: Preterax and Diamicron MR Controlled Evaluation,[25] and Veterans Affairs Diabetes Trial[26]) have failed to show any differences in CVD mortality despite improving glycemic control. The ACCORD trial showed increased mortality with intensive diabetes intervention (ie, lower targets for HbA$_{1c}$). Recently, novel agents in the newest classes of diabetes treatments (ie, glucagon-like peptide 1 [GLP-1] receptor analogs and sodium-glucose transporter-2 inhibitors) have shown CVD benefits in high-risk patients[27–32] in high-quality randomized, placebo-controlled trials (**Table 3**).

POTENTIAL CARDIOVASCULAR DISEASE RISK REDUCTION FOLLOWING METABOLIC SURGERY
Mortality Reduction and Metabolic Surgery

High-quality randomized controlled trials have been performed for metabolic surgery in management of poorly controlled diabetes, but no randomized surgical trials exist with CVD endpoints. Observational studies examining the effects of metabolic surgery suggest improved CVD outcomes (**Table 4**). The Swedish Obese Subjects (SOS) study, a prospective, matched cohort study, demonstrated that metabolic surgery compared with conventional treatment in obese subjects improved surrogate markers, including new-onset diabetes, hypertriglyceridemia, low high-density lipoprotein (HDL) cholesterol, and hypertension.[33] Consistent with these benefits, macrovascular complications (ie, MI, CVA, and lower extremity amputation) were reduced 32% with surgery[34] and mortality was decreased 53%.[35] A frequently cited caveat to the SOS study is that the surgery cohort includes vertical banded gastroplasty (66%) and adjustable gastric banding (18%), operations that rarely are performed in contemporary metabolic surgery. Most investigators would argue, however, that the operations used currently (eg, Roux-en-Y gastric bypass and sleeve gastrectomy) likely are more effective than the operations performed in the SOS study.

Table 3
Notable nonsurgical trials examining morbidity and mortality in patients with diabetes

Trial	Study Type	Patient Population	Primary Endpoint	Follow-up	Intervention(s)	Sample Size (Intervention vs Control)	Findings
Da Qing Diabetes Prevention Study[132]	RCT	Patients with IGT	CV mortality, all-cause mortality, diabetes incidence	23 y	Lifestyle intervention vs standard care	430 vs 138	CV mortality (41% decrease), all-cause mortality (29% decrease), diabetes incidence (45% decrease)
PREDIMED study[11]	RCT	Patients with high risk for CV events and/or diabetes	Composite (MI, CVA, or CV mortality)	4.8 y median	Dietary interventions (Mediterranean with EVOO vs Mediterranean with nuts vs control/low-fat diet)	2543 vs 2454 vs 2450	Stopped prematurely EVOO vs control (2.1% decrease) Nuts vs control (1.7% decrease)
Malmö study[133]	Nonrandomized	Patients with NGT and IGT	All-cause mortality	12 y	Diet and exercise	6389 NGT vs 288 IGT-intervention vs 135 IGT vs 144 diabetes	IGT patients with intervention had similar mortality to NGT patients
LEADER trial[27]	RCT	Patients with high risk for CV events and diabetes	Composite (MI, CVA, or CV mortality)	3.8 y	GLP-1 receptor agonist vs placebo	4668 vs 4672	Primary endpoint lower liraglutide vs placebo (13% decrease)
PROactive 10 trial[134]	RCT	Patients with high risk for CV events and diabetes	Composite (MI, CVA, or CV mortality)	2.9 y	Thiazolidinedione vs placebo	2605 vs 2633	Primary endpoint lower pioglitazone vs placebo (18% decrease)

Trial	Type	Population	Primary Endpoint	Duration	Intervention	N	Results
EMPA-REG OUTCOME trial[28]	RCT	Patients with high risk for CV events and diabetes	Composite (MI, CVA, or CV Mortality)	3.1 y	SGLT2 inhibitor vs placebo	4687 vs 2333	Primary endpoint lower empagliflozin vs placebo (13% decrease)
SUSTAIN-6 trial[135]	RCT	Patients with high risk for CV events and diabetes	Composite (MI, CVA, or CV mortality)	2.1 y	GLP-1 receptor agonist vs placebo	1648 vs 1649	No difference in primary endpoint
DAPA-HF trial[29]	RCT	Patients with NYHA class II, III, or IV CHF with or without diabetes	Composite (worsening CHF or CV mortality)	1.5 y	SGLT2 inhibitor vs placebo	2373 vs 2371	Primary endpoint lower dapagliflozin vs placebo (26% decrease) Improvements regardless of diabetes status
CANVAS Program[30]	Combined data from 2 RCTs	Patients with high risk for CV events and diabetes	Composite (MI, CVA, or CV mortality)	3.6 y	SGLT2 inhibitor vs placebo	5795 vs 4347	Primary endpoint lower canagliflozin vs placebo (14% decrease)
CREDENCE trial[31]	RCT	Patients with albuminuric CKD and diabetes	Composite (ESRD, doubling of creatinine, or CV mortality)	2.6 y	SGLT2 inhibitor vs placebo	2202 vs 2199	Terminated early Primary endpoint lower canagliflozin vs placebo (20% decrease)
REWIND trial[32]	RCT	Patients with high risk for CV events and diabetes	Composite (MI, CVA, or CV mortality)	5.4 y	GLP-1 receptor agonist vs placebo	4949 vs 4952	Primary endpoint lower dulaglutide vs placebo (12% decrease)
PIONEER 6 trial[136]	Noninferiority RCT	Patients with high risk for CV events, CKD, or CV risk	Composite (MI, CVA, or CV mortality)	1.3 y	GLP-1 receptor agonist vs Placebo	1591 vs 1592	Semaglutide not inferior compared with placebo

Abbreviations: CHF, congestive heart failure; CKD, chronic kidney disease; EVOO, extravirgin olive oil; IGT, impaired glucose tolerance; NGT, normal glucose tolerance; NYHA, New York Heart Association; RCT, randomized clinical trial; SGLT2, sodium glucose transporter 2.
Data from Refs.[11,27–32,132–136]

Table 4
Surgical studies examining mortality in patients undergoing metabolic surgery

N	Year	Study Type	First Author	Journal	Sample Size (Surgery vs Control)	Mortality Relative Risk Reduction (%)
1	1997	Retrospective cohort	MacDonald KG	J Gastro Surg[137]	154 vs 78	68
2	2004	Retrospective cohort	Christou NV	Ann Surg[138]	1035 vs 5746	89
3	2004	Retrospective cohort	Flum DR	J Am Coll Surg[139]	3328 vs 66,109	33
4	2007	Retrospective cohort	Adams TD	N Engl J Med[37]	7925 vs 7925	40
5	2007	Retrospective cohort	Busetto L	Surg Obes Relat Dis[140]	821 vs 821	60
6	2007	Retrospective cohort	Peeters A	Ann Surg[141]	966 vs 2119	72
7	2007	Prospective observational	Sjöström L	N Engl J Med[142]	2010 vs 2037	29
8	2007	Retrospective cohort	Sowemimo OA	Surg Obes Relat Dis[143]	908 vs 112	82
9	2008	Retrospective cohort	Perry CD	Ann Surg[144]	11,903 vs 11,903	50
10	2010	Retrospective cohort	Marsk R	Br J Surg[145]	1216 vs 5327	30
11	2011	Retrospective cohort	Maciejewski MK[a]	JAMA[146]	850 vs 41,244	36
12	2012	Retrospective cohort	Johnson RJ	Am Surg[147]	349 vs 903	40
13	2013	Retrospective cohort	Scott JD	Surg Obes Relat Dis[148]	4747 vs 3066/1,327[a]	19–55
14	2015	Retrospective cohort	Arterburn DE[b]	JAMA[149]	2500 vs 7462	53
15	2015	Prospective observational	Eliasson B	Lancet Diab Endo[150]	6132 vs 6132	58
16	2015	Retrospective cohort	Guidry CA	Am J Surg[151]	430 vs 5232	52
17	2016	Retrospective cohort	Davidson LE	JAMA Surg[152]	7925 vs 7925	40
18	2016	Retrospective cohort	Flanagan E	Am Surg[153]	363 vs 100	68
19	2017	Retrospective cohort	Lent MR	Diabetes Care[154]	3242 vs 2428	56
20	2018	Retrospective cohort	Pontiroli AE	Cardiovasc Diabetol[155]	385 vs 681	48/54
21	2018	Retrospective cohort	Reges O	JAMA[156]	8385 vs 25,155	50
22	2018	Retrospective cohort	Fisher DP	JAMA[36]	5301 vs 14,934	67
23	2019	Retrospective cohort	Moussa OM	Ann Surg[157]	8655 vs 178,406[#]	51

24	2019	Retrospective cohort	Kauppila JH	Gastroenterology[158]	49,977 vs 494,842	37
25	2019	Retrospective cohort	Ceriani V	Int J Obes[159]	472 vs 1405	36
26	2019	Retrospective cohort	Aminian A	JAMA[38]	2287 vs 11,435	41
27	2020	Retrospective cohort	Singh P	Br J Surg[160]	5170 vs 9995	30
28	2020	Retrospective cohort	Moussa O	Eur Heart J[161]	3701 vs 3701	75
29	2020	Retrospective cohort	Liakopoulos V	Diabetes Care[162]	5321 vs 5321	42
30	2020	Retrospective cohort	Sheetz KH	JAMA Surg[163]	1597 vs 4750	31
31	2020	Retrospective cohort	Doumouras AG	Ann Intern Med[164]	13,679 vs 13,679	32
32	2020	Retrospective cohort	Stenberg E	PLoS Med[165]	11,863 vs 26,199	16

[a] Not significant reduction after propensity matching.
[b] The follow-up study to Maciejewski and colleagues[146] reported significant mortality reduction after metabolic surgery.[149]
Data from Refs.[36–38,137–167]

Even though the SOS study has its drawbacks, the findings are similar to other large, retrospective studies[36,37] examining the effects of metabolic surgery on major CV outcomes. In a cohort of Roux-en-Y gastric bypass patients, Adams and colleagues[37] showed that surgery was associated with a 40% decreased all-cause mortality compared with a control group over a 7-year average follow-up that was matched for age, sex, and body mass index. In another well-controlled observational study in patients with type 2 diabetes mellitus, Fisher and colleagues[36] demonstrated that metabolic surgery was associated with a significant reduction in the incidence of macrovascular events (40% decrease; hazard ratio [HR] 0.60 [95% CI, 0.42–0.86]) and a lower incidence of CAD (36% decrease; HR 0.64 [95% CI, 0.42–0.99]) after 5 years. The study also showed a 67% reduction in all-cause mortality at 5 years (HR 0.33 [95% CI, 0.21–0.52]). Most recently, Aminian and colleagues[38] demonstrated in a large cohort study of patients with obesity and diabetes that all-cause mortality was decreased significantly (41%; HR 0.59 [95% CI, 0.48–0.72]) with metabolic surgery compared with a nonsurgical control group after 8 years. Metabolic surgery was associated with a significant benefit for the primary outcome (**Fig. 2**A), which was a composite of major CV endpoints (ie, all-cause mortality, coronary artery events, cerebrovascular events, heart failure, nephropathy, and atrial fibrillation). In this same study, metabolic surgery reduced the secondary endpoint, a composite of MI, CVA, and all-cause mortality (**Fig. 2**B). Despite a lack of prospective, randomized clinical trials, these observational studies strongly suggest a CV mortality benefit from metabolic surgery.

Morbidity Reduction and Metabolic Surgery

Obesity and type 2 diabetes mellitus are associated with a broad risk that includes not only macrovascular complications (eg, MI, CVA, and mortality), but also additional CV outcomes (**Fig. 3**). Similar to reductions in all-cause mortality, evidence suggests that

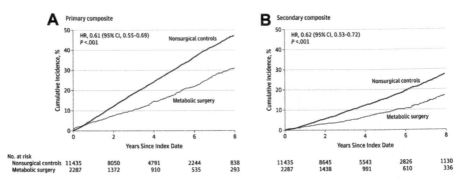

Fig. 2. Eight-year cumulative incidence (Kaplan-Meier) for 2 composite endpoints. (*A*) The primary endpoint was the incidence of extended major adverse CV events (MACE: composite of 6 outcomes), defined as first occurrence of coronary artery events, cerebrovascular events, heart failure, atrial fibrillation, nephropathy, and all-cause mortality, recording the first occurrence after the index date as the event date. (*B*) The secondary composite end points included 3-component MACE (all-cause mortality, MI, and ischemic stroke), recording the first occurrence after the index date as the event date. For both end points, the median observation time was 4.0 years (interquartile range [IQR], 2.1 to 6.1) for nonsurgical patients and 3.3 years (IQR, 1.2–6.3) for surgical patients. HR indicates HR. Figure redrawn from Aminian and colleagues. (*Adapted from* Aminian A, Zajichek A, Arterburn DE, et al. Association of metabolic surgery with major adverse cardiovascular outcomes in patients with type 2 diabetes and obesity. JAMA. 2019;322(13):1271-12; with permission.)

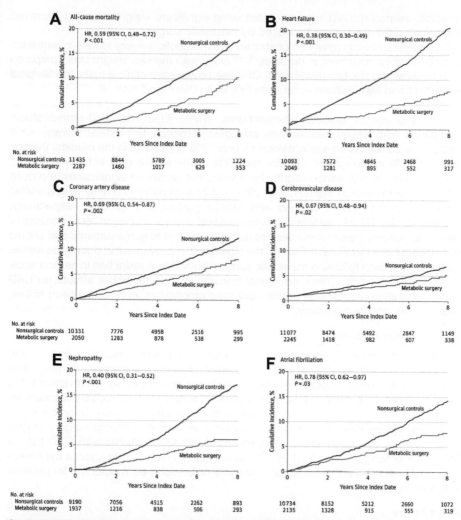

Fig. 3. Eight-year cumulative incidence estimates (Kaplan-Meier) for 6 individual endpoints. For each 5 individual outcomes (except all-cause mortality), any patient with a history of that outcomes prior to the index date was eliminated from risk assessment only for that outcome. For each 5 individual outcomes (except all-cause mortality), any patient with a history of that outcome prior to the index date was eliminated from risk assessment only for that outcome. (*A*) For all-cause mortality, median observation time was 4.0 years (IQR, 2.1 to 6.1) in the nonsurgical group and 3.3 years (IQR, 1.2–6.3) in the surgical group; (*B*) for heart failure, 4.1 years (IQR, 2.2–6.2) and 3.3 years (IQR, 1.1–6.4); (*C*) for CAD, 4.0 years (IQR, 2.1–6.1) and 3.3 years (IQR, 1.1–6.4); (*D*) for nephropathy, 4.1 years (IQR, 2.2–6.2) and 3.3 years (IQR, 1.1–6.3); (*E*) for cerebrovascular disease and (*F*) atrial fibrillation, 4.0 years (IQR, 2.1–6.1) and 3.3 years (IQR, 1.1–6.3). Figure redrawn from Aminian and colleagues. (*Adapted from* Aminian A, Zajichek A, Arterburn DE, et al. Association of metabolic surgery with major adverse cardiovascular outcomes in patients with type 2 diabetes and obesity. JAMA. 2019;322(13):1271-12; with permission.)

morbidity related to CVD is reduced following significant weight loss and improved cardiometabolic risk factors produced by metabolic surgery.

Several clinical trials have demonstrated that metabolic surgery results in remission or significant improvement in diabetes[39–42] along with marked weight loss compared with medical and lifestyle treatments. Of these prospective clinical trials, the Surgical Treatment and Medications Potentially Eradicate Diabetes Efficiently (STAMPEDE[39]) trial examined diabetes remission as the primary endpoint (ie, HgbA$_{1c}$ <6% with or without the use of diabetes medications). STAMPEDE was a 3-armed study, comparing both sleeve gastrectomy and gastric bypass to medical therapy. At 1 year, diabetes remission was obtained by only 12% of patients in the medical therapy arm but 42% in the gastric bypass and 37% in the sleeve gastrectomy groups.[43] These improvements waned slightly by 5 years but remained significantly improved compared with medical therapy, with 29% and 23% of patients maintaining diabetes remission in the gastric bypass and sleeve gastrectomy groups, respectively, compared with 5% of patients receiving medical therapy.[39] Regardless, benefits of metabolic surgery persist even despite diabetes relapse in some patients and should not be considered a failure.[44] Overall, the significant improvement in obesity as well as diabetes remission following metabolic surgery likely drives reduction in several additional CVD outcomes. These additional benefits include favorable effects on CAD events, including reduction in revascularization procedures, congestive heart failure, dysrhythmia, and nephropathy.

Coronary Artery Disease

Observational evidence suggests an association between metabolic surgery and reduction in CAD events in obese patients following metabolic surgery (see **Fig. 3**C). Atherogenic lipoprotein levels, which are linked closely to atherosclerotic heart disease are improved following metabolic surgery.[45,46] Surrogate markers for coronary atherosclerosis, such as coronary calcium scores, are more favorable in patients undergoing metabolic surgery.[47] Patients undergoing bariatric surgery require fewer coronary revascularization procedures.[48] Although patients with CAD have a higher risk of surgical complications,[49] this risk should be weighed against the potential benefits associated with metabolic surgery on the long-term outcome for patients with existing CAD.

Heart Failure

Obesity is associated with cardiac dysfunction, even in the absence of diabetes, and many bariatric patients have significantly impaired diastolic function. Furthermore, some patients with severe obesity can develop heart failure with reduced ejection fraction—obesity cardiomyopathy.[50] Observational studies demonstrate a reduction in incidence of heart failure[38] following metabolic surgery, consistent with previous studies demonstrated that marked weight loss is associated with a reduced incidence of heart failure.[51–53] Shimada and colleagues[54] found metabolic surgery reduced postoperative emergency department and heart failure –related hospitalization in 524 patients with preoperative heart failure. For patients with diastolic dysfunction, metabolic surgery improves heart failure–related symptoms, reverses cardiac remodeling, and improves diastolic relaxation.[55] Metabolic surgery also is associated with improved systolic function,[56–58] which may be secondary to structural and/or positive metabolic changes within the myocardium.[59–61] Regardless of the mechanism, concurrent improvement in other CVD risk factors secondary to marked weight loss (ie, hypertension and glycemic control) also likely contribute to the reported improvements in cardiac function/outcomes.[62]

Dysrhythmia

Atrial fibrillation is highly prevalent in patients with diabetes and obesity and confers an increased risk of morbidity and mortality.[63–65] A recent meta-analysis showed that atrial fibrillation was associated with increased risk for several forms of CV morbidity and all-cause mortality (46% increase).[52] The strongest association was observed between atrial fibrillation and heart failure, with a nearly 5-fold increase in risk.[63] Weight loss prior to ablation procedures is associated with significantly decreased rates of atrial fibrillation recurrence.[66,67] Because body weight is associated strongly with failure of ablation procedures, metabolic surgery in obese patients with atrial fibrillation has been proposed to improve the potential therapeutic efficacy of ablation.[68,69]

Nonsurgical studies have examined whether weight loss with lifestyle intervention can reduce risk of developing atrial fibrillation. Despite modest weight loss in Look AHEAD, there was no risk reduction for developing atrial fibrillation,[70] and a meta-analysis of other studies reporting at least 5% nonsurgical weight loss also showed no benefit.[71] In surgical studies examining atrial fibrillation, the SOS cohort showed that individuals post–metabolic surgery had a lower of incidence for atrial fibrillation,[72] consistent with the concept that more robust weight loss is required to show risk reduction. Other observational studies have demonstrated 22% relative risk reduction after surgery compared with nonsurgical controls,[38] which was replicated in a recent small, prospective trial.[73]

Nephropathy

Nephropathy is another source of significant morbidity and mortality that may be favorably influenced by metabolic surgery. In patients with nephropathy secondary to diabetic kidney disease, improved glycemic control following surgery appears to slow the progression of diabetic kidney disease. Approximately half of patients also exhibit resolution of albuminuria and show improved estimated glomerular filtration rate.[74,75] This improvement in nephropathy recently has been demonstrated in a prospective, randomized trial comparing metabolic surgery with best medical therapy.[76] In that study, surgical complications were not increased despite the higher preoperative risk of these patients prior to metabolic surgery.

In addition to improved insulin sensitivity and glycemic and blood pressure control postoperatively, obesity intrinsically predisposes to obesity-related glomerulopathy that also may be alleviated by the marked weight loss following metabolic surgery.[77] The beneficial effects of metabolic surgery on renal function in patients with obesity and diabetes have been reproduced by other retrospective matched cohorts[78] as well as in the SOS study.[79]

WHAT DRIVES CARDIOVASCULAR RISK REDUCTION FOLLOWING METABOLIC SURGERY?

Although the potential benefits of metabolic surgery on CV morbidity and mortality have not yet been tested directly in randomized clinical trials, observational evidence suggests that surgery potentially is superior to nonsurgical management of obesity and diabetes. These findings likely reflect the robust sustained weight loss produced by metabolic surgery compared with other therapies for obesity.

The large effects of surgery on weight loss leads to the prevailing hypothesis that much of the benefit of metabolic surgery is secondary to weight reduction. Many diseases are known to improve with weight loss and these diseases typically improve significantly with metabolic surgery (eg, diabetes, hypertension, and dyslipidemia). Weight loss also is associated with improved whole-body insulin sensitivity[80] that improves glucose tolerance and glycemic control, which subsequently leads to improved lipid trafficking, dyslipidemia, and decreased systemic inflammation.[81–83] Long-term weight loss coupled with improved insulin sensitivity also likely acts to improve hepatic steatosis and nonalcoholic fatty liver disease.

Although obesity-associated diseases are significantly improved following marked weight loss, there is considerable evidence that some of the benefits observed with metabolic surgery are independent of weight loss.[84–86] Effects on diabetes status can occur rapidly on obese patients following metabolic surgery prior to major weight loss. These effects are observed within days to weeks of surgery, with early improvement in hepatic insulin sensitivity preceding changes in skeletal muscle.[87] In addition to rapid changes in insulin sensitivity, there are effects on appetite and food preference/taste/smell,[88–92] intestinal hormones[93,94] and bile acid metabolism and signaling.[95,96] Some of these changes may be secondary to altered nutrient transport, either by increased delivery of undigested food to the small intestine and/or by a lack of ability to transport fuels from the intestinal lumen.[97] These weight-independent changes also likely induce other changes within the intestine, including intestinal adaptation/remodeling[98–100] and beneficial changes in the gut microbiome.[96,101] There are more recently described changes in cholesterol metabolism[102–105] that also may contribute to favorable effects. Additional evidence for weight loss-independent effects is observed in patients who regain a significant amount of weight following metabolic surgery, but in whom the metabolic benefits persist despite increased body weight.[106]

A review of all these changes is beyond the scope of this review; however, the historical attribution of malabsorption as the mechanism of benefit after metabolic surgery largely has been disproved as the mediator of the observed weight loss and metabolic improvements. Even though there is a slight increase in fat malabsorption following some procedures (eg, duodenal switch more than Roux-en-Y gastric bypass), there is good evidence that malabsorption is not driving the weight loss.[107–110] Similarly, mechanical restriction has been disproved as well by several studies,[111–113] which clearly implicates hormonal and other metabolic factors as responsible for weight loss and metabolic improvements. Several excellent reviews have summarized the likely mechanisms of benefit for metabolic surgery on weight loss and metabolism.[114–116]

KNOWLEDGE GAPS AND FUTURE DIRECTIONS

The potential benefits of metabolic surgery on CV risk reduction are a topic of particular interest with numerous unanswered questions. Despite an increasing amount of rigorous basic science and clinical research on the improvements following metabolic surgery, the exact mechanisms leading to decreased reduction in CVD events are not understood completely. Similarly, whether or not one operation may be superior to another for CVD risk reduction anf whether procedure selection for individual patients should vary to maximize individual patient benefit need to be explored. Certainly, many of the metabolic benefits observed in these patients are at least in part driven by the marked weight loss postoperatively. There is uncertainty, however, whether increased CV risk reduction continues to parallel increased weight loss or whether a minimum or maximum weight loss threshold exists for CVD risk reduction.

Although these are fruitful areas for further research, a large knowledge gap is the absence of a randomized clinical trial designed to compare the effects on CV outcomes between metabolic surgery and the current best medical therapy. Nonsurgical studies have explored pharmacologic and lifestyle therapies to reduce CV risk with minimal or no CV benefit despite improvements in several anthropometric and laboratory parameters. Although retrospective and prospective observational studies have demonstrated improved CV outcomes with metabolic surgery, only a randomized clinical trial can unequivocally demonstrate the effectiveness of metabolic surgery. Until such a trial is conducted, skeptics will continue to doubt the effectiveness of metabolic surgery and patients may be denied access to this potentially life-saving treatment with substantial CV risk reduction.

SUMMARY

The pandemics of obesity and diabetes are continuing to worsen and are slowly degrading the progress made in the past century on CV morbidity and mortality. The best available data suggest that metabolic surgery may be the ideal treatment of obesity and associated type 2 diabetes mellitus. Randomized trials to sufficiently answer this question are needed, because previous nonsurgical trials have demonstrated that modest weight loss with lifestyle and/or pharmacologic approaches does not improve major CVD outcomes. Even though these benefits have not been documented in randomized, clinical trials, currently available evidence, and expert consensus suggest that metabolic surgery is a viable and effective therapy with CVD benefits that likely will be confirmed in future prospective clinical trials.

DISCLOSURE

Dr. Nissen reported receiving grants from Abbvie, AstraZeneca, Amgen, Eli Lilly, Esperion, Medtronic, MyoKardia, Novartis, Pfizer, and Silence Therapeutics. Dr. Aminian reported receiving grant from Medtronic. No other disclosures were reported.

REFERENCES

1. Heron M. Deaths: leading causes for 2017. Natl Vital Stat Rep 2019;68(6):1–77.
2. Preston SH, Vierboom YC, Stokes A. The role of obesity in exceptionally slow US mortality improvement. Proc Natl Acad Sci 2018;115(5):957–61.
3. Ford ES, Capewell S. Coronary heart disease mortality among young adults in the u.s. from 1980 through 2002 concealed leveling of mortality rates. J Am Coll Cardiol 2007;50(22):2128–32.
4. Woolf SH, Schoomaker H. Life Expectancy and Mortality Rates in the United States, 1959-2017. Jama 2019;322(20):1996–2016.
5. Murphy SL, Xu J, Kochanek KD, et al. Mortality in the United States, 2017. Nchs Data Brief 2018;(328):1–8.
6. Xu J, Murphy SL, Kockanek KD, et al. Mortality in the United States, 2018. Nchs Data Brief 2020;(355):1–8.
7. Rubino F, Nathan DM, Eckel RH, et al. Metabolic surgery in the treatment algorithm for type 2 diabetes: a joint statement by international diabetes organizations. Diabetes care 2016;39(6):861–77.
8. Jensen MD, Ryan DH, Apovian CM, et al. 2013 AHA/ACC/TOS guideline for the management of overweight and obesity in adults: a report of the American College of Cardiology/American Heart Association Task Force on Practice Guidelines and The Obesity Society. J Am Coll Cardiol 2013;63(25 Pt B):2985–3023.
9. Nabel EG, Braunwald E. A tale of coronary artery disease and myocardial infarction. N Engl J Med 2012;366(1):54–63.
10. Jonas MA, Oates JA, Ockene JK, et al. Statement on smoking and cardiovascular disease for health care professionals. Am Heart Assoc Circ 1992;86(5):1664–9.

11. Estruch R, Ros E, Salas-Salvadó J, et al. Primary Prevention of Cardiovascular Disease with a Mediterranean Diet Supplemented with Extra-Virgin Olive Oil or Nuts. N Engl J Med 2018;378(25):e34.

12. Collaboration PS. Age-specific relevance of usual blood pressure to vascular mortality: a meta-analysis of individual data for one million adults in 61 prospective studies. Lancet 2002;360(9349):1903–13.

13. Hebert PR, Gaziano JM, Chan KS, et al. Cholesterol Lowering With Statin Drugs, Risk of Stroke, and Total Mortality: An Overview of Randomized Trials. Jama 1997;278(4):313.

14. Collaboration ERF, Angelantonio ED, Kaptoge S, et al. Association of cardiometabolic multimorbidity with mortality. Jama 2015;314(1):52.

15. Collaboration ERF, Sarwar N, Gao P, et al. Diabetes mellitus, fasting blood glucose concentration, and risk of vascular disease: a collaborative meta-analysis of 102 prospective studies. Lancet 2010;375(9733):2215–22.

16. Aminian A, Zajichek A, Arterburn DE, et al. Predicting 10-Year Risk of End-Organ Complications of Type 2 Diabetes With and Without Metabolic Surgery: A Machine Learning Approach. Diabetes Care 2020;43(4):852–9.

17. Group TLAR. Cardiovascular Effects of Intensive Lifestyle Intervention in Type 2 Diabetes. N Engl J Med 2013;369(2):145–54.

18. Wing RR, Lang W, Wadden TA, et al. Benefits of modest weight loss in improving cardiovascular risk factors in overweight and obese individuals with type 2 diabetes. Diabetes care 2011;34(7):1481–6.

19. Group LAR. Association of the magnitude of weight loss and changes in physical fitness with long-term cardiovascular disease outcomes in overweight or obese people with type 2 diabetes: a post-hoc analysis of the Look AHEAD randomised clinical trial. Lancet Diabetes Endocrinol 2016;4(11):913–21.

20. Nathan DM, Group DR. The diabetes control and complications trial/epidemiology of diabetes interventions and complications study at 30 years: overview. Diabetes Care 2014;37(1):9–16.

21. Implications of the United Kingdom Prospective Diabetes Study. Diabetes Care 2002;25(Supplement 1):S28–32.

22. Group UPDS (UKPDS). Effect of intensive blood-glucose control with metformin on complications in overweight patients with type 2 diabetes (UKPDS 34). UK Prospective Diabetes Study (UKPDS) Group. Lancet Lond Engl 1998;352(9131):854–65.

23. Holman RR, Paul SK, Bethel MA, et al. 10-Year Follow-up of Intensive Glucose Control in Type 2 Diabetes. N Engl J Med 2008;359(15):1577–89.

24. Action to Control Cardiovascular Risk in Diabetes Study Group, Gerstein HC, Miller ME, et al. Effects of intensive glucose lowering in type 2 diabetes. N Engl J Med 2008;358(24):2545–59.

25. Heller SR. A Summary of the ADVANCE Trial. Diabetes Care 2009;32(Suppl 2):S357–61.

26. Duckworth W, Abraira C, Moritz T, et al. Glucose control and vascular complications in veterans with type 2 diabetes. N Engl J Med 2009;360(2):129–39.

27. Marso SP, Daniels GH, Brown-Frandsen K, et al. Liraglutide and cardiovascular outcomes in type 2 diabetes. N Engl J Med 2016;375(4):311–22.

28. Zinman B, Wanner C, Lachin JM, et al. Empagliflozin, Cardiovascular Outcomes, and Mortality in Type 2 Diabetes. N Engl J Med 2015;373(22):2117–28.

29. McMurray JJV, Solomon SD, Inzucchi SE, et al. Dapagliflozin in Patients with Heart Failure and Reduced Ejection Fraction. N Engl J Med 2019;381(21):1995–2008.

30. Neal B, Perkovic V, Mahaffey KW, et al. Canagliflozin and Cardiovascular and Renal Events in Type 2 Diabetes. N Engl J Med 2017;377(7):644–57.

31. Perkovic V, Jardine MJ, Neal B, et al. Canagliflozin and Renal Outcomes in Type 2 Diabetes and Nephropathy. N Engl J Med 2019;380(24):2295–306.

32. Gerstein HC, Colhoun HM, Dagenais GR, et al. Dulaglutide and cardiovascular outcomes in type 2 diabetes (REWIND): a double-blind, randomised placebo-controlled trial. Lancet 2019;394(10193):121–30.

33. Sjöström L, Lindroos A-K, Peltonen M, et al. Lifestyle, diabetes, and cardiovascular risk factors 10 years after bariatric surgery. N Engl J Med 2004;351(26): 2683–93.

34. Sjöström L, Peltonen M, Jacobson P, et al. Association of bariatric surgery with long-term remission of type 2 diabetes and with microvascular and macrovascular complications. JAMA 2014;311(22):2297–304.

35. Sjöström L, Peltonen M, Jacobson P, et al. Bariatric Surgery and Long-term Cardiovascular Events. JAMA 2012;307(1):56–65.

36. Fisher DP, Johnson E, Haneuse S, et al. Association Between Bariatric Surgery and Macrovascular Disease Outcomes in Patients With Type 2 Diabetes and Severe Obesity. Jama 2018;320(15):1570–82.

37. Adams TD, Gress RE, Smith SC, et al. Long-term mortality after gastric bypass surgery. N Engl J Med 2007;357(8):753–61.

38. Aminian A, Zajichek A, Arterburn DE, et al. Association of metabolic surgery with major adverse cardiovascular outcomes in patients with type 2 diabetes and obesity. JAMA 2019;322(13):1271–82.

39. Schauer PR, Bhatt DL, Kirwan JP, et al. Bariatric Surgery versus Intensive Medical Therapy for Diabetes — 5-Year Outcomes. N Engl J Med 2017;376(7): 641–51.

40. Peterli R, Wölnerhanssen BK, Peters T, et al. Effect of Laparoscopic Sleeve Gastrectomy vs Laparoscopic Roux-en-Y Gastric bypass on weight loss in patients with morbid obesity: the sm-boss randomized clinical trial. JAMA 2018;319(3): 255–65.

41. Salminen P, Helmiö M, Ovaska J, et al. Effect of Laparoscopic Sleeve Gastrectomy vs Laparoscopic Roux-en-Y Gastric Bypass on Weight Loss at 5 Years Among Patients With Morbid Obesity: The SLEEVEPASS Randomized Clinical Trial. JAMA 2018;319(3):241–54.

42. Ruiz-Tovar J, Carbajo MA, Jimenez JM, et al. Long-term follow-up after sleeve gastrectomy versus Roux-en-Y gastric bypass versus one-anastomosis gastric bypass: a prospective randomized comparative study of weight loss and remission of comorbidities. Surg Endosc 2019;33(2):401–10.

43. Schauer PR, Kashyap SR, Wolski K, et al. Bariatric Surgery versus Intensive Medical Therapy in Obese Patients with Diabetes. N Engl J Med 2012; 366(17):1567–76.

44. Aminian A, Vidal J, Salminen P, et al. Late relapse of diabetes after bariatric surgery: not rare, but not a failure. Diabetes Care 2020;dc191057. https://doi.org/10.2337/dc19-1057.

45. Bhatt DL, Aminian A, Kashyap SR, et al. Cardiovascular biomarkers after metabolic surgery versus medical therapy for diabetes. J Am Coll Cardiol 2019;74(2): 261–3.

46. Padilla N, Maraninchi M, Béliard S, et al. Effects of bariatric surgery on hepatic and intestinal lipoprotein particle metabolism in obese, nondiabetic humans. Arterioscler Thromb Vasc Biol 2014;34(10):2330–7.

47. Priester T, Ault TG, Davidson L, et al. Coronary calcium scores 6 years after bariatric surgery. Obes Surg 2015;25(1):90–6.
48. Michaels AD, Mehaffey JH, Hawkins RB, et al. Bariatric surgery reduces long-term rates of cardiac events and need for coronary revascularization: a propensity-matched analysis. Surg Endosc 2019;34(6):2638–43.
49. Pirlet C, Biertho L, Poirier P, et al. Comparison of short and long term cardiovascular outcomes after bariatric surgery in patients with vs without coronary artery disease. Am J Cardiol 2019;125(1):40–7.
50. Kindel TL, Strande JL. Bariatric surgery as a treatment for heart failure: review of the literature and potential mechanisms. Surg Obes Relat Dis 2018;14(1): 117–22.
51. Benotti PN, Wood GC, Carey DJ, et al. Gastric Bypass Surgery Produces a Durable Reduction in Cardiovascular Disease Risk Factors and Reduces the Long-Term Risks of Congestive Heart Failure. J Am Heart Assoc 2017;6(5). https://doi.org/10.1161/jaha.116.005126.
52. Jamaly S, Carlsson L, Peltonen M, et al. Surgical obesity treatment and the risk of heart failure. Eur Heart J 2019;40(26):2131–8.
53. Sundström J, Bruze G, Ottosson J, et al. Weight Loss and Heart Failure: A Nationwide Study of Gastric Bypass Surgery Versus Intensive Lifestyle Treatment. Circulation 2017;135(17):1577–85.
54. Shimada YJ, Tsugawa Y, Brown DFM, et al. Bariatric surgery and emergency department visits and hospitalizations for heart failure exacerbation: population-based, self-controlled series. J Am Coll Cardiol 2016;67(8):895–903.
55. Mikhalkova D, Holman SR, Jiang H, et al. Bariatric surgery-induced cardiac and lipidomic changes in obesity-related heart failure with preserved ejection fraction: gastric bypass: HFpEF and Lipidomic Effects. Obesity 2017;26(2):284–90.
56. Vest AR, Patel P, Schauer PR, et al. Clinical and Echocardiographic Outcomes After Bariatric Surgery in Obese Patients With Left Ventricular Systolic Dysfunction. Circ Hear Fail 2016;9(3):e002260.
57. Leichman JG, Wilson EB, Scarborough T, et al. Dramatic reversal of derangements in muscle metabolism and left ventricular function after bariatric surgery. Am J Med 2008;121(11):966–73.
58. Ramani GV, McCloskey C, Ramanathan RC, et al. Safety and efficacy of bariatric surgery in morbidly obese patients with severe systolic heart failure. Clin Cardiol 2008;31(11):516–20.
59. Lin CH, Kurup S, Herrero P, et al. Myocardial oxygen consumption change predicts left ventricular relaxation improvement in obese humans after weight loss. Obesity 2011;19(9):1804–12.
60. Nijhawan S, Richards W, O'Hea MF, et al. Bariatric surgery rapidly improves mitochondrial respiration in morbidly obese patients. Surg Endosc 2013; 27(12):4569–73.
61. Aggarwal R, Harling L, Efthimiou E, et al. The effects of bariatric surgery on cardiac structure and function: a systematic review of cardiac imaging outcomes. Obes Surg 2015;26(5):1030–40.
62. Aleassa EM, Khorgami Z, Kindel TL, et al. Impact of bariatric surgery on heart failure mortality. Surg Obes Relat Dis 2019;15(7):1189–96.
63. Odutayo A, Wong CX, Hsiao AJ, et al. Atrial fibrillation and risks of cardiovascular disease, renal disease, and death: systematic review and meta-analysis. BMJ 2016;354:i4482.

64. Huxley RR, Filion KB, Konety S, et al. Meta-analysis of cohort and case-control studies of type 2 diabetes mellitus and risk of atrial fibrillation. Am J Cardiol 2011;108(1):56–62.
65. Tedrow UB, Conen D, Ridker PM, et al. The long- and short-term impact of elevated body mass index on the risk of new atrial fibrillation the WHS (women's health study). J Am Coll Cardiol 2010;55(21):2319–27.
66. Donnellan E, Wazni O, Kanj M, et al. Outcomes of atrial fibrillation ablation in morbidly obese patients following bariatric surgery compared with a nonobese cohort. Circ Arrhythmia Electrophysiol 2019;12(10):e007598.
67. Donnellan E, Wazni O, Elshazly M, et al. Impact of Bariatric Surgery on Atrial Fibrillation Type. Circ Arrhythmia Electrophysiol 2020;13(2). https://doi.org/10.1161/circep.119.007626.
68. Middeldorp ME, Lau DH, Sanders P. Is bypassing traditional weight-loss the answer for atrial fibrillation? Circ Arrhythmia Electrophysiol 2019;12(10):e007864.
69. Kadhim K, Middeldorp ME, Hendriks JM, et al. Bariatric surgery and atrial fibrillation: does the end justify the means? Europace 2019;21(10):1454–6.
70. Alonso A, Bahnson JL, Gaussoin SA, et al. Effect of an intensive lifestyle intervention on atrial fibrillation risk in individuals with type 2 diabetes: the Look AHEAD randomized trial. Am Heart J 2015;170(4):770–7.e5.
71. Jones NR, Taylor KS, Taylor CJ, et al. Weight change and the risk of incident atrial fibrillation: a systematic review and meta-analysis. Heart 2019;105(23):1799–805.
72. Jamaly S, Carlsson L, Peltonen M, et al. Bariatric Surgery and the Risk of New-Onset Atrial Fibrillation in Swedish Obese Subjects. J Am Coll Cardiol 2016;68(23):2497–504.
73. Yılmaz M, Altın C, Tekin A, et al. Assessment of Atrial Fibrillation and Ventricular Arrhythmia Risk after Bariatric Surgery by P Wave/QT Interval Dispersion. Obes Surg 2017;28(4):932–8.
74. Young L, Hanipah ZN, Brethauer SA, et al. Long-term impact of bariatric surgery in diabetic nephropathy. Surg Endosc 2018;33(5):1654–60.
75. Imam TH, Fischer H, Jing B, et al. Estimated GFR Before and After Bariatric Surgery in CKD. Am J Kidney Dis 2017;69(3):380–8.
76. Cohen RV, Pereira TV, Aboud CM, et al. Effect of gastric bypass vs best medical treatment on early-stage chronic kidney disease in patients with type 2 diabetes and obesity: a randomized clinical trial. JAMA Surg 2020;155(8):e200420.
77. D'Agati VD, Chagnac A, Vries APJ de, et al. Obesity-related glomerulopathy: clinical and pathologic characteristics and pathogenesis. Nat Rev Nephrol 2016;12(8):453–71.
78. O'Brien R, Johnson E, Haneuse S, et al. Microvascular Outcomes in Patients With Diabetes After Bariatric Surgery Versus Usual Care: A Matched Cohort Study. Ann Intern Med 2018;169(5):300.
79. Carlsson LMS, Sjöholm K, Karlsson C, et al. Long-term incidence of microvascular disease after bariatric surgery or usual care in patients with obesity, stratified by baseline glycaemic status: a post-hoc analysis of participants from the Swedish Obese Subjects study. Lancet Diabetes Endocrinol 2017;5(4):271–9.
80. Bradley D, Magkos F, Eagon JC, et al. Matched weight loss induced by sleeve gastrectomy or gastric bypass similarly improves metabolic function in obese subjects. Obesity (Silver Spring) 2014;22(9):2026–31.
81. Shulman GI. Ectopic fat in insulin resistance, dyslipidemia, and cardiometabolic disease. N Engl J Med 2014;371(12):1131–41.

82. Coimbra S, Reis F, Ferreira C, et al. Weight loss achieved by bariatric surgery modifies high-density lipoprotein subfractions and low-density lipoprotein oxidation towards atheroprotection. Clin Biochem 2018;63:46–53.

83. Gómez-Martin JM, Balsa JA, Aracil E, et al. Beneficial changes on plasma apolipoproteins A and B, high density lipoproteins and oxidized low density lipoproteins in obese women after bariatric surgery: comparison between gastric bypass and sleeve gastrectomy. Lipids Health Dis 2018;17(1):145.

84. Flynn CR, Albaugh VL, Abumrad NN. Metabolic effects of bile acids: potential role in bariatric surgery. Cell Mol Gastroenterol Hepatol 2019. https://doi.org/10.1016/j.jcmgh.2019.04.014.

85. Albaugh VL, Flynn CR, Cai S, et al. Early Increases in Bile Acids Post Roux-en-Y Gastric Bypass Are Driven by Insulin-Sensitizing, Secondary Bile Acids. J Clin Endocrinol Metab 2015;100(9):E1225–33.

86. Goncalves D, Barataud A, Vadder FD, et al. Bile Routing Modification Reproduces Key Features of Gastric Bypass in Rat. Ann Surg 2015;262(6):1006–15.

87. Dunn JP, Abumrad NN, Breitman I, et al. Hepatic and peripheral insulin sensitivity and diabetes remission at 1 month after Roux-en-Y gastric bypass surgery in patients randomized to omentectomy. Diabetes care 2012;35(1):137–42.

88. Kenler HA, Brolin RE, Cody RP. Changes in eating behavior after horizontal gastroplasty and Roux-en-Y gastric bypass. Am J Clin Nutr 1990;52(1):87–92.

89. Roux CW le, Bueter M, Theis N, et al. Gastric bypass reduces fat intake and preference. Am J Physiol Regul Integr Comp Physiol 2011;301(4):R1057–66.

90. Zheng H, Shin AC, Lenard NR, et al. Meal patterns, satiety, and food choice in a rat model of Roux-en-Y gastric bypass surgery. Am J Physiol Regul Integr Comp Physiol 2009;297(5):R1273–82.

91. Hajnal A, Zharikov A, Polston JE, et al. Alcohol reward is increased after Roux-en-Y gastric bypass in dietary obese rats with differential effects following ghrelin antagonism. PLoS One 2012;7(11):e49121.

92. Hajnal A, Kovacs P, Ahmed T, et al. Gastric bypass surgery alters behavioral and neural taste functions for sweet taste in obese rats. Am J Physiol Gastrointest Liver Physiol 2010;299(4):G967–79.

93. Breitman I, Isbell JM, Saliba J, et al. Effects of proximal gut bypass on glucose tolerance and insulin sensitivity in humans. Diabetes care 2013;36(4):e57.

94. Tamboli RA, Antoun J, Sidani RM, et al. Metabolic responses to exogenous ghrelin in obesity and early after R oux-en- Y gastric bypass in humans. Diabetes Obes Metab 2017;19(9):1267–75.

95. Ryan KK, Tremaroli V, Clemmensen C, et al. FXR is a molecular target for the effects of vertical sleeve gastrectomy. Nature 2014;509(7499):183–8.

96. Albaugh VL, Banan B, Antoun J, et al. Role of Bile Acids and GLP-1 in mediating the metabolic improvements of bariatric surgery. Gastroenterology 2019;156(4):1041–51.e4.

97. Baud G, Daoudi M, Hubert T, et al. Bile Diversion in Roux-en-Y Gastric Bypass Modulates Sodium-Dependent Glucose Intestinal Uptake. Cell Metabolism 2016;1–14. https://doi.org/10.1016/j.cmet.2016.01.018.

98. Kohli R, Kirby M, Setchell KDR, et al. Intestinal adaptation after ileal interposition surgery increases bile acid recycling and protects against obesity-related comorbidities. Am J Physiol Gastrointest Liver Physiol 2010;299(3):G652–60.

99. Cavin J-B, Bado A, Gall ML. Intestinal Adaptations after Bariatric Surgery: Consequences on Glucose Homeostasis. Trends Endocrinol Metab 2017;28(5):354–64.

100. Saeidi N, Meoli L, Nestoridi E, et al. Reprogramming of intestinal glucose meta-bolism and glycemic control in rats after gastric bypass. Science 2013; 341(6144):406–10.
101. Flynn CR, Albaugh VL, Cai S, et al. Bile diversion to the distal small intestine has comparable metabolic benefits to bariatric surgery. Nat Commun 2015;6(1): 7715.
102. Lorkowski SW, Brubaker G, Rotroff DM, et al. Bariatric Surgery Improves HDL function examined by apoa1 exchange rate and cholesterol efflux capacity in patients with obesity and type 2 diabetes. Biomol 2020;10(4):551.
103. Zvintzou E, Skroubis G, Chroni A, et al. Effects of bariatric surgery on HDL struc-ture and functionality: results from a prospective trial. J Clin Lipidol 2014;8(4): 408–17.
104. Maraninchi M, Padilla N, Béliard S, et al. Impact of bariatric surgery on apolipo-protein C-III levels and lipoprotein distribution in obese human subjects. J Clin Lipidol 2017;11(2):495–506.e3.
105. Graessler J, Bornstein TD, Goel D, et al. Lipidomic profiling before and after Roux-en-Y gastric bypass in obese patients with diabetes. Pharmacogenomics J 2014;14(3):201–7.
106. Aminian A, Jamal M, Augustin T, et al. Failed Surgical Weight Loss Does Not Necessarily Mean Failed Metabolic Effects. Diabetes Technol Ther 2015; 17(10):682–4.
107. Carswell KA, Vincent RP, Belgaumkar AP, et al. The effect of bariatric surgery on intestinal absorption and transit time. Obes Surg 2014;24(5):796–805.
108. Kumar R, Lieske JC, Collazo-Clavell ML, et al. Fat malabsorption and increased intestinal oxalate absorption are common after roux-en-Y gastric bypass sur-gery. Surgery 2011;149(5):654–61.
109. Odstrcil EA, Martinez JG, Ana CAS, et al. The contribution of malabsorption to the reduction in net energy absorption after long-limb Roux-en-Y gastric bypass. Am J Clin Nutr 2010;92(4):704–13.
110. Mulla CM, Middelbeek RJW, Patti ME. Mechanisms of weight loss and improved metabolism following bariatric surgery. Ann N Y Acad Sci 2017;384(Pt 2):766.
111. Grayson BE, Schneider KM, Woods SC, et al. Improved rodent maternal meta-bolism but reduced intrauterine growth after vertical sleeve gastrectomy. Sci Transl Med 2013;5(199):199ra112.
112. Hao Z, Mumphrey MB, Townsend RL, et al. Reprogramming of defended body weight after Roux-En-Y gastric bypass surgery in diet-induced obese mice. Obesity (Silver Spring) 2016. https://doi.org/10.1002/oby.21400.
113. Stefater MA, Sandoval DA, Chambers AP, et al. Sleeve gastrectomy in rats im-proves postprandial lipid clearance by reducing intestinal triglyceride secretion. Gastroenterology 2011;141(3):939–49.e1-4.
114. Albaugh VL, Flynn CR, Tamboli RA, et al. Recent advances in metabolic and bariatric surgery. F1000Research 2016;5:978.
115. Gimeno RE, Briere DA, Seeley RJ. Leveraging the Gut to Treat Metabolic Dis-ease. Cell Metab 2020. https://doi.org/10.1016/j.cmet.2020.02.014.
116. Evers SS, Sandoval DA, Seeley RJ. The Physiology and Molecular Underpin-nings of the Effects of Bariatric Surgery on Obesity and Diabetes. Annu Rev Physiol 2016;79(1). annurev-physiol-022516-034423.
117. Kannel WB, McGee D, Gordon T. A general cardiovascular risk profile: The Fra-mingham study. Am J Cardiol 1976;38(1):46–51.
118. Anderson KM, Wilson PW, Odell PM, et al. An updated coronary risk profile. A statement for health professionals. Circulation 1991;83(1):356–62.

119. Wilson PWF, D'Agostino RB, Levy D, et al. Prediction of Coronary Heart Disease Using Risk Factor Categories. Circulation 1998;97(18):1837–47.
120. Conroy RM, Pyörälä K, Fitzgerald AP, et al. Estimation of ten-year risk of fatal cardiovascular disease in Europe: the SCORE project. Eur Heart J 2003; 24(11):987–1003.
121. Ridker PM, Buring JE, Rifai N, et al. Development and Validation of Improved Algorithms for the Assessment of Global Cardiovascular Risk in Women: The Reynolds Risk Score. Jama 2007;297(6):611.
122. Hippisley-Cox J, Coupland C, Vinogradova Y, et al. Derivation and validation of QRISK, a new cardiovascular disease risk score for the United Kingdom: prospective open cohort study. BMJ 2007;335(7611):136.
123. Hippisley-Cox J, Coupland C, Vinogradova Y, et al. Predicting cardiovascular risk in England and Wales: prospective derivation and validation of QRISK2. BMJ 2008;336(7659):1475.
124. Hippisley-Cox J, Coupland C, Robson J, et al. Derivation, validation, and evaluation of a new QRISK model to estimate lifetime risk of cardiovascular disease: cohort study using QResearch database. BMJ 2010;341(dec09 1):c6624.
125. Muntner P, Colantonio LD, Cushman M, et al. Validation of the atherosclerotic cardiovascular disease Pooled Cohort risk equations. Jama 2014;311(14): 1406–15.
126. Lloyd-Jones DM, Huffman MD, Karmali KN, et al. Estimating Longitudinal Risks and Benefits From Cardiovascular Preventive Therapies Among Medicare Patients: The Million Hearts Longitudinal ASCVD Risk Assessment Tool: A Special Report From the American Heart Association and American College of Cardiology. Circulation 2017;135(13):e793–813.
127. Jaspers NEM, Blaha MJ, Matsushita K, et al. Prediction of individualized lifetime benefit from cholesterol lowering, blood pressure lowering, antithrombotic therapy, and smoking cessation in apparently healthy people. Eur Heart J 2019; 41(11):1190–9.
128. James WPT, Caterson ID, Coutinho W, et al. Effect of Sibutramine on Cardiovascular Outcomes in Overweight and Obese Subjects. N Engl J Med 2010; 363(10):905–17.
129. Caterson ID, Finer N, Coutinho W, et al. Maintained intentional weight loss reduces cardiovascular outcomes: results from the Sibutramine Cardiovascular OUTcomes (SCOUT) trial. Diabetes Obes Metab 2012;14(6):523–30.
130. Bohula EA, Scirica BM, Inzucchi SE, et al. Effect of lorcaserin on prevention and remission of type 2 diabetes in overweight and obese patients (CAMELLIA-TIMI 61): a randomised, placebo-controlled trial. Lancet 2018;392(10161):2269–79.
131. Nissen SE, Wolski KE, Prcela L, et al. Effect of Naltrexone-Bupropion on Major Adverse Cardiovascular Events in Overweight and Obese Patients With Cardiovascular Risk Factors: A Randomized Clinical Trial. Jama 2016;315(10): 990–1004.
132. Li G, Zhang P, Wang J, et al. Cardiovascular mortality, all-cause mortality, and diabetes incidence after lifestyle intervention for people with impaired glucose tolerance in the Da Qing Diabetes Prevention Study: a 23-year follow-up study. Lancet Diabetes Endocrinol 2014;2(6):474–80.
133. Eriksson K-F, Lindgärde F. No excess 12-year mortality in men with impaired glucose tolerance who participated in the Malmö Preventive Trial with diet and exercise. Diabetologia 1998;41(9):1010–6.
134. Wilcox R, Kupfer S, Erdmann E, et al. Effects of pioglitazone on major adverse cardiovascular events in high-risk patients with type 2 diabetes: results from

PROspective pioglitAzone Clinical Trial In macro Vascular Events (PROactive 10). Am Heart J 2008;155(4):712–7.

135. Marso SP, Bain SC, Consoli A, et al. Semaglutide and Cardiovascular Outcomes in Patients with Type 2 Diabetes. N Engl J Med 2016;375(19):1834–44.

136. Husain M, Birkenfeld AL, Donsmark M, et al. Oral Semaglutide and Cardiovascular Outcomes in Patients with Type 2 Diabetes. N Engl J Med 2019;381(9): 841–51.

137. MacDonald KG, Long SD, Swanson MS, et al. The gastric bypass operation reduces the progression and mortality of non-insulin-dependent diabetes mellitus. J Gastrointest Surg 1997;1(3):213–20.

138. Christou NV, Sampalis JS, Liberman M, et al. Surgery decreases long-term mortality, morbidity, and health care use in morbidly obese patients. Ann Surg 2004; 240(3):416–24.

139. Flum DR, Dellinger EP. Impact of gastric bypass operation on survival: A population-based analysis. J Am Coll Surg 2004;199(4):543–51.

140. Favretti F, Segato G, Ashton D, et al. Laparoscopic Adjustable Gastric Banding in 1,791 Consecutive Obese Patients: 12-Year Results. Obes Surg 2007;17(2): 168–75.

141. Peeters A, O'Brien PE, Laurie C, et al. Substantial intentional weight loss and mortality in the severely obese. Ann Surg 2007;246(6):1028–33.

142. Sjöström L, Narbro K, Sjöström CD, et al. Effects of bariatric surgery on mortality in Swedish Obese Subjects. N Engl J Med 2007;357(8):741–52.

143. Sowemimo OA, Yood SM, Courtney J, et al. Natural history of morbid obesity without surgical intervention. Surg Obes Relat Dis 2007;3(1):73–7.

144. Perry CD, Hutter MM, Smith DB, et al. Survival and Changes in Comorbidities After Bariatric Surgery. Ann Surg 2008;247(1):21–7.

145. Marsk R, Näslund E, Freedman J, et al. Bariatric surgery reduces mortality in Swedish men. Br J Surg 2010;97(6):877–83.

146. Maciejewski ML, Livingston EH, Smith VA, et al. Survival Among High-Risk Patients After Bariatric Surgery. JAMA 2011;305(23):2419–26.

147. Johnson RJ, Johnson BL, Blackhurst DW, et al. Bariatric surgery is associated with a reduced risk of mortality in morbidly obese patients with a history of major cardiovascular events. Am Surg 2012;78(6):685–92.

148. Scott JD, Johnson BL, Blackhurst DW, et al. Does bariatric surgery reduce the risk of major cardiovascular events? A retrospective cohort study of morbidly obese surgical patients. Surg Obes Relat Dis 2013;9(1):32–9.

149. Arterburn DE, Olsen MK, Smith VA, et al. Association Between Bariatric Surgery and Long-term Survival. JAMA 2015;313(1):62–70.

150. Eliasson B, Liakopoulos V, Franzén S, et al. Cardiovascular disease and mortality in patients with type 2 diabetes after bariatric surgery in Sweden: a nationwide, matched, observational cohort study. Lancet Diabetes Endocrinol 2015; 3(11):847–54.

151. Guidry CA, Davies SW, Sawyer RG, et al. Gastric bypass improves survival compared with propensity-matched controls: a cohort study with over 10-year follow-up. Am J Surg 2015;209(3):463–7.

152. Davidson LE, Adams TD, Kim J, et al. Association of patient age at gastric bypass surgery with long-term all-cause and cause-specific mortality. JAMA Surg 2016. https://doi.org/10.1001/jamasurg.2015.5501.

153. Flanagan E, Ghaderi I, Overby DW, et al. Reduced survival in bariatric surgery candidates delayed or denied by lack of insurance approval. Am Surg 2016; 82(2):166–70.

154. Lent MR, Benotti PN, Mirshahi T, et al. All-Cause and Specific-Cause Mortality Risk After Roux-en-Y Gastric Bypass in Patients With and Without Diabetes. Diabetes Care 2017;40(10):1379–85.
155. Pontiroli AE, Zakaria AS, Fanchini M, et al. A 23-year study of mortality and development of co-morbidities in patients with obesity undergoing bariatric surgery (laparoscopic gastric banding) in comparison with medical treatment of obesity. Cardiovasc Diabetol 2018;17(1):161.
156. Reges O, Greenland P, Dicker D, et al. Association of Bariatric Surgery Using Laparoscopic Banding, Roux-en-Y Gastric Bypass, or Laparoscopic Sleeve Gastrectomy vs Usual Care Obesity Management With All-Cause Mortality. Jama 2018;319(3):279.
157. Moussa OM, Erridge S, Chidambaram S, et al. Mortality of the Severely Obese: A Population Study. Ann Surg 2019;269(6):1087–91.
158. Kauppila JH, Tao W, Santoni G, et al. Effects of Obesity Surgery on Overall and Disease-specific Mortality in a 5-Country, Population-based Study. Gastroenterology 2019;1–29. https://doi.org/10.1053/j.gastro.2019.03.048.
159. Ceriani V, Sarro G, Micheletto G, et al. Long-term mortality in obese subjects undergoing malabsorptive surgery (biliopancreatic diversion and biliointestinal bypass) versus medical treatment. Int J Obes 2018;43(6):1147–53.
160. Singh P, Subramanian A, Adderley N, et al. Impact of bariatric surgery on cardiovascular outcomes and mortality: a population-based cohort study. Br J Surg 2020;107(4):432–42.
161. Moussa O, Ardissino M, Heaton T, et al. Effect of bariatric surgery on long-term cardiovascular outcomes: a nationwide nested cohort study. Eur Heart J 2020. https://doi.org/10.1093/eurheartj/ehaa069.
162. Liakopoulos V, Franzén S, Svensson A-M, et al. Renal and Cardiovascular Outcomes After Weight Loss From Gastric Bypass Surgery in Type 2 Diabetes: Cardiorenal Risk Reductions Exceed Atherosclerotic Benefits. Diabetes Care 2020; 43(6):1276–84.
163. Sheetz KH, Gerhardinger L, Dimick JB, et al. Bariatric Surgery and Long-term Survival in Patients With Obesity and End-stage Kidney Disease. JAMA Surg 2020;155(7). https://doi.org/10.1001/jamasurg.2020.0829.
164. Doumouras AG, Hong D, Lee Y, et al. Association Between Bariatric Surgery and All-Cause Mortality: A Population-Based Matched Cohort Study in a Universal Health Care System. Ann Intern Med 2020. https://doi.org/10.7326/m19-3925.
165. Stenberg E, Cao Y, Marsk R, et al. Association between metabolic surgery and cardiovascular outcome in patients with hypertension: A nationwide matched cohort study. PLoS Med 2020;17(9):e1003307.
166. Aminian A, Nissen SE. Success (but Unfinished) Story of Metabolic Surgery. Diabetes Care 2020;43(6):1175–7.
167. Aminian A, Aleassa EM, Bhatt DL, et al. Bariatric surgery is associated with a lower rate of death after myocardial infarction and stroke: A nationwide study. Diabetes Obes Metab 2019;21(9):2058–67.

Obesity, Bariatric Surgery, and Hip/Knee Arthroplasty Outcomes

Katelyn M. Mellion, MD[a], Brandon T. Grover, DO[b],*

KEYWORDS

- Bariatric surgery • Lower extremity osteoarthritis • Arthroplasty • Outcomes

KEY POINTS

- Osteoarthritis is a common comorbidity in patients with obesity.
- Obesity contributes to the development and progression of osteoarthritis due to structural/mechanical factors as well as changes in the proinflammatory hormonal milieu caused by metabolic syndrome.
- Although there is no consensus on the timing of bariatric surgery relative to total joint arthroplasty (TJA) in patients with obesity, several studies suggest a benefit of weight loss prior to TJA.

INTRODUCTION

Osteoarthritis is highly prevalent in the United States. Approximately 26% of the total adult population is projected to have arthritis by 2040.[1] Osteoarthritis results in more functional loss than any other disease and results in more hospital charges than pneumonia, stroke, or complications from diabetes.[2,3] Obesity is an independent risk factor for osteoarthritis.[4] The risk for knee osteoarthritis has been shown to be several times greater for individuals with obesity compared with those with normal weight.[5] Changes in both biomechanics and the systemic inflammatory milieu attributed to obesity contribute to this increased risk.[6]

More than 1 million total knee and total hip replacement procedures are performed each year in the United States, with an increasing number performed on patients with obesity.[7–9] Unfortunately, patients with obesity are at a higher risk of complication after total joint arthroplasty (TJA) than patients with a normal weight.[7,10] The American Association of Hip and Knee Surgeons suggests weight loss prior to TJA for patients with body mass index (BMI) greater than 40 kg/m².[11] For patients in this weight

[a] Department of Medical Education, Advanced Gastrointestinal Minimally Invasive Surgery and Bariatric Fellowship, Gundersen Health System, 1900 South Avenue C05-001, La Crosse, WI 54601, USA; [b] Department of Surgery, Gundersen Health System, 1900 South Avenue C05-001, La Crosse, WI 54601, USA
* Corresponding author.
E-mail address: btgrover@gundersenhealth.org

Surg Clin N Am 101 (2021) 295–305
https://doi.org/10.1016/j.suc.2020.12.011
0039-6109/21/© 2020 Elsevier Inc. All rights reserved.

surgical.theclinics.com

category, bariatric surgery is the only known method for reliable and sustained weight loss as well as comorbidity resolution.[12] This article reviews the impact of obesity and weight loss on osteoarthritis and TJA outcomes. Then the literature on the impact of bariatric surgery on the symptoms and progression of osteoarthritis as well as TJA outcomes is reviewed. Finally, ongoing trials and future directions for research in this area are discussed.

IMPACT OF OBESITY ON LOWER LIMB OSTEOARTHRITIS

Obesity is an independent risk factor for osteoarthritis.[4] According to a 2018 report by the Centers for Disease Control and Prevention, individuals with obesity were twice as likely to be diagnosed with arthritis compared with individuals with normal weight.[13] Similarly, a Norwegian study found men and women with obesity had an 8-fold and 5-fold risk of requiring total hip arthroplasty (THA), respectively, compared with underweight individuals.[14] Several studies have suggested a direct relationship between BMI and the presence of osteoarthritis. In a Finnish study of male and female farmers, aged 40 to 64 years, a 40% increased risk of knee osteoarthritis was found for every 3.8-kg/m^2 increase of BMI within a 10-year follow-up.[15]

Joint wear and tear secondary to mechanical and structural factors classically have been suggested as the mechanism for osteoarthritis. Joint load during walking is related directly to body weight. Contact forces in the hip during walking have been shown to be 2-times to 3-times body weight,[16] and knee-joint loads during walking and stair climbing have been shown to be even higher than loads across the hip joint.[17] Gait disturbances also are common in patients with obesity, including altered lower extremity biomechanics for walking, standing, and rising from a sitting position. These adaptations in gait lead to alterations in the regions of the articular cartilage within the joint that bears the load,[18] which can lead to changes in the composition, structure, and mechanical characteristics of articular cartilage.[19–21]

Although mechanical and structural factors surely contribute to the development of osteoarthritis, recent studies suggest they cannot solely account for the relationship between obesity and osteoarthritis.[22] For example, in a systematic review and meta-analysis by Long and colleagues,[23] increased fat mass was associated with non–weight-bearing (hand joint) osteoarthritis. Because obesity has been shown to be associated with a chronic inflammatory state, the inflammatory factors associated with obesity may contribute to the development of osteoarthritis. Patients with obesity have a higher adipocyte mass compared with normal-weight individuals. Adipocytes are known to be metabolically active cells that secrete a multitude of factors, collectively termed, *adipocytokines*. Because many of these adipocytokines are thought to play a role in cartilage homeostasis, the changes in the adipocytokine milieu in the obese population are thought to contribute to the degradation of cartilage and, therefore, the development of osteoarthritis.[24]

Adipocytokines of interest include leptin, resistin, visfatin, lipocalin-2, and apelin (**Fig. 1**).[22,25]

Leptin, a satiety hormone produced by adipocytes, is known to be present in both plasma and synovial fluid in higher concentrations in individuals with obesity.[26] Furthermore, increased expression of leptin in cartilage, subchondral bone, synovial tissues, and osteophytes has been associated with increased severity of osteoarthritis seen radiographically.[24,27] Leptin interacts with proinflammatory cytokines to influence both chondrocytes (to increase the production of several inflammatory factors, growth factors and matrix metalloproteinases)[25] and chondrogenic progenitor cells (by altering their ability to maintain cartilage homeostasis and replace damaged

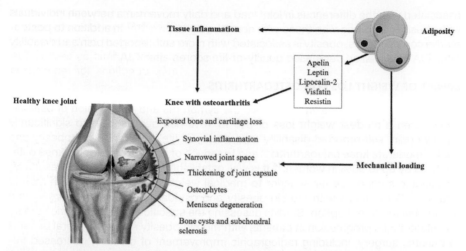

Fig. 1. Illustration depicting the effects of increased fat mass on cartilage hemostasis. (*Adapted from* Uhalte E, Wilkinson JM, Southam L, et al. Pathways to understanding the genomic aetiology of osteoarthritis. Hum Mol Genet. 2017;26(R2):R193-R201; with permission.)

tissue).[24] Resistin is a proinflammatory adipocytokine that has been associated with increased levels of other cytokines and with increased osteoblast proliferation. Resistin concentrations are higher in patients with osteoarthritis compared with healthy controls; however, the exact mechanism of how resistin contributes to the development of osteoarthritis is unknown.[25] Visfatin is more prevalent in both the serum and synovial fluid of patients with osteoarthritis, where it increases degradation of joint connective tissue and extracellular matrix.[25] Lipocalin-2 is expressed in joint tissues and found in elevated levels in patients with obesity as well as in patients with osteoarthritis. Increased levels have been correlated with fracture risk in elderly patients. This hormone has been shown to stimulate pro-osteoclastogenic factors, inhibit antiosteoclastogenic factors, and reduce chondrocyte proliferation.[25] Apelin is a proinflammatory adipokine that increases expression of catabolic factors in chondrocytes and decreases proteoglycan in articular cartilage. It is found in elevated levels in the synovial fluid of individuals with osteoarthritis. Furthermore, increased levels of apelin have been associated with increased osteoarthritis disease severity.[25]

IMPACT OF OBESITY ON ARTHROPLASTY

The standard of care for end-stage knee and hip osteoarthritis is TJA. The risk of both short-term and long-term complications of these procedures increases with increasing patient BMI.[16,28] Short-term postoperative complications likely are related to both increased intraoperative technical difficulty as well as the increased incidence of comorbidities in patients with obesity. TJA in patients with obesity has been associated with an increase in technical errors, surgeon-reported difficulty, and problems that occur during surgery compared with patients with a normal weight.[29–31] Obesity also is associated with an increased risk of surgical site infections, respiratory complications, thromboembolic events, and hospital length of stay.[30–37] Long-term complications, such as accelerated bare surface wear, early prosthesis failure, implant loosening, need for revisional joint surgery, and component malposition, likely are associated with the differences in joint load and daily movements between individuals with obesity compared with those with normal weight.[35,36,38–41] In addition to postoperative complications, obesity is associated with more self-reported pain and disability after TJA[42] as well as decreased quality-of-life scores after TJA.[41]

IMPACT OF WEIGHT LOSS ON OSTEOARTHRITIS

Weight loss has been shown to improve the symptoms and progression of osteoarthritis. Even a modest weight loss of 5% to 10% has been shown to significantly improve pain, self-reported disability, and quality of life in patients with obesity and mild to moderate knee osteoarthritis[43] and to reduce of odds of developing knee osteoarthritis by up to 50% in women.[44] It is well established that the long-term results after bariatric surgery are far superior to medical weight loss in patients with morbid obesity.[12] For patients with morbid obesity and osteoarthritis, bariatric surgery is a reasonable treatment option. Studies assessing the specific effect of bariatric surgery on osteoarthritis progression in patients with morbid obesity suggest several benefits to bariatric surgery, including radiographic improvement of disease, decreased frequency and intensity of joint pain, improved physical function, and improved range of motion.[45–48] There are several studies that suggest resolution of arthropathy on long-term follow-up after bariatric surgery alone.[49,50]

Given the mechanisms for the development of osteoarthritis in patients with morbid obesity, the symptom improvements realized after weight loss in this population are not surprising. After bariatric surgery and weight loss, patients experience improvements in postural stability and sway during walking, which may decrease the magnitude and frequency of abnormal joint loads.[51] Significant improvements have also been noted in physical function as measured by the Western Ontario and McMaster Universities Arthritis Index (WOMAC).[52,53] In addition to improved gait mechanics and decreased joint load, bariatric surgery also has been shown to alter levels of several adipocytokines within the first year after bariatric surgery. For example, the decrease in leptin following bariatric surgery has been shown to correspond directly to the reduction in osteoarthritic knee pain.[54] Some studies suggest, however, that weight loss leads to increased torque across joints due to the increased stride length and gait velocity that accompany weight loss,[55,56] with some suggestion that higher weight loss after bariatric surgery could increase the likelihood of undergoing TJA.[57] Although the likelihood of undergoing TJA does not indicate that the patient necessarily has worse osteoarthritis, given these data, low-velocity and low-impact exercise may be warranted in the first year after weight loss surgery in order to prevent increased stress on the hip and knee joints.[58]

BARIATRIC SURGERY AND TOTAL ARTHROPLASTY

There is some debate regarding the timing of bariatric surgery with respect to TJA. There has been speculation that the increased mobility allowed by TJA in the obese population may allow more efficient nonsurgical weight loss or, even better, weight loss after bariatric surgery if TJA is performed first. The available evidence, however, does not support this. Despite increased mobility after TJA, most patients maintain their preoperative weight and some patients actually gain weight postoperatively.[58] TJA is not suggested as a treatment of significant weight loss. As a simple fact, even patients without osteoarthritis and intact mobility struggle to lose weight without surgery. This suggests that patients are unlikely to realize long-term weight loss benefit from TJA.

The American Association of Hip and Knee Surgeons strongly recommends consideration for weight loss prior to TJA in patients with BMI greater than 40 kg/m^2 due to the increased risk of complications, poorer functional outcomes, and increased cost of TJA in patients with morbid obesity compared with patients with normal weight.[11] Because bariatric surgery has been shown the only reliable method of long-term weight loss and comorbidity resolution for patients with morbid obesity,[12] some practitioners recommend bariatric surgery prior to TJA in this patient population. Studies investigating the effect of bariatric surgery on TJA outcomes show mixed results; however, there generally are several benefits to performing bariatric surgery prior to TJA, which are discussed.

Although there are a handful of systematic reviews evaluating the effect of bariatric surgery prior to TJA, these all include some variable combination of the same several primary studies.[4,59,60] Of the studies that offered comparisons between patients undergoing TJA with and without prior bariatric surgery, most suggested benefits to surgical weight loss prior to TJA.

A large study by Werner and colleagues,[61] using a Medicare database with 78,036 patients, found a decreased rate of 90-day major and minor complications in patients with morbid obesity who underwent bariatric surgery compared with patients with morbid obesity who did not undergo bariatric surgery prior to total knee arthroplasty (TKA). Similarly, a retrospective study of patients undergoing elective TKA or THA between 1997 and 2011 in New York utilized propensity matching to compare TJA outcomes in patients with morbid obesity who did and did not undergo bariatric surgery prior to arthroplasty. They compared 2636 patients in each arm who underwent TKA and found those after bariatric surgery had decreased in-hospital complications, decreased 90-day complication rate, and a similar revision rate. They also compared 792 patients in each arm who underwent THA and found those after bariatric surgery had decreased in-hospital complications with similar revision and dislocation risks.[62] A study from Mayo Clinic by Watts and colleagues[63] compared the outcome of THA in 42 patients with morbid obesity who previously underwent bariatric surgery and 94 patients who did not, in a matched cohort study. They found a decrease in reoperations and revisions for patients who underwent bariatric surgery prior to THA.[63] Kulkarni and colleagues[64] similarly found that patients with morbid obesity who underwent bariatric surgery prior to TJA had 3.5-times lower likelihood of wound infection and 7-times lower likelihood of hospital readmission compared with those who underwent TJA alone. Nearing and colleagues[65] found that operative time and length of hospital stay were decreased for patients who had arthroplasty performed after bariatric surgery with similar rates of early complications and late reinterventions.

There are potential advantages to performing bariatric surgery prior to TJA other than postoperative outcomes, such as potential increased access to care and decreased costs. Many rural facilities refer patients with obesity to tertiary medical centers to undergo TJA. This requires increased transportation costs and difficulty with follow-up. If patients with osteoarthritis are able to lose weight with bariatric surgery, they may be able to undergo TJA at an institution closer to home, improving access to care and eliminating some of the complexities of follow-up.[58] A study by Springer and colleagues found that a majority of patients with BMI greater than 40 kg/m^2 and end-stage osteoarthritis who are required to lose weight prior to TJA are most likely to remain morbidly obese and never undergo TJA.[58] Only 20% of the 289 patients in this study underwent bariatric surgery, suggesting that increasing the availability of resources and coordinated care could facilitate patients' weight loss and treatment of their osteoarthritis.[66]

There also are studies that have found worse TJA outcomes after bariatric surgery. Martin and colleagues utilized the Mayo Clinic Joint Registry to find that patients who underwent bariatric surgery prior to TKA had an increased risk of reoperation compared with patients with a similar prebariatric surgery BMI, although there were no differences in rates of complications, revisional surgery, or periprosthetic joint infection.[67] The most common reason for reoperation in this group was for limitation of movement, which was treated with manipulation under general anesthesia. It may be that these patients were candidates for such manipulation, whereas other patients with a higher BMI were not and remained with limited mobility. Another possibility, however, could be poorer healing in patients after bariatric surgery due to protein malnutrition or vitamin deficiencies.[67] Nickel and colleagues[68] analyzed 39,014 patients from the Medicare database in a similar study to compare patients with obesity who underwent bariatric surgery prior to TJA to both morbidly obese patients and normal weight patients who did not have prior bariatric surgery. Because the group of patients who had bariatric surgery prior to TJA in this study had significantly more comorbidities (including anemia, cardiovascular disease, pulmonary disease, liver disease, ulcers, polysubstance abuse, psychiatric disorders, and tobacco abuse) compared with the other groups, it is difficult to draw meaningful conclusions from this study, which did find higher medical and surgical complication rates in this group at 30-days', 90-days', and 2-years' follow-up.[68] Lee and colleagues[69] identified patients aged 65 years and older who had undergone THA or TKA from a sample from Medicare part B data, from 1999 to 2012, to evaluate the risks of multiple comorbidities, including having bariatric surgery up to 24 months prior, at 0.5 year, 1 year, 2 years, and 5 years postoperatively. Bariatric surgery prior to THA was not associated with an increased overall risk for revision but was associated with an increased risk for revision for periprosthetic infection. Patients undergoing TKA following bariatric surgery were at increased overall risk for revision but not at increased risk for revision for periprosthetic infection. Patients in the bariatric surgery group in this study were being compared with all patients who did not undergo bariatric surgery within the last 24 months. There was no comparison of comorbidities between these 2 groups, which makes drawing conclusions from this data difficult.[69]

Differences in timing between bariatric surgery and TJA may partially account for the mixed outcomes reported on patients who undergo bariatric surgery prior to TJA. Some studies have been done to try to identify the ideal time to perform TJA with respect to bariatric surgery. Severson and colleagues[70] found the best outcomes in patients who underwent TKA more than 2 years after bariatric surgery. These patients had shorter anesthesia time, total operative time, and tourniquet time compared with patients who underwent TKA prior to bariatric surgery or less than 2 years after bariatric surgery. There was no difference in 90-day complication rates and duration of hospital stay among the groups.[70] Schwarzkopf and colleagues[71] used the Healthcare Cost and Utilization Project California State Inpatient Database to identify patients who underwent TJA following bariatric surgery from 2007 to 2011. They found patients undergoing THA more than 6 months after bariatric surgery were significantly less likely to have a 90-day readmission compared with patients undergoing THA within 6 months of bariatric surgery.[71] Liu and colleagues[72] used the New York Statewide Planning and Research Cooperative System database to evaluate the effect of patients who underwent TKA less than 2 years after bariatric surgery compared with patients with morbid obesity and patients without morbid obesity undergoing TKA. They found bariatric surgery was not a risk factor for nonelective readmissions at 30-days', 90 days, or 1 year and that there was no difference in overall cost between patients with morbid obesity who did or did not undergo bariatric surgery.[72] Given these data, it is reasonable to wait until a patient has reached a stable weight (usually 6–24 months after bariatric surgery) to perform TJA.

A few studies have looked specifically at the costs of performing bariatric surgery prior to TJA. The results from these studies are also mixed. In a retrospective study from the Mayo Clinic, Kremers and colleagues[9] showed that for every 5-unit increase in BMI over 30 kg/m^2, hospitalization cost increased \$300 and \$650 for TKA and for revisional TKA, respectively. This was found despite adjusting for comorbidities and complications.[9] In a study by McLawhorn and colleagues,[73] the cost of performing bariatric surgery prior to TKA in patients with morbid obesity and osteoarthritis was compared with the cost of performing TKA alone in BMI-matched patients. Cost calculations included costs of treatment, complications, 90-day follow-up, and quality-adjusted life-years. This study determined that the extra cost per quality-adjusted life-year in the population with prior bariatric surgery was \$13,910, which the investigators deemed cost-effective.[73]

FUTURE PERSPECTIVES

There currently are no prospective or randomized controlled trials on the effect of bariatric surgery on TJA outcomes. Further research is required to determine the optimal timing for bariatric surgery relative to TJA, the ideal metabolic surgical procedure for patients with osteoarthritis, the percentage of morbidly obese patients who may avoid TJA after having bariatric surgery, and the effect of increased mobility and exercise capability on patients with osteoarthritis after bariatric surgery.

The Surgical Weight-Loss to Improve Functional Status Trajectories Following Total Knee Arthroplasty (NCT02598531) trial is the first prospective, controlled, multicenter trial comparing TKA outcomes between in patients with severe obesity who undergo TKA with and without prior bariatric surgery. This trial currently is recruiting patients.[74]

CLINICS CARE POINTS

- Osteoarthritis is a common comorbidity in patients with obesity.
- Obesity contributes to the development and progression of osteoarthritis due to structural/mechanical factor as well as to changes in the proinflammatory hormonal milieu caused by metabolic syndrome.
- Although there is no consensus on the timing of bariatric surgery relative to TJA in the obese population, several studies suggest benefit to weight loss prior to TJA.

DISCLOSURE

The authors gratefully acknowledge grant support provided by the Foundation for Surgical Fellowships for the Minimally Invasive Bariatric Surgery and Advanced Laparoscopy Fellowship.

REFERENCES

1. Hootman JM, Helmick CG, Barbour KE, et al. Updated projected prevalence of self-reported doctor-diagnosed arthritis and arthritis-attributable activity limitation among US adults, 2015-2040. Arthritis Rheumatol 2016;68(7):1582–7.
2. Guccione AA, Felson DT, Anderson JJ, et al. The effects of specific medical conditions on the functional limitations of elders in the Framingham Study. Am J Public Health 1994;84(3):351–8.

3. Teichtahl AJ, Wluka AE, Wang Y, et al. Obesity and adiposity are associated with the rate of patella cartilage volume loss over 2 years in adults without knee osteoarthritis. Ann Rheum Dis 2009;68(6):909–13.

4. Gu A, Cohen JS, Malahias MA, et al. The effect of bariatric surgery prior to lower-extremity total joint arthroplasty: a systematic review. HSS J 2019;15(2):190–200.

5. Toivanen AT, Heliovaara M, Impivaara O, et al. Obesity, physically demanding work and traumatic knee injury are major risk factors for knee osteoarthritis–a population-based study with a follow-up of 22 years. Rheumatology (Oxford) 2010;49(2):308–14.

6. Koonce RC, Bravman JT. Obesity and osteoarthritis: more than just wear and tear. J Am Acad Orthop Surg 2013;21(3):161–9.

7. Belmont PJ Jr, Goodman GP, Waterman BR, et al. Thirty-day postoperative complications and mortality following total knee arthroplasty: incidence and risk factors among a national sample of 15,321 patients. J Bone Joint Surg Am 2014; 96(1):20–6.

8. Fehring TK, Odum SM, Griffin WL, et al. The obesity epidemic: its effect on total joint arthroplasty. J Arthroplasty 2007;22(6 Suppl 2):71–6.

9. Kremers HM, Visscher SL, Kremers WK, et al. The effect of obesity on direct medical costs in total knee arthroplasty. J Bone Joint Surg Am 2014;96(9):718–24.

10. Salih S, Sutton P. Obesity, knee osteoarthritis and knee arthroplasty: a review. BMC Sports Sci Med Rehabil 2013;5(1):25.

11. Workgroup of the American Association of Hip and Knee Surgeons Evidence Based Committee. Obesity and total joint arthroplasty: a literature based review. J Arthroplasty 2013;28(5):714–21.

12. Torgerson JS, Sjostrom L. The Swedish Obese Subjects (SOS) study–rationale and results. Int J Obes Relat Metab Disord 2001;25(Suppl 1):S2–4.

13. Centers for Disease Control and Prevention. Arthritis-related statistics. U.S. Department of Health & Human Services; 2018. Available at: https://www.cdc.gov/arthritis/data_statistics/arthritis-related-stats.htm. Accessed December 20, 2019.

14. Flugsrud GB, Nordsletten L, Espehaug B, et al. Risk factors for total hip replacement due to primary osteoarthritis: a cohort study in 50,034 persons. Arthritis Rheum 2002;46(3):675–82.

15. Manninen P, Riihimaki H, Heliovaara M, et al. Overweight, gender and knee osteoarthritis. Int J Obes Relat Metab Disord 1996;20(6):595–7.

16. Bergmann G, Deuretzbacher G, Heller M, et al. Hip contact forces and gait patterns from routine activities. J Biomech 2001;34(7):859–71.

17. Taylor WR, Heller MO, Bergmann G, et al. Tibio-femoral loading during human gait and stair climbing. J Orthop Res 2004;22(3):625–32.

18. Runhaar J, Koes BW, Clockaerts S, et al. A systematic review on changed biomechanics of lower extremities in obese individuals: a possible role in development of osteoarthritis. Obes Rev 2011;12(12):1071–82.

19. Maly MR, Costigan PA, Olney SJ. Contribution of psychosocial and mechanical variables to physical performance measures in knee osteoarthritis. Phys Ther 2005;85(12):1318–28.

20. Mundermann A, Dyrby CO, Andriacchi TP. Secondary gait changes in patients with medial compartment knee osteoarthritis: increased load at the ankle, knee, and hip during walking. Arthritis Rheum 2005;52(9):2835–44.

21. Rejeski WJ, Craven T, Ettinger WH Jr, et al. Self-efficacy and pain in disability with osteoarthritis of the knee. J Gerontol B Psychol Sci Soc Sci 1996;51(1):P24–9.

22. Sowers MR, Karvonen-Gutierrez CA. The evolving role of obesity in knee osteo-arthritis. Curr Opin Rheumatol 2010;22(5):533–7.
23. Long H, Xie D, Zeng C, et al. Association between body composition and osteo-arthritis: A systematic review and meta-analysis. Int J Rheum Dis 2019;22(12): 2108–18.
24. Francisco V, Pino J, Campos-Cabaleiro V, et al. Obesity, fat mass and immune system: role for leptin. Front Physiol 2018;9:640.
25. Francisco V, Perez T, Pino J, et al. Biomechanics, obesity, and osteoarthritis. The role of adipokines: When the levee breaks. J Orthop Res 2018;36(2):594–604.
26. Dumond H, Presle N, Terlain B, et al. Evidence for a key role of leptin in osteoar-thritis. Arthritis Rheum 2003;48(11):3118–29.
27. Simopoulou T, Malizos KN, Iliopoulos D, et al. Differential expression of leptin and leptin's receptor isoform (Ob-Rb) mRNA between advanced and minimally affected osteoarthritic cartilage; effect on cartilage metabolism. Osteoarthritis Cartilage 2007;15(8):872–83.
28. Andersen RE, Crespo CJ, Bartlett SJ, et al. Relationship between body weight gain and significant knee, hip, and back pain in older Americans. Obes Res 2003;11(10):1159–62.
29. Dorr LD, Boiardo RA. Technical considerations in total knee arthroplasty. Clin Or-thop Relat Res 1986;205:5–11.
30. Jarvenpaa J, Kettunen J, Kroger H, et al. Obesity may impair the early outcome of total knee arthroplasty. Scand J Surg 2010;99(1):45–9.
31. Nunez M, Lozano L, Nunez E, et al. Good quality of life in severely obese total knee replacement patients: a case-control study. Obes Surg 2011;21(8):1203–8.
32. Jamsen E, Nevalainen P, Eskelinen A, et al. Obesity, diabetes, and preoperative hyperglycemia as predictors of periprosthetic joint infection: a single-center anal-ysis of 7181 primary hip and knee replacements for osteoarthritis. J Bone Joint Surg Am 2012;94(14):e101.
33. Bozic KJ, Lau E, Kurtz S, et al. Patient-related risk factors for periprosthetic joint infection and postoperative mortality following total hip arthroplasty in Medicare patients. J Bone Joint Surg Am 2012;94(9):794–800.
34. Mantilla CB, Horlocker TT, Schroeder DR, et al. Risk factors for clinically relevant pulmonary embolism and deep venous thrombosis in patients undergoing pri-mary hip or knee arthroplasty. Anesthesiology 2003;99(3):552–60 [discussion: 555A].
35. Chee YH, Teoh KH, Sabnis BM, et al. Total hip replacement in morbidly obese pa-tients with osteoarthritis: results of a prospectively matched study. J Bone Joint Surg Br 2010;92(8):1066–71.
36. Foran JR, Mont MA, Rajadhyaksha AD, et al. Total knee arthroplasty in obese pa-tients: a comparison with a matched control group. J Arthroplasty 2004;19(7): 817–24.
37. Vincent HK, Vincent KR. Obesity and inpatient rehabilitation outcomes following knee arthroplasty: a multicenter study. Obesity (Silver Spring) 2008;16(1):130–6.
38. Abdel MP, Bonadurer GF 3rd, Jennings MT, et al. Increased Aseptic Tibial Fail-ures in Patients With a BMI >/=35 and well-aligned total knee arthroplasties. J Arthroplasty 2015;30(12):2181–4.
39. Kerkhoffs GM, Servien E, Dunn W, et al. The influence of obesity on the compli-cation rate and outcome of total knee arthroplasty: a meta-analysis and system-atic literature review. J Bone Joint Surg Am 2012;94(20):1839–44.

40. Watts CD, Houdek MT, Wagner ER, et al. Morbidly obese vs nonobese aseptic revision total hip arthroplasty: surprisingly similar outcomes. J Arthroplasty 2016;31(4):842–5.
41. Barrett M, Prasad A, Boyce L, et al. Total hip arthroplasty outcomes in morbidly obese patients: A systematic review. EFORT Open Rev 2018;3(9):507–12.
42. Pozzobon D, Ferreira PH, Blyth FM, et al. Can obesity and physical activity predict outcomes of elective knee or hip surgery due to osteoarthritis? A meta-analysis of cohort studies. BMJ Open 2018;8(2):e017689.
43. Chu IJH, Lim AYT, Ng CLW. Effects of meaningful weight loss beyond symptomatic relief in adults with knee osteoarthritis and obesity: a systematic review and meta-analysis. Obes Rev 2018;19(11):1597–607.
44. Felson DT, Anderson JJ, Naimark A, et al. Obesity and knee osteoarthritis. The Framingham Study. Ann Intern Med 1988;109(1):18–24.
45. Groen VA, van de Graaf VA, Scholtes VA, et al. Effects of bariatric surgery for knee complaints in (morbidly) obese adult patients: a systematic review. Obes Rev 2015;16(2):161–70.
46. Abu-Abeid S, Wishnitzer N, Szold A, et al. The influence of surgically-induced weight loss on the knee joint. Obes Surg 2005;15(10):1437–42.
47. Hooper MM, Stellato TA, Hallowell PT, et al. Musculoskeletal findings in obese subjects before and after weight loss following bariatric surgery. Int J Obes (Lond) 2007;31(1):114–20.
48. Peltonen M, Lindroos AK, Torgerson JS. Musculoskeletal pain in the obese: a comparison with a general population and long-term changes after conventional and surgical obesity treatment. Pain 2003;104(3):549–57.
49. Nelson LG, Lopez PP, Haines K, et al. Outcomes of bariatric surgery in patients > or =65 years. Surg Obes Relat Dis 2006;2(3):384–8.
50. Moon Han S, Kim WW, Oh JH. Results of laparoscopic sleeve gastrectomy (LSG) at 1 year in morbidly obese Korean patients. Obes Surg 2005;15(10):1469–75.
51. Ponta ML, Gozza M, Giacinto J, et al. Effects of obesity on posture and walking: study prior to and following surgically induced weight loss. Obes Surg 2014;24(11):1915–20.
52. Bragge T, Lyytinen T, Hakkarainen M, et al. Lower impulsive loadings following intensive weight loss after bariatric surgery in level and stair walking: a preliminary study. Knee 2014;21(2):534–40.
53. Hortobagyi T, Herring C, Pories WJ, et al. Massive weight loss-induced mechanical plasticity in obese gait. J Appl Physiol (1985) 2011;111(5):1391–9.
54. Chen SX, Bomfim FA, Youn HA, et al. Predictors of the effect of bariatric surgery on knee osteoarthritis pain. Semin Arthritis Rheum 2018;48(2):162–7.
55. Vartiainen P, Bragge T, Lyytinen T, et al. Kinematic and kinetic changes in obese gait in bariatric surgery-induced weight loss. J Biomech 2012;45(10):1769–74.
56. Vincent HK, Ben-David K, Conrad BP, et al. Rapid changes in gait, musculoskeletal pain, and quality of life after bariatric surgery. Surg Obes Relat Dis 2012;8(3):346–54.
57. Trofa D, Smith EL, Shah V, et al. Total weight loss associated with increased physical activity after bariatric surgery may increase the need for total joint arthroplasty. Surg Obes Relat Dis 2014;10(2):335–9.
58. Springer BD, Carter JT, McLawhorn AS, et al. Obesity and the role of bariatric surgery in the surgical management of osteoarthritis of the hip and knee: a review of the literature. Surg Obes Relat Dis 2017;13(1):111–8.

59. Stavrakis AI, Khoshbin A, McLawhorn AS, et al. Bariatric surgery prior to total joint arthroplasty, does it decrease the risk of obesity related perioperative complications? Curr Rheumatol Rep 2018;20(2):7.

60. Smith TO, Aboelmagd T, Hing CB, et al. Does bariatric surgery prior to total hip or knee arthroplasty reduce post-operative complications and improve clinical outcomes for obese patients? Systematic review and meta-analysis. Bone Joint J 2016;98-B(9):1160–6.

61. Werner BC, Kurkis GM, Gwathmey FW, et al. Bariatric surgery prior to total knee arthroplasty is associated with fewer postoperative complications. J Arthroplasty 2015;30(9 Suppl):81–5.

62. McLawhorn AS, Levack AE, Lee YY, et al. Bariatric surgery improves outcomes after lower extremity arthroplasty in the morbidly obese: A propensity score-matched analysis of a New York Statewide Database. J Arthroplasty 2018; 33(7):2062–9.e4.

63. Watts CD, Martin JR, Houdek MT, et al. Prior bariatric surgery may decrease the rate of re-operation and revision following total hip arthroplasty. Bone Joint J 2016;98-B(9):1180–4.

64. Kulkarni A, Jameson SS, James P, et al. Does bariatric surgery prior to lower limb joint replacement reduce complications? Surgeon 2011;9(1):18–21.

65. Nearing EE 2nd, Santos TM, Topolski MS, et al. Benefits of bariatric surgery before elective total joint arthroplasty: is there a role for weight loss optimization? Surg Obes Relat Dis 2017;13(3):457–62.

66. Giori NJ, Amanatullah DF, Gupta S, et al. Risk reduction compared with access to care: quantifying the trade-off of enforcing a body mass index eligibility criterion for joint replacement. J Bone Joint Surg Am 2018;100(7):539–45.

67. Martin JR, Watts CD, Taunton MJ. Bariatric surgery does not improve outcomes in patients undergoing primary total knee arthroplasty. Bone Joint J 2015;97-B(11): 1501–5.

68. Nickel BT, Klement MR, Penrose CT, et al. Lingering risk: bariatric surgery before total knee arthroplasty. J Arthroplasty 2016;31(9 Suppl):207–11.

69. Lee GC, Ong K, Baykal D, et al. Does prior bariatric surgery affect implant survivorship and complications following primary total hip arthroplasty/total knee arthroplasty? J Arthroplasty 2018;33(7):2070–4.e1.

70. Severson EP, Singh JA, Browne JA, et al. Total knee arthroplasty in morbidly obese patients treated with bariatric surgery: a comparative study. J Arthroplasty 2012;27(9):1696–700.

71. Schwarzkopf R, Lavery JA, Hooper J, et al. Bariatric surgery and time to total joint arthroplasty: does it affect readmission and complication rates? Obes Surg 2018; 28(5):1395–401.

72. Liu JX, Paoli AR, Mahure SA, et al. Preoperative bariatric surgery and the risk of readmission following total joint replacement. Orthopedics 2018;41(2):107–14.

73. McLawhorn AS, Southren D, Wang YC, et al. Cost-effectiveness of bariatric surgery prior to total knee arthroplasty in the morbidly obese: a computer model-based evaluation. J Bone Joint Surg Am 2016;98(2):e6.

74. Surgical Weight-Loss to Improve Functional Status Trajectories Following Total Knee Arthroplasty (SWIFT Trial). 2019. Available at: https://clinicaltrials.gov/ct2/show/NCT02598531. Accessed December 25, 2019.

Ventral Hernia Management in Obese Patients

Diana E. Peterman, MD, Jeremy A. Warren, MD*

KEYWORDS

- Ventral hernia repair • Ventral hernia repair in obesity • Preoperative weight loss
- Neoadjuvant bariatric surgery

KEY POINTS

- Obesity increases the risk for elective open ventral hernia repair.
- Preoperative weight loss, by medical or surgical means, is ideal before proceeding with ventral hernia repair, although is not achievable by many patients.
- The risk of incarceration while awaiting weight loss must be considered, because outcomes for emergency hernia repair are significantly worse than elective hernia repair.
- Significant delay in ventral hernia repair while awaiting weight loss may have a negative impact on patient quality of life.
- Surgeon judgment and patient goals and expectations are key to tailoring the approach for ventral hernia repair in obese patients.

INTRODUCTION

The prevalence of obesity (body mass index [BMI] $\geq$30 kg/m^2) continues to increase in the United States, now accounting for 42.4% of adults, and severe obesity (BMI >40 kg/m^2) now stands at 9.2%.[1] There is a clear association between obesity and rate of primary ventral, inguinal, and incisional hernia formation. Regner and colleagues[2] reviewed the National Surgical Quality Improvement Program (NSQIP) data, finding that approximately 60% of 106,968 patients who underwent elective ventral hernia repair (VHR) were obese. Goodenough and colleagues[3] identified a BMI greater than or equal to 25 kg/m^2 as an independent predictor of incisional hernia. Lau and colleagues[4] identified a progressively increasing risk of ventral hernia (VH) formation with each BMI stratum: BMI 25 kg/m^2 to 29.9 kg/m^2, odds ratio (OR) 1.63; BMI 30 kg/m^2 to 39.9 kg/m^2, OR 2.62; 40 kg/m^2 to 49.9 kg/m^2, OR 3.91; and 50 kg/m^2 to 59.9 kg/m^2, OR 4.85. A similar study found that a BMI of greater than or equal to 30 kg/m^2 conferred nearly double the risk of VH.[5]

Department of Surgery, Division of Minimal Access & Bariatric Surgery, Prisma Health-Upstate, University of South Carolina School of Medicine Greenville, 701 Grove Road, ST 3, Greenville, SC 29607, USA
* Corresponding author.
E-mail address: Jeremy.warren@prismahealth.org

Surg Clin N Am 101 (2021) 307–321
https://doi.org/10.1016/j.suc.2020.12.014
0039-6109/21/© 2020 Elsevier Inc. All rights reserved.

Obesity negatively affects surgical outcomes after VHR and abdominal wall reconstruction (AWR) due to increased risk of surgical site infection (SSI) or surgical site occurrence (SSO), recurrence, and perioperative complications associated with obesity-related comorbidities, such as diabetes, cardiovascular disease, and sleep apnea. Although preoperative weight loss can ameliorate these risks, it often is difficult to achieve, potentially resulting in higher rates of emergency VHR in already complex, high-risk patients. The optimal algorithm for VHR in obese patients remains elusive. Recently published guidelines on bariatric and hernia surgery from the American Society for Metabolic and Bariatric Surgery cite 47 studies, of which only 1 was level 1b evidence, with the remainder level III or lower.[6] The risk of elective VHR varies greatly between repair techniques and must be weighed against patient quality of life (QOL), hernia-related symptoms, risk of incarceration, and the ability to achieve optimal weight loss prior to repair.

OUTCOMES OF VENTRAL HERNIA REPAIR IN OBESE PATIENTS

Numerous studies implicate obesity in perioperative complications, including higher intraoperative blood loss, prolonged operative time, cardiopulmonary complications, thromboembolic events, SSO, SSI, and incisional hernia formation or recurrence (Table 1).[7–9] Novitsky and colleagues[10] reported increased risk of wound events, pulmonary complications, myocardial infarction, shock, prolonged hospitalization, and nonroutine discharge to other facilities OR with home-health (as opposed to routine discharge to home) in obese patients after VHR. They strongly advocate for preoperative weight loss. A risk stratification system developed using NSQIP data found that a BMI of greater than 35 kg/m^2 confers nearly double the risk of SSO.[11] Pernar and colleagues[9] reported significantly higher postoperative wound complications in patients with BMI greater than or equal to 40 kg/m^2 undergoing open VHR (OVHR), suggesting these patients should undergo preemptive bariatric surgery (BS) to maximize weight loss prior. Anecdotally, many surgeons cite a BMI of 40 kg/m^2 to 45 kg/m^2 as a cutoff for offering elective VHR.

Obesity also likely increases the risk of hernia recurrence. In a follow-up analysis of a randomized controlled trial (RCT) comparing onlay, suture repair, and autograft VHR, Sauerland and colleagues[12] found that obesity was the strongest predictor of hernia recurrence, increasing with each unit of BMI. Kaminski[13] followed patients after gastric restrictive procedure and concurrent VHR, reporting hernia recurrence from 33% in patients still weighing greater than 250 lbs (113kg) compared with 5% in patients who achieved a weight of less than 200 lb. Lower hernia recurrence also was seen in patients with antecedent BS compared with a propensity score matched cohort of obese patients without prior BS (24% vs 6.7%, respectively).[14] In contrast, Giordano and colleagues[15] reported no increase in recurrence in patients after open AWR with component separation. Obesity was not an independent risk factor for recurrence for patients undergoing open retromuscular VHR (RMVHR) in data from the authors' institution.[16] Alizai and colleagues[17] showed no difference in recurrence between obese and nonobese patients (7.9% vs 7.0%, respectively) undergoing laparoscopic VHR (LVHR) or open sublay repair. In a review of 185 patients, Smolevitz and colleagues[18] found no difference in hernia recurrence or complication rates in patients with a BMI greater than or equal to 40 kg/m^2 compared with BMI less than 40 kg/m^2 who underwent elective OVHR with anterior component separation.

OPTIONS FOR VENTRAL HERNIA REPAIR

Differences in reported outcomes are due to disparate comparator groups, small single-institution studies, registry-based data that lack discrete data on hernia

Table 1
Effect of obesity on ventral hernia repair outcomes

Author (Year)	Body Mass Index (kg/m²)	N	Ventral Hernia Repair Technique	Surgical Site Infection (%)	Surgical Site Occurrence (%)	Hernia Recurrence (%)	Other Morbidity (%)
Fekkes et al,[23] 2015	<25	1481	OVHR (1,239)	6.3%	0.6%[a]	NR	NR
			LVHR (242)	1.2%	0%		
	25–30	2492	OVHR (1,960)	6.4%	0.6%		
			LVHR (532)	2.4%	0.2%		
	30–35	2136	OVHR (1,662)	7.8%	0.9%		
			LVHR (474)	3.7%	0.2%		
	35–40	1135	OVHR (858)	7.8%	1.1%		
			LVHR (277)	4.1%	0%		
	>40	987	OVHR (761)	11.9%	2.9%		
			LVHR (226)	4.8%	0.4%		
Regner et al,[2] 2015							Reported at least 1 complication
	20–25	5883	OVHR (5,883)	1.7%	NR	NR	2.7%
			LVHR (1,328)	0.5%			1%
	25–30	12,398	OVHR (12,398)	2.3%			3.2%
			LVHR (3,229)	0.8%			1.7%
	30–35	11,097	OVHR (11,097)	3.4%			4.4%
			LVHR (3,426)	1.2%			2.1%
	35–40	6215	OVHR (6,215)	5.0%			6.2%
			LVHR (2,212)	1.2%			1.8%
	≥40	5457	OVHR (5,457)	8.0%			9.6%
			LVHR (2,238)	2.1%			3.0%

(continued on next page)

Table 1
(continued)

Author (Year)	Body Mass Index (kg/m²)	N	Ventral Hernia Repair Technique	Surgical Site Infection (%)	Surgical Site Occurrence (%)	Hernia Recurrence (%)	Other Morbidity (%)
Alizai et al,[17] 2017							Morbidity not specified
	< 30	109	Lap IPOM (47)	2.8%	14.7%	7.9%	8.5%
			Open sublay (62)				32.5%
	≥ 30	69	Lap IPOM (41)	5.8%	30.4%	7.0%	22%
			Open sublay (28)				53.6%
Giordano et al,[15] 2017	< 30	235	Open underlay or sublay	11.1%[b]	14.9%	7.7%	NR
	30–35	140		16.3%	26.4%	11.4%	
	≥ 35	136		17.7%	36.8%	10.3%	

Abbreviation: NR, not reported.
[a] Wound disruption/dehiscence.
[b] Combined based on reported infection cellulitis, infection abscess, mesh infection.
Data from Refs.[2,15,17,23]

characteristics and surgical technique, and substantial differences in outcomes between surgical approach for VHR. Additionally, BMI may not be the only, or even the most important, metric for predicting complications in obese patients. Visceral adiposity, waist circumference, morphometric fat distribution, and waist-to-hip ratio may be more reliable predictors of complications.[6,19] For patients who do not have access to BS, are unsuccessful in achieving adequate weight loss, or with complex or highly symptomatic hernias, repair may be warranted despite obesity.

Laparoscopic Versus Open Ventral Hernia Repair

LVHR typically is performed via a transabdominal approach with placement of mesh in an intraperitoneal position (intraperitoneal onlay mesh [IPOM]), secured with tacks and/or sutures, with or without defect closure. Comparative studies consistently demonstrate lower SSI and other wound complications compared with OVHR, and LVHR generally is preferred for obese patients.[2,20–23] It is important to distinguish the repair techniques reported in these trials. Although LVHR technique is fairly uniform, OVHR outcomes can vary widely by approach. For example, Itani and colleagues[22] performed an RCT of open onlay versus LVHR, a trial that was terminated due to higher wound complications with open repair. Onlay mesh repair, however, is associated with the highest risk of wound complications of OVHR techniques due to disruption of the abdominal wall blood supply and extensive subcutaneous dissection.[24–26] For comparison, an RCT by Eker and colleagues[27] found no difference in wound complications or hernia recurrence between LVHR and open sublay VHR.

Although uncommon, intraperitoneal mesh does present the possibility of secondary mesh complications in the event of subsequent abdominal operations. In the authors' experience with management of mesh infections, approximately 40% of patients had an intervening abdominal operation, and infected intraperitoneal mesh almost universally requires explantation.[28] Additionally, large hernia defects are less amenable to LVHR, with higher risks of recurrence or mesh eventration and poor QOL.[20,29–31]

Open Abdominal Wall Reconstruction

Despite potential for higher complications, AWR with component separation can provide excellent functional outcomes.[32,33] The type of myofascial release performed is important. The Rives-Stoppa repair, properly considered a rectus abdominis myofascial release, is the basis for most AWR. Additional myofascial release can be achieved via an anterior approach and external oblique release (Ramirez component separation[34]), which carries significant wound morbidity due to disruption of the abdominal wall blood supply. Transversus abdominis release (TAR)[35] uses a posterior approach, resulting in significantly fewer wound complications compared with external oblique release while still providing significant advancement of the rectus abdominis for AWR.[33,36–38]

Robotic Ventral Hernia Repair

Robotic VHR provides an excellent alternative with promising early results. Robotic rRMVHR (rRMVHR), with or without TAR, facilitates AWR with extraperitoneal mesh placement by a minimally invasive approach. Retrospective comparison of rRMVHR to LVHR demonstrated similar rate of SSI with a shorter length of stay (LOS). Mean BMI in both groups was 35 kg/m^2.[39] Compared with open RMVHR, rRMVHR shortens the hospital LOS, also potentially lowering the rate of SSI. Again, the mean BMI in this study was class 1 obesity (33 kg/m^2).[40] The latest iteration of rRMVHR, the extended-view totally extraperitoneal,[41] approach is an especially attractive option and is the authors' preferred approach. The authors' experience with this approach in 178 patients with a mean BMI of 36.2 kg/m² resulted in SSI of 2.8%, mean LOS of 1 day, and 54% of cases performed as outpatient procedures (unpublished data, Warren JA, 2019). Review of the authors' entire robotic experience (n = 408) demonstrates similar outcomes for robotic VHR in patients with BMI greater than 40 (n = 114) to those with BMI less than 40 (n = 294): rate of SSI is 5.3% versus 3.7% (P = .490) and SSO is 58.8% versus 46.9% (P = .031), with almost all SSOs being seromas and more patients requiring percutaneous drainage in the lower BMI group (unpublished data). Current follow-up in the literature is too short to adequately assess recurrence from rRMVHR. Although not yet conclusive, this represents an excellent option for definitive AWR in obese patients, particularly when weight loss is not achievable.

PREOPERATIVE WEIGHT LOSS

Ideally, the risk posed by obesity can be mitigated by preoperative weight loss, with most recommending a BMI of less than 40 kg/m² prior to VHR.[9,42–45] Options for achieving optimal preoperative BMI include self-directed weight loss, medical weight loss through multidisciplinary approach, pharmacotherapy, endoscopic interventions, or surgical weight loss.

Medical Weight Loss

Patient counseling on weight loss alone is insufficient. Ssentongo and colleagues[44] found this approach failed to produce significant weight loss, with increase in BMI in 19% of patients prior to surgery. Multidisciplinary programs are more successful. Rosen and colleagues[45] used a protein-sparing modified fast in collaboration with medical weight loss specialist, resulting in significant weight loss and decrease in BMI of 9 kg/m² over an average of 17 months. Chan and colleagues[46] reported a 12% BMI reduction in patients undergoing VHR after participation in a program limiting intake to 1500 calories per day. In an RCT of obese VH patients randomized to prehabilitation with targeted nutritional education and physical therapy versus standard patient counseling, Liang and colleagues[47] saw a trend toward greater weight loss with prehabilitation but a higher rate of dropout, potentially due to greater time commitment. There was a trend toward lower wound complications in prehabilitation patients and in those achieving weight loss by either method, but this was not statistically significant.[47] Finally, pharmacotherapy for obesity can achieve a 5% to 10% weight reduction at 1 year. This approach is time intensive and minimally effective and carries a high attrition rate of up to 40% due to adverse events or side-effects.[48,49]

Surgical Weight Loss

Unequivocally, surgical weight loss is superior to medical management in achieving sustained weight loss and remission or improvement in comorbid disease.[50,51] Neoadjuvant BS can reduce the risk of hernia recurrence, wound complications, and medical morbidity.[14,52] When performing BS in the presence of a VH, management of the hernia defect is an important consideration. Eid and colleagues[53] reported 37.5% of patients receiving BS with deferred VHR presented with small bowel obstruction due to incarceration, leading them to recommend concurrent repair with absorbable/biologic mesh. Subsequent study suggested a tailored approach, leaving chronically incarcerated omentum in situ to effectively prevent incarceration, primary closure for smaller defects, or permanent mesh repair for larger defects.[54]

RISK OF DEFERRED VENTRAL HERNIA REPAIR

Unfortunately, not all patients have access to or willingness to receive BS, or to delay VHR, to achieve weight loss prior to repair.[55] Delays of up to 18 months may be needed for patients to have BS and reach optimal weight loss, and nonsurgical weight loss may take even longer. This delay can have an impact on patient QOL and carries a risk of incarceration, necessitating emergency VHR in an already high-risk population. These factors must be considered.

Presence of a VH has a negative impact on QOL as measured by several functional parameters, and VHR results in significant improvement in patient satisfaction.[32,33,56–59] Additionally, there is a risk of incarceration during the period of watchful waiting (WW). In the study by Liang and colleagues,[47] 4 patients (6.8%) in the prehabilitation group presented with incarceration requiring emergency VHR. Kokotovic and colleagues[60] emergency repair at 4% over 5 years, with a crossover rate from WW to elective repair of 19% for incisional hernias. Verhelst and colleagues[61] compared 255 patients with VHR (n = 151) versus WW (n = 104). Crossover from WW to VHR was 33%, 24% (7.6% of total WW group) of whom required emergent VHR. Patients in the crossover group had a higher incidence of intraoperative bowel perforation (13%), enterocutaneous fistula (7%), and mortality (5.8%) than those that received operative treatment initially.[61]

RISK OF EMERGENCY VENTRAL HERNIA REPAIR

Emergent VHR is associated with higher mortality, increased risk of bowel resection, longer LOS, higher rate of readmission and reoperation, and increased SSI compared with elective repair, and morbidity is higher still in obese patients.[62,63] Repair without mesh is more likely with emergency VHR, increasing recurrence risk.[62] In an NSQIP study of 39,822 VHR patients, 56% of all patients were obese. Emergency VHR was required in 7.4% of patients, of whom 68.9% were obese, with BMI greater than 40 kg/m^2 conferring a 3-times higher risk of requiring emergent repair. Emergent VHR is less likely to utilize mesh; increases risk of SSI, return to the operating room, dehiscence, and mortality; and doubles the overall surgical complications in obese patients.[64]

Hernia characteristics help predict the risk of incarceration. Review of the Danish Hernia Database revealed female gender, older age, umbilical hernia defects between 2 cm and 7 cm, and incisional hernia defects up to 7 cm increased risk of emergency VHR.[63] Fueter and colleagues[65] compared the hernia sac to defect diameters, the hernia-neck ratio (HNR), as a predictor of incarceration. An HNR greater than or equal to 2.5 was associated with a 53-fold increase risk of complications, and patients presenting with incarceration had a significantly larger HNR (3.33 vs 1.76, respectively), concluding that WW may not be appropriate for these patients.[65]

Finally, there is a risk of progression of hernia complexity while awaiting VHR. Jensen and colleagues[66] followed 35 patients with incisional hernia for an average of 30 weeks between initial assessment and VHR. During this time, the median defect area increased significantly from 117.3 cm^2 to 150.4 cm^2. For already large hernias, this may increase the risk of complications during subsequent VHR and may result in suboptimal repair if fascial closure is not achievable. These studies question the wisdom of mandated preoperative weight loss in all patients, suggesting a more tailored approach is warranted.

Table 2
Outcomes of concurrent bariatric surgery and ventral hernia repair

Author (Year)	N	Bariatric Procedure	Ventral Hernia Repair Technique	Reoperation	Morbidity	Surgical site infection	Recurrence
Spaniolas et al,[75] 2015	503	RYGB (433) SG (70)	NR	3.5% 2.9%	8.3% 8.6%	5.1% 1.4%	NR
Khorgami et al,[76] 2017	988	RYGB (544) SG (444)	OVHR (322) or LVHR (666)	24 (4.4%) 9 (2%)	36 (6.6%) 12 (2.7%)	17 (1.7%)	NR
		RYGB (544) SG (444)	None	6 (1.1%) 0 (0%)	16 (2.9%) 11 (2.5%)	18 (1.8%)	
Sharma et al,[70] 2017	159	RYGB (105) SG (50) AGB (4)	Primary (115) Mesh (44)	NR	10 (8.7%) 10 (22.7%)	NR	28 14
Krivan et al,[73] 2019	106	RYGB or SG	LVHR (59) OVHR (47)	NR	NR	1 (1.7%) 5 (10.6%)	5 (8.5%) 7 (14.9%)

Abbreviations: AGB, adjustable gastric band; NR, not reported; RYGBP, Roux-en-Y gastric bypass; SG, sleeve gastrectomy.
Data from Refs.[68,71,73,74]

CONCURRENT VENTRAL HERNIA REPAIR AND BARIATRIC SURGERY

Presented with the risks of elective VHR or WW in obese patients, VHR at the time of BS is an attractive option. Several studies indicate this is safe and effective (**Table 2**).[53,54,67–70] Krivan and colleagues[71] reported hernia recurrence of 11.3% in their population of concurrent BS with VHR, comparable to nonbariatric patients (12.7%), with low wound morbidity. A recent systematic review demonstrated VH recurrence after concurrent VHR and BS was just 1.1% with synthetic mesh repair, 14.3% with biologic mesh repair, and 25.7% with suture repair and no increase in 30-day wound morbidity.[72] Spaniolas and colleagues[73] identified 503 NSQIP patients that underwent laparoscopic BS with VHR, finding a higher risk of SSI but no difference in overall morbidity. Conversely, Khorgami and colleagues,[74] also using NSQIP data, showed concomitant VHR and laparoscopic BS had an increased 30-day morbidity regardless of the type of bariatric procedure or method of VHR. Propensity-matched data from the Metabolic and Bariatric Surgery Accreditation and Quality Improvement Program (MBSAQIP) compared laparoscopic BS with and without concomitant VHR, finding that concurrent VHR had a higher risk of major complications (5.8% vs 3.8%, respectively) with no difference in mortality.[75]

NSQIP and MBSAQIP data cannot account for specifics of VHR technique, morphology of the hernia, or long-term outcomes. The major concern with concurrent BS and VHR is the potential for intraperitoneal mesh complications when placed during clean-contaminated procedures. Risk of mesh infection is low, but intraperitoneal mesh is more likely than extraperitoneal mesh to require removal in the event of infection.[28] Patients with large, complex hernias not amenable to standard laparoscopic repair probably should be staged, because the risk of concurrent OVHR with open or laparoscopic BS can affect the outcomes of both the bariatric procedure and VHR, and incarceration risk is relatively lower.

HERNIA PREVENTION

Morbidity associated with VH has led many to advocate hernia prevention during laparotomy. Small-bite laparotomy closure (5-mm bites, 5-mm advance using a 2–0 slowly absorbable suture) reduces the risk of incisional hernia from 21% to 13%.[76] Several studies demonstrate the safety and efficacy of prophylactic mesh placement at the time of laparotomy closure in high-risk patients, significantly

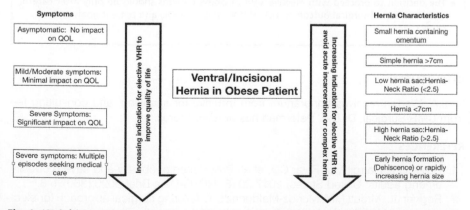

Fig. 1. Weighing patient symptoms and hernia characteristics for clinical decision making in obese patients with VH.

reducing the incidence of incisional hernia.[77–80] Meta-analysis shows an 85% risk reduction in incisional hernia with prophylactic mesh placement in at-risk patients undergoing midline laparotomy with comparable risk of complications.[77] Cost-utility analysis demonstrated that prophylactic mesh augmentation in high risk patients is more cost effective than primary suture closure.[5] Despite data supporting prophylactic mesh, most US surgeons are reluctant to adopt this practice due to perceived risk of mesh-related complications, unfamiliarity with technique, perceived poor generalizability to their patient population, and lack of reimbursement.[81,82]

SUMMARY

Obese patients with VH present a complex clinical scenario in which the ideal treatment, namely preoperative weight loss, may not be feasible or safe. Based on the available evidence and personal experience in a high-volume hernia practice in which 13% of patients have a BMI greater than or equal to 40 kg/m^2, VHR can be offered to patients that are ineligible for BS, are highly symptomatic, or have a hernia morphology that portends higher potential risk for incarceration (**Fig. 1**). Robotic VHR is preferred when possible, which can mitigate the risk of wound complications while still accomplishing complete AWR, providing excellent functional outcomes and acceptable risk of hernia recurrence. For patients with minimal symptoms, weight loss always is encouraged, and patients routinely are referred for medical or surgical weight loss with close follow-up to monitor their weight, hernia anatomy, and symptoms. Ultimately, the art of medicine must prevail through careful consideration of risk versus benefit and careful alignment of patient expectations with realistic outcomes.

CLINICS CARE POINTS

- Outcomes of VHR in obese patients is suboptimal, primarily due to higher rates of wound complications.
- Preoperative weight loss does improve outcomes of elective VHR but may come at the expense of poor QOL and the risk of acute incarceration while awaiting adequate weight loss.
- When considering elective VHR in obese patients, minimally invasive approach is preferred, and robotic AWR may represent an ideal solution.
- The decision to proceed with elective VHR in obese patients should be only after careful consideration of surgical outcomes, risk of WW, patient QOL, and patient goals and expectations,

DISCLOSURES

Dr J.A. Warren receives honorarium from Intuitive for speaking, and consulting fee from CMR Surgical. Dr D.E. Peterman has no disclosures.

REFERENCES

1. Hales CM, Carroll MD, Fryar CD, et al. Prevalence of obesity and severe obesity among adults: United States, 2017-2018. NCHS Data Brief 2020;(360):1–8.
2. Regner JL, Mrdutt MM, Munoz-Maldonado Y. Tailoring surgical approach for elective ventral hernia repair based on obesity and national surgical quality improvement program outcomes. Am J Surg 2015;210(6):1024–9, discussion1029–30.

3. Goodenough CJ, Ko TC, Kao LS, et al. Development and validation of a risk stratification score for ventral incisional hernia after abdominal surgery: hernia expectation rates in intra-abdominal surgery (the HERNIA Project). J Am Coll Surg 2015;220(4):405–13.

4. Lau B, Kim H, Haigh PI, et al. Obesity increases the odds of acquiring and incarcerating noninguinal abdominal wall hernias. Am Surg 2020;78(10):1118–21.

5. Fischer JP, Basta MN, Mirzabeigi MN, et al. A risk model and cost analysis of incisional hernia after elective, abdominal surgery based upon 12,373 cases: the case for targeted prophylactic intervention. Ann Surg 2015;263(5):1010–7.

6. Menzo EL, Hinojosa M, Carbonell A, et al. American society for metabolic and bariatric surgery and american hernia society consensus guideline on bariatric surgery and hernia surgery. Surg Obes Relat Dis 2018;14(9):1221–32.

7. Tjeertes EKM, Tjeertes EEKM, Hoeks SE, et al. Obesity–a risk factor for postoperative complications in general surgery? BMC Anesthesiol 2015;15(1):112–7.

8. Owei L, Swendiman RA, Torres-Landa S, et al. Impact of body mass index on minimally invasive ventral hernia repair: an ACS-NSQIP analysis. Hernia 2019; 23(5):899–907.

9. Pernar LIM, Pernar CH, Dieffenbach BV, et al. What is the BMI threshold for open ventral hernia repair? Surg Endosc 2017;31(3):1311–7.

10. Novitsky YW, Orenstein SB. Effect of patient and hospital characteristics on outcomes of elective ventral hernia repair in the United States. Hernia 2013;17(5): 639–45.

11. Fischer JP, Wink JD, Tuggle CT, et al. Wound risk assessment in ventral hernia repair: generation and internal validation of a risk stratification system using the ACS-NSQIP. Hernia 2015;19(1):103–11.

12. Sauerland S, Korenkov M, Kleinen T, et al. Obesity is a risk factor for recurrence after incisional hernia repair. Hernia 2004;8(1):42–6.

13. Kaminski DL. The role of gastric restrictive procedures in treating ventral hernias in morbidly obese patients. Int J Surg Investig 2000;2(2):159–64.

14. Chandeze M-M, Moszkowicz D, Beauchet A, et al. Ventral hernia surgery in morbidly obese patients, immediate or after bariatric surgery preparation: Results of a case-matched study. Surg Obes Relat Dis 2019;15(1):83–8.

15. Giordano SA, Garvey PB, Baumann DP, et al. The impact of body mass index on abdominal wall reconstruction outcomes: a comparative study. Plast Reconstr Surg 2017;139(5):1234–44.

16. Cobb WS, Warren JA, Ewing JA, et al. Open retromuscular mesh repair of complex incisional hernia: predictors of wound events and recurrence. J Am Coll Surg 2015;220(4):606–13.

17. Alizai PH, Andert A, Lelaona E, et al. Impact of obesity on postoperative complications after laparoscopic and open incisional hernia repair - a prospective cohort study. Int J Surg 2017;48:220–4.

18. Smolevitz J, Jacobson R, Thaqi M, et al. Outcomes in complex ventral hernia repair with anterior component separation in class III obesity patients. Am J Surg 2018;215(3):458–61.

19. Aquina CT, Rickles AS, Probst CP, et al. Visceral obesity, not elevated BMI, is strongly associated with incisional hernia after colorectal surgery. Dis Colon Rectum 2015;58(2):220–7.

20. Bittner R, Bain K, Bansal VK, et al. Update of Guidelines for laparoscopic treatment of ventral and incisional abdominal wall hernias (International Endohernia Society (IEHS))-Part A. Surg Endosc 2019;33(10):3069–139.

21. Warren JA, Love M. Incisional hernia repair: minimally invasive approaches. Surg Clin North Am 2018;98(3):537–59.
22. Itani KMF, Hur K, Kim LT, et al. Comparison of laparoscopic and open repair with mesh for the treatment of ventral incisional hernia: a randomized trial. Arch Surg 2010;145(4):322–8, discussion328.
23. Fekkes JF, Velanovich V. Amelioration of the effects of obesity on short-term postoperative complications of laparoscopic and open ventral hernia repair. Surg Laparosc Endosc Percutan Tech 2015;25(2):151–7.
24. Timmermans L, de Goede B, van Dijk SM, et al. Meta-analysis of sublay versus onlay mesh repair in incisional hernia surgery. Am J Surg 2014;207(6):980–8.
25. Venclauskas L, Maleckas A, Kiudelis M. One-year follow-up after incisional hernia treatment: results of a prospective randomized study. Hernia 2010;14(6):575–82.
26. Albino FP, Patel KM, Nahabedian MY, et al. Does mesh location matter in abdominal wall reconstruction? A systematic review of the literature and a summary of recommendations. Plast Reconstr Surg 2013;132(5):1295–304.
27. Eker HH, Hansson BME, Buunen M, et al. Laparoscopic vs. open incisional hernia repair: a randomized clinical trial. JAMA Surg 2013;148(3):259–63.
28. Warren JA, Love M, Cobb WS, et al. Factors affecting salvage rate of infected prosthetic mesh. Am J Surg 2020. https://doi.org/10.1016/j.amjsurg.2020.01.028.
29. Nardi M, Millo P, Brachet Contul R, et al. Laparoscopic ventral hernia repair with composite mesh: analysis of risk factors for recurrence in 185 patients with 5 years follow-up. Int J Surg 2017;40:38–44.
30. Carter SA, Hicks SC, Brahmbhatt R, et al. Recurrence and pseudorecurrence after laparoscopic ventral hernia repair: predictors and patient-focused outcomes. Am Surg 2014;80(2):138–48.
31. Liang MK, Clapp M, Li LT, et al. Patient Satisfaction, chronic pain, and functional status following laparoscopic ventral hernia repair. World J Surg 2013;37(3):530–7.
32. Haskins IN, Prabhu AS, Jensen KK, et al. Effect of transversus abdominis release on core stability: short-term results from a single institution. Surgery 2019;165(2):412–6.
33. Blair LJ, Cox TC, Huntington CR, et al. The effect of component separation technique on quality of life (QOL) and surgical outcomes in complex open ventral hernia repair (OVHR). Surg Endosc 2017;31(9):3539–46.
34. Ramirez OM, Ruas E, Dellon AL. "Components separation" method for closure of abdominal-wall defects: an anatomic and clinical study. Plast Reconstr Surg 1990;86(3):519.
35. Novitsky YW, Elliott HL, Orenstein SB, et al. Transversus abdominis muscle release: a novel approach to posterior component separation during complex abdominal wall reconstruction. Am J Surg 2012;204(5):709–16.
36. Pauli EM, Rosen MJ. Open ventral hernia repair with component separation. Surg Clin North Am 2013;93(5):1111–33.
37. Wegdam JA, Thoolen JMM, Nienhuijs SW, et al. Systematic review of transversus abdominis release in complex abdominal wall reconstruction. Hernia 2018;148(3):544–611.
38. Sneiders D, Yurtkap Y, Kroese LF, et al. Anatomical study comparing medialization after Rives-Stoppa, anterior component separation, and posterior component separation. Surgery 2019. https://doi.org/10.1016/j.surg.2018.11.013.
39. Warren JA, Cobb WS, Ewing JA, et al. Standard laparoscopic versus robotic retromuscular ventral hernia repair. Surg Endosc 2017;31(1):324–32.

40. Carbonell AM, Warren JA, Prabhu AS, et al. Reducing length of stay using a robotic-assisted approach for retromuscular ventral hernia repair: a comparative analysis from the americas hernia society quality collaborative. Ann Surg 2018; 267(2):210–7.
41. Belyansky I, Reza Zahiri H, Sanford Z, et al. Early operative outcomes of endoscopic (eTEP access) robotic-assisted retromuscular abdominal wall hernia repair. Hernia 2018;22(5):837–47.
42. Liang MK, Holihan JL, Itani K, et al. Ventral hernia management: expert consensus guided by systematic review. Ann Surg 2016. https://doi.org/10.1097/SLA.0000000000001701.
43. Petro CC, Prabhu AS. Preoperative planning and patient optimization. Surg Clin North Am 2018;98(3):483–97.
44. Ssentongo P, DeLong CG, Ssentongo AE, et al. Exhortation to lose weight prior to complex ventral hernia repair: nudge or noodge? Am J Surg 2020;219(1):136–9.
45. Rosen MJ, Aydogdu K, Grafmiller K, et al. A multidisciplinary approach to medical weight loss prior to complex abdominal wall reconstruction: is it feasible? J Gastrointest Surg 2015;19(8):1399–406.
46. Chan G, Chan CK. A review of incisional hernia repairs: preoperative weight loss and selective use of the mesh repair. Hernia 2005;9(1):37–41.
47. Liang MK, Bernardi K, Holihan JL, et al. Modifying risks in ventral hernia patients with prehabilitation: a randomized controlled trial. Ann Surg 2018;268(4):674–80.
48. Khera R, Murad MH, Chandar AK, et al. Association of pharmacological treatments for obesity with weight loss and adverse events: a systematic review and meta-analysis. JAMA 2016;315(22):2424–34.
49. Pilitsi E, Farr OM, Polyzos SA, et al. Pharmacotherapy of obesity: available medications and drugs under investigation. Metabolism 2019;92:170–92.
50. Schauer PR, Bhatt DL, Kirwan JP, et al. Bariatric surgery versus intensive medical therapy for diabetes - 5-year outcomes. N Engl J Med 2017;376(7):641–51.
51. Billeter AT, Scheurlen KM, Probst P, et al. Meta-analysis of metabolic surgery versus medical treatment for microvascular complications in patients with type 2 diabetes mellitus. Br J Surg 2018;105(3):168–81.
52. Newcomb WL, Polhill JL, Chen AY, et al. Staged hernia repair preceded by gastric bypass for the treatment of morbidly obese patients with complex ventral hernias. Hernia 2008;12(5):465–9.
53. Eid GM, Mattar SG, Hamad G, et al. Repair of ventral hernias in morbidly obese patients undergoing laparoscopic gastric bypass should not be deferred. Surg Endosc 2004;18(2):207–10.
54. Datta T, Eid G, Nahmias N, et al. Management of ventral hernias during laparoscopic gastric bypass. Surg Obes Relat Dis 2008;4(6):754–7.
55. Sadhasivam S, Larson CJ, Lambert PJ, et al. Refusals, denials, and patient choice: reasons prospective patients do not undergo bariatric surgery. Surg Obes Relat Dis 2007;3(5):531–5, discussion535–6.
56. Cherla DV, Moses ML, Viso CP, et al. Impact of abdominal wall hernias and repair on patient quality of life. World J Surg 2018;42(1):19–25.
57. Feng MP, Baucom RB, Broman KK, et al. Early repair of ventral incisional hernia may improve quality of life after surgery for abdominal malignancy: a prospective observational cohort study. Hernia 2019;23(1):81–90.
58. Rogmark P, Smedberg S, Montgomery A. Long-term follow-up of retromuscular incisional hernia repairs: recurrence and quality of life. World J Surg 2017; 42(4):974–80.

59. Langbach O, Bukholm I, Benth JŠ, et al. Long-term quality of life and functionality after ventral hernia mesh repair. Surg Endosc 2016;30(11):5023–33.
60. Kokotovic D, Sjølander H, Gögenur I, et al. Watchful waiting as a treatment strategy for patients with a ventral hernia appears to be safe. Hernia 2016;20(2):1–7.
61. Verhelst J, Timmermans L, van de Velde M, et al. Watchful waiting in incisional hernia: is it safe? Surgery 2015;157(2):297–303.
62. Altom LK, Snyder CW, Gray SH, et al. Outcomes of emergent incisional hernia repair. Am Surg 2011;77(8):971–6.
63. Helgstrand F, Rosenberg J, Kehlet H, et al. Outcomes after emergency versus elective ventral hernia repair: a prospective nationwide study. World J Surg 2013;37(10):2273–9.
64. Mrdutt MM, Munoz-Maldonado Y, Regner JL. Impact of obesity on postoperative 30-day outcomes in emergent open ventral hernia repairs. Am J Surg 2016; 212(6):1068–75.
65. Fueter T, Schäfer M, Fournier P, et al. The hernia-neck-ratio (HNR), a novel predictive factor for complications of umbilical hernia. World J Surg 2016;40(9): 2084–90.
66. Jensen KK, Arnesen RB, Christensen JK, et al. Large incisional hernias increase in size. J Surg Res 2019;244:160–5.
67. Raziel A, Sakran N, Szold A, et al. Concomitant bariatric and ventral/incisional hernia surgery in morbidly obese patients. Surg Endosc 2014;28(4):1209–12.
68. Sharma G, Boules M, Punchai S, et al. Outcomes of concomitant ventral hernia repair performed during bariatric surgery. Surg Endosc 2017;31(4):1573–82.
69. Chan DL, Talbot ML, Chen Z, et al. Simultaneous ventral hernia repair in bariatric surgery. ANZ J Surg 2014;84(7–8):581–3.
70. Praveenraj P, Gomes RM, Kumar S, et al. Concomitant bariatric surgery with laparoscopic intra-peritoneal onlay mesh repair for recurrent ventral hernias in morbidly obese patients: an evolving standard of care. Obes Surg 2016;26(6): 1191–4.
71. Krivan MS, Giorga A, Barreca M, et al. Concomitant ventral hernia repair and bariatric surgery: a retrospective analysis from a UK-based bariatric center. Surg Endosc 2019;33(3):705–10.
72. Lazzati A, Nassif GB, Paolino L. Concomitant ventral hernia repair and bariatric surgery: a systematic review. Obes Surg 2018;28(9):2949–55.
73. Spaniolas K, Kasten KR, Mozer AB, et al. Synchronous ventral hernia repair in patients undergoing bariatric surgery. Obes Surg 2015;25(10):1864–8.
74. Khorgami Z, Haskins IN, Aminian A, et al. Concurrent ventral hernia repair in patients undergoing laparoscopic bariatric surgery: a case-matched study using the national surgical quality improvement program database. Surg Obes Relat Dis 2017;13(6):997–1002.
75. Moolla M, Dang J, Modasi A, et al. Concurrent laparoscopic ventral hernia repair with bariatric surgery: a propensity-matched analysis. J Gastrointest Surg 2020; 24(1):58–66.
76. Deerenberg EB, Harlaar JJ, Steyerberg EW, et al. Small bites versus large bites for closure of abdominal midline incisions (STITCH): a double-blind, multicentre, randomised controlled trial. Lancet 2015;386(10000):1254–60.
77. Borab ZM, Shakir S, Lanni MA, et al. Does prophylactic mesh placement in elective, midline laparotomy reduce the incidence of incisional hernia? A systematic review and meta-analysis. Surgery 2017;161(4):1149–63.
78. Jairam AP, Timmermans L, Eker HH, et al. Prevention of incisional hernia with prophylactic onlay and sublay mesh reinforcement versus primary suture only in

midline laparotomies (PRIMA): 2-year follow-up of a multicentre, double-blind, randomised controlled trial. Lancet 2017;390(10094):567–76.

79. García-Ureña MÁ, López-Monclús J, Hernando LAB, et al. Randomized controlled trial of the use of a large-pore polypropylene mesh to prevent incisional hernia in colorectal surgery. Ann Surg 2015;261(5):876–81.

80. Muysoms FE, Detry O, Vierendeels T, et al. Prevention of Incisional hernias by prophylactic mesh-augmented reinforcement of midline laparotomies for abdominal aortic aneurysm treatment: a randomized controlled trial. Ann Surg 2016; 263(4):638–45.

81. Holland J, Chesney T, Dossa F, et al. Do North American colorectal surgeons use mesh to prevent parastomal hernia? A survey of current attitudes and practice. Can J Surg 2019;62(6):426–35.

82. López Cano M, Harris HW, Fisher JP, et al. Practice patterns and attitudes of surgeons on the use of prophylactic mesh to prevent parastola hernia: a cross-sectional survey. Wound Manag Prev 2019;65(9):14–23.

Addiction Transfer and Other Behavioral Changes Following Bariatric Surgery

Afton M. Koball, PhD, ABPP[a,*], Gretchen Ames, PhD, ABPP[b],
Rachel E. Goetze, PhD[c]

KEYWORDS

- Addiction transfer • Behavior changes • Psychological evaluation

KEY POINTS

- Addiction transfer is controversial and not well-supported by current literature.
- Numerous positive and "negative" behavior changes occur after bariatric surgery.
- Psychological evaluation and ongoing follow-up care from a trained behavioral health provider is essential in assessing and providing education about potential risks.

INTRODUCTION

It is well-known that bariatric surgery is the most successful tool for treatment of morbid obesity.[1] Despite its important treatment implications for obesity and related comorbidities, bariatric surgery requires several behavioral changes that warrant comprehensive evaluation and support before and after surgery. This article outlines emerging scientific and anecdotal evidence for addiction transfer after bariatric surgery. Other common behavioral changes that impact adherence, weight loss, and psychiatric risk after surgery are also reviewed.

ADDICTION TRANSFER

"Addiction transfer" theory (ie, "cross addiction," "addiction shift," or "symptom substitution")[2] in those undergoing bariatric surgery has existed colloquially for many years and refers to the belief that individuals can shift or transfer an addiction from one substance (eg, food) to another (eg, alcohol) after surgery.[3] This theory has gained interest over the last decade as researchers and clinicians have become more aware of the alarming incidence of alcohol problems and addiction-related deaths after

[a] Behavioral Medicine, Gundersen Health System, 1900 South Avenue, La Crosse, WI 54601, USA; [b] Mayo Clinic, 4500 San Pablo Road, Jacksonville, FL 32224, USA; [c] VA Maine Healthcare System-Togus, 1 VA Center, Augusta, ME 04330, USA
* Corresponding author.
E-mail address: amkoball@gundersenhealth.org

Surg Clin N Am 101 (2021) 323–333
https://doi.org/10.1016/j.suc.2020.12.005
0039-6109/21/© 2021 Elsevier Inc. All rights reserved.

bariatric surgery.[2,4,5] Despite the ubiquity of this phenomenon, little scientific research has supported its existence, and more recent studies have even disputed it.[2] Nevertheless, this phenomenon is commonly misunderstood and often feared by those seeking or who have had bariatric surgery and similarly by some providers.

Alcohol Use

It is now well-understood that individuals undergoing bariatric surgery are at an increased risk of developing problems with alcohol use postoperatively. Several reviews have highlighted this literature over the past decade[2,6] and indicate that the prevalence of alcohol misuse and/or alcohol use disorder (AUD) development postoperatively ranges (see Ivezaj and associates[2]). Moreover, individuals who have had bariatric surgery are overrepresented in substance use programs, highlighting the significant impacts on patient's quality of life after surgery.[7]

In the first 1 to 2 years after surgery, data on alcohol use are mixed.[8–10] In the long term, however, a preponderance of the literature now indicates increasing risk of problematic alcohol use.[2,10–12] Previous research has suggested that those having Roux-en-Y gastric bypass are more susceptible to problems than those who have other restrictive surgeries, although more recent research contradicts this finding.[10] Especially concerning is the frequency of de novo alcohol concerns.[11,13]

Several risk factors for problematic alcohol use have been identified including male sex, younger age, smoking, regular alcohol use before surgery, lower social support, and surgery type (ie, Roux-en-Y gastric bypass); some research has suggested that surgery type plus differential patient characteristics are predictive of AUD risk.[10] The mechanisms behind problematic alcohol use development after surgery are not entirely understood; however, a significant body of research has emerged, which highlights several neural and pharmacokinetic predictors from both animal and human studies (see Ivezaj and associates[2] for a thorough review).

In its 2016 position statement on alcohol use and bariatric surgery, the American Society for Metabolic and Bariatric Surgery[14] concluded that (1) patients should be thoroughly screened and educated about alcohol risks, (2) active AUDs are considered a contraindication for bariatric surgery, and (3) a period of sustained abstinence before surgery is recommended for those with active or historical AUDs. It is commonly recommended that patients who have undergone bariatric surgery avoid alcohol lifelong postoperatively to decrease the risk of future problematic alcohol use.

Other Substance Use

Substance use problems and disorders can develop after bariatric surgery, although this phenomenon has been less researched and the findings are mixed. Many studies combine data on illegal drug use with alcohol use, making it difficult to hypothesize about postsurgery drug use specifically. Moreover, cannabis, which is now recreationally and/or medically legal in many states, is often included with illicit drug use, despite being more prevalent and potentially having different impacts. Illicit drug use and/or cannabis use may increase after surgery,[12,15] although the data are mixed.[16] An increased risk of illicit drug use after bariatric surgery is associated with male sex, younger age, smoking, regular alcohol use, having a low income, antidepressant use, and a history of psychiatric hospitalization.[12]

Opioid Use

The risk of increased use of and addiction to opioid medications has been similarly documented after bariatric surgery. Opioids are often used at higher rates after bariatric surgery in both individuals who were and were not prescribed these medications preoperatively.[17–19] One study found that 77% of patients who used opioids before surgery continued their use long term, with use increasing in years 1 to 3.[20] In more recent studies, opioid use was decreased at 6 months, followed by an increase by 7 years postoperative (20% of patients using), suggesting a nonlinear progression of use.[21,22]

Peptide and pharmacokinetic changes in the speed and degree of absorption seem to drive increased opioid use after bariatric surgery. Tolerance to opioids, increased pain sensitivity with opiate use, as well as fewer pain management options postoperatively have all been identified as potential mechanisms of increased opiate use after surgery.[22] In efforts to decrease the frequency of problematic opioid use after bariatric surgery, the Metabolic and Bariatric Surgery Accreditation and Quality Improvement Program has focused its most recent quality improvement initiative in this area with the Bariatric Surgery Targeting Opioids program.

Support for Addiction Transfer Theory

As described elsewhere in this article, several physiologic and metabolic reasons for addiction after surgery have been identified. Reward deficiency syndrome has been described as a potential mechanism for addiction transfer after bariatric surgery.[23] It hypothesizes that compulsive overeating and obesity act as "protective factors" against the reinforcing properties of substances (eg, alcohol), and draw parallels with nonbariatric research, which indicates some support for neurogenetic changes in dopamine, predisposing certain people to addictive behaviors and/or obesity.[23] Unfortunately, no specific research has examined reward deficiency syndrome in those having had bariatric surgery. Similarly, Brunault and colleagues[24] discuss the frequency with which liver transplant patients develop obesity. They speculate that those with a history of AUD may transfer their addiction to food after liver transplantation, thereby increasing obesity risk.[24] Similarly, their review does not include specific tests of this theory in postbariatric surgery patients.

Although little research has documented support for addiction transfer theory, it has been so widely described by individuals who have had bariatric surgery (in 1 study, >80% of patients who had undergone bariatric surgery identified addiction transfer/substitution as a reason for substance use development after surgery[25]) that it is also worthwhile to consider that research has not fully examined this idea adequately. Believing the experiences of patients is important, and when overlooked can be catastrophic. Alcohol problems postoperatively, for example, were described by patients for many years and met with some skepticism by providers[26] until comprehensive studies began to find empirical support for their claims.

Criticisms of Addiction Transfer Theory

There are several problematic assumptions about the addiction transfer theory that highlight its inaccuracies. This theory assumes that all or most individuals with obesity are addicted to food and this is the primary cause of their obesity. As is now well-understood, obesity develops from a multifactorial set of forces, including genetic, metabolic, environmental, and behavioral variables, rather than solely owing to overeating and physical inactivity. Similarly, not everyone who experiences obesity is addicted to food[2]; this belief system has arisen from biased attitudes about the personal responsibility and volitional control of body weight.

In a recent review, Ivezaj and colleagures[2] discuss several additional criticisms of addiction transfer theory. First, few studies have demonstrated a link between food addiction, loss of control (LOC) eating, or binge eating and problems with alcohol or other substances after surgery, as might be expected if addiction transfer were occurring. Second, problematic alcohol use tends to develop beyond the first 1 to 2 years after surgery; if addiction transfer were truly occurring, one would expect that patients would begin to struggle with nonfood addictions nearly immediately. Third, there is clear evidence for addiction development to vary by surgery type, suggesting physiologic and metabolic factors (rather than addiction transfer) as the primary driver for postsurgery problems with addiction.

OTHER BEHAVIORAL CHANGES

Bariatric surgery results in numerous positive behavioral changes that lead to weight loss and improved quality of life after surgery. The most striking changes in behavior often occur within the first 1 to 2 years after surgery, and many persist lifelong. Despite these positive changes, unhealthy behaviors that warrant further evaluation and intervention can also develop after surgery.

Problematic Eating Behaviors

Although problematic eating behaviors like binge eating disorder (BED) or LOC eating, graze eating, and food addiction are common among patients seeking bariatric surgery, research has consistently shown that the presence of these behaviors before surgery is not reliably associated with suboptimal weight loss.[27–32] Research has also shown that problematic eating behaviors often improve significantly the first 1 to 2 years after surgery,[33,34] although their long-term durability is less clear. Some patients experience recurrence of maladaptive eating within the first year after surgery, whereas others may develop new onset problems.[28,32,35,36] The majority of patients who experience weight regain after surgery report problematic eating behaviors that either recur after improvement or are new-onset problems.[32,36]

Binge eating and loss of control eating

The prevalence of BED among patients seeking bariatric surgery is approximately 10%.[37] The prominent features of BED are "eating, in a discrete period of time (eg, within any 2-h period), an amount of food that is, larger than most would eat in similar period of time under similar circumstances and lack of control over eating during the episode."[38] Operationalizing binge eating after bariatric surgery is difficult given the anatomic changes that limit quantity of food consumption.[39] LOC eating has been shown to be predictive of poorer initial weight loss and/or weight regain.[30,36,40,41] LOC eating observed in the first 3 postoperative years may be the most important predictor of less than optimal weight loss,[35,36,40] and its severity may be the best predictor of psychological stress or impairment after surgery.[31]

Grazing eating

Although presently there is no consistent definition of graze eating in the literature, it seems to include the concepts of continuous unplanned eating episodes unrelated to hunger or satiety and the association of graze eating with LOC eating.[31,41,42] There is consensus in the literature that graze eating typically improves in the short term after surgery, yet may reoccur and be a potential risk factor for less than optimal long-term weight loss.[36,40]

Food addiction

The current definition of food addiction is consistent with *Diagnostic and Statistical Manual of Mental Disorders*, 5th edition, criteria for substance-related and addiction disorders.[43] In the current literature, self-reported food addiction varies and is associated with higher levels of mood disorders and eating disordered behaviors.[44] Food addiction, although prevalent before surgery, does not seem to impact weight loss in the first 12-month after bariatric surgery.[45] The proposed shared mechanisms between food addiction and BED/LOC eating are reward system dysfunction, cravings, impulsivity, and emotion dysregulation.[46] Conversely, withdrawal and tolerance may be unique to food addiction, whereas dietary restraint, overevaluation of weight and shape, and body image dissatisfaction are more characteristic of eating disorders,[47] although there is considerable overlap between these constructs.

Sedentary Behavior

Physical activity after bariatric surgery has been associated with improved weight loss outcomes.[48] Physical activity recommendations after bariatric surgery encourage individuals to aim for 300 minutes of structured exercise each week with strength training incorporated 2 to 3 times weekly; however, there is little guidance regarding how to best implement and support these recommendations.[49] Although individuals often voice the intention of increasing physical activity after bariatric surgery, these presurgical goals are often overestimates of achieved postsurgical activity levels.[50] Notably, sedentary behavior is one of the most common areas of nonadherence after bariatric surgery and some patients experience a decrease from presurgical levels of physical activity.[51] Perhaps because bariatric surgery is a robust intervention resulting in large weight loss, patients may become complacent about consistent adherence with a physical activity regimen.

Self-Harm and Suicide

Several large studies and literature reviews have investigated the incidence of deliberate self-harm and suicide after bariatric surgery.[52–54] A recent systematic review and meta-analysis concluded that after bariatric surgery patients had a greater risk of suicide (2.7/1000 patients) compared with age-, sex-, and body mass index-matched patients who did not have bariatric surgery.[54] Data from the Swedish Obese Subjects study found the risk of self-harm and suicide was doubled for patients who underwent bariatric surgery compared with nonsurgical controls. Predictors of suicide and nonfatal self-harm after surgery include being male, having a psychiatric disorder history before surgery, and sleep difficulties.[1,52] The severity of psychiatric problems before surgery, poor psychosocial adjustment to life after surgery, a lack of improvement in quality of life, persistent mobility restriction, and less than expected weight loss or weight regain also seem to be important factors for suicide risk.[55]

DISCUSSION

Recognizing the risks of addiction, problematic eating behaviors, sedentary behavior, and self-harm or suicide is critical in improving patient quality of life after bariatric surgery. There are several ways these goals can be achieved within bariatric surgery teams, including thorough assessment and education in presurgical psychological evaluations and postsurgery intervention and support.

Presurgical Psychological Evaluation

Bariatric behavioral health providers play an important role in multidisciplinary bariatric surgery teams, and principal among their responsibilities is identifying behavioral and psychosocial factors that may negatively impact bariatric surgery course. The central role of the bariatric behavioral health provider is making presurgical treatment recommendations to patients and the multidisciplinary team aimed at optimizing bariatric surgery readiness, outcomes, and long-term success.[56]

Updated in 2016, the American Society for Metabolic and Bariatric Surgery recommendations for prebariatric surgery psychological evaluation outlines domains most important to evaluate before surgery, including many of the behaviors reviewed in this article.[56] Presurgical psychological evaluation provides an opportunity to educate patients about risks associated with recurring or new onset problems and to build a positive and trusted relationship that may enhance the patient's willingness to engage in postsurgical multidisciplinary team visits and seek behavioral support as needed.[56]

Postsurgical Intervention and Support

After bariatric surgery, difficulty following surgical recommendations and participating in long-term follow-up is common.[57] Attending postsurgical appointments with bariatric surgery team members may be an especially important variable to consider for maintained success after bariatric surgery.[58] For individuals who experience weight regain after bariatric surgery, structured behavioral programs are associated with greater weight loss, improved mood, and reduced binge eating behaviors.[59]

The importance of long-term follow-up after bariatric surgery has been recommended owing to the risk for nonadherence to the postoperative regime, limited weight loss or weight regain, problematic eating behaviors, substance use, psychosocial challenges, changes in mood, and suicide risk.[56] These recommendations reiterate that behavior change and maintenance after bariatric surgery is a dynamic process that can wane over time, making long-term psychosocial follow-up, especially important as a part of a multidisciplinary approach to providing ongoing high-quality care. Bariatric surgery support groups have also been shown to be important in postsurgery outcomes and are required by programs accredited by Metabolic and Bariatric Surgery Accreditation and Quality Improvement Program.[60,61] Frequently, these support groups are accessed online and/or through social media platforms like Facebook, which has been identified by those seeking and who have had bariatric surgery as their preferred place to search for bariatric surgery-related information.[62] Ensuring that bariatric teams have a virtual method of supporting their patients postoperatively is important given that misinformation of nutrition-related content is common in these groups.[63]

Motivational Interviewing

Motivational interviewing is style of communication that fosters collaborative conversations between health care providers and patients.[64] When used with individuals before or after bariatric surgery, the aim is to strengthen motivation, commitment to lifestyle change, and confidence in making and maintaining healthy behavioral changes in the long term. Interventions including motivational interviewing have been associated with greater reductions in weight,[65,66] increased physical activity, and improved dietary behaviors.[67–69] When incorporated before bariatric surgery, motivational interviewing strategies have been associated with more realistic goal setting and improved program retention.[70,71] For those experiencing weight regain after surgery, a combination of motivational interviewing and cognitive behavioral therapy has been found to increase confidence, motivation, and behavioral adherence with postsurgical recommendations.[72]

CLINICS CARE POINTS

- Addiction transfer is controversial and not well-supported by current literature. Rather, development of addiction after surgery seems driven by neural, peptide, and pharmacokinetic changes resulting from the surgery itself.

- Numerous positive and "negative" behavior changes including addiction, problematic eating, sedentary behavior, and self-harm/suicide occur after bariatric surgery, several in the first 1 to 3 years, and many remain risk factors lifelong.

- Psychological evaluation from a trained behavioral health provider is essential in assessing and providing education about these risks. Similarly, behavioral health providers and other team members (eg, dietitians, bariatricians) are critical for providing intervention and support postoperatively.

- Motivational interviewing skills can be used by all members of a bariatric team preoperatively and postoperatively to reduce ambivalence, evoke motivation for change, and build trusting relationships with patients.

DISCLOSURER

The authors have nothing to disclose.

REFERENCES

1. Sjostrom L. Review of the key results from the Swedish Obese Subjects (SOS) trial - a prospective controlled intervention study of bariatric surgery. J Intern Med 2013;273(3):219–34.
2. Ivezaj V, Benoit SC, Davis J, et al. Changes in alcohol use after metabolic and bariatric surgery: predictors and mechanisms. Curr Psychiatry Rep 2019; 21(9):85.
3. McFadden KM. Cross-addiction: from morbid obesity to substance abuse. Bariatr Nurs Surg Patient Care 2010;5:145–78.
4. Kanji S, Wong E, Akioyamen L, et al. Exploring pre-surgery and post-surgery substance use disorder and alcohol use disorder in bariatric surgery: a qualitative scoping review. Int J Obes (Lond) 2019;43(9):1659–74.
5. White GE, Courcoulas AP, King WC. Drug- and alcohol-related mortality risk after bariatric surgery: evidence from a 7-year prospective multicenter cohort study. Surg Obes Relat Dis 2019;15(7):1160–9.
6. Spadola CE, Wagner EF, Dillon FR, et al. Alcohol and drug use among postoperative bariatric patients: a systematic review of the emerging research and its implications. Alcohol Clin Exp Res 2015;39(9):1582–601.
7. Saules KK, Wiedemann A, Ivezaj V, et al. Bariatric surgery history among substance abuse treatment patients: prevalence and associated features. Surg Obes Relat Dis 2010;6(6):615–21.
8. Wee CC, Mukamal KJ, Huskey KW, et al. High-risk alcohol use after weight loss surgery. Surg Obes Relat Dis 2014;10(3):508–13.
9. Coluzzi I, Iossa A, Spinetti E, et al. Alcohol consumption after laparoscopic sleeve gastrectomy: 1-year results. Eat Weight Disord 2019;24(6):1131–6.
10. Ibrahim N, Alameddine M, Brennan J, et al. New onset alcohol use disorder following bariatric surgery. Surg Endosc 2019;33(8):2521–30.
11. King WC, Chen JY, Mitchell JE, et al. Prevalence of alcohol use disorders before and after bariatric surgery. JAMA 2012;307(23):2516–25.
12. King WC, Chen JY, Courcoulas AP, et al. Alcohol and other substance use after bariatric surgery: prospective evidence from a U.S. multicenter cohort study. Surg Obes Relat Dis 2017;13(8):1392–402.
13. Wiedemann AA, Saules KK, Ivezaj V. Emergence of New Onset substance use disorders among post-weight loss surgery patients. Clin Obes 2013;3(6): 194–201.

14. Parikh M, Johnson JM, Ballem N, et al. ASMBS position statement on alcohol use before and after bariatric surgery. Surg Obes Relat Dis 2016;12(2):225–30.

15. Vidot DC, Prado G, De La Cruz-Munoz N, et al. Postoperative marijuana use and disordered eating among bariatric surgery patients. Surg Obes Relat Dis 2016; 12(1):171–8.

16. Conason A, Teixeira J, Hsu CH, et al. Substance use following bariatric weight loss surgery. JAMA Surg 2013;148(2):145–50.

17. Maciejewski ML, Smith VA, Berkowitz TSZ, et al. Long-term opioid use after bariatric surgery. Surg Obes Relat Dis 2020;16(8):1100–10.

18. Heinberg LJ, Pudalov L, Alameddin H, et al. Opioids and bariatric surgery: a review and suggested recommendations for assessment and risk reduction. Surg Obes Relat Dis 2019;15(2):314–21.

19. Wallen S, Szabo E, Palmetun-Ekback M, et al. Use of opioid analgesics before and after gastric bypass surgery in Sweden: a population-based study. Obes Surg 2018;28(11):3518–23.

20. Raebel MA, Newcomer SR, Reifler LM, et al. Chronic use of opioid medications before and after bariatric surgery. JAMA 2013;310(13):1369–76.

21. King WC, Chen JY, Belle SH, et al. Change in pain and physical function following bariatric surgery for severe obesity. JAMA 2016;315(13):1362–71.

22. King WC, Chen JY, Belle SH, et al. Use of prescribed opioids before and after bariatric surgery: prospective evidence from a U.S. multicenter cohort study. Surg Obes Relat Dis 2017;13(8):1337–46.

23. Blum K, Bailey J, Gonzalez AM, et al. Neuro-Genetics of Reward Deficiency Syndrome (RDS) as the root cause of "addiction transfer": a new phenomenon common after bariatric surgery. J Genet Syndr Gene Ther 2011;2012(1). S2-001.

24. Brunault P, Salame E, Jaafari N, et al. Why do liver transplant patients so often become obese? The addiction transfer hypothesis. Med Hypotheses 2015; 85(1):68–75.

25. Ivezaj V, Saules KK, Wiedemann AA. "I didn't see this coming.": why are postbariatric patients in substance abuse treatment? Patients' perceptions of etiology and future recommendations. Obes Surg 2012;22(8):1308–14.

26. Sogg S. Alcohol misuse after bariatric surgery: epiphenomenon or "Oprah" phenomenon? Surg Obes Relat Dis 2007;3(3):366–8.

27. Conceicao E, Bastos AP, Brandao I, et al. Loss of control eating and weight outcomes after bariatric surgery: a study with a Portuguese sample. Eat Weight Disord 2014;19(1):103–9.

28. Nasirzadeh Y, Kantarovich K, Wnuk S, et al. Binge eating, loss of control over eating, emotional eating, and night eating after bariatric surgery: results from the Toronto bari-PSYCH Cohort Study. Obes Surg 2018;28(7):2032–9.

29. Mitchell JE, King WC, Courcoulas A, et al. Eating behavior and eating disorders in adults before bariatric surgery. Int J Eat Disord 2015;48(2):215–22.

30. Pinto-Bastos A, de Lourdes M, Brandao I, et al. Weight loss trajectories and psychobehavioral predictors of outcome of primary and reoperative bariatric surgery: a 2-year longitudinal study. Surg Obes Relat Dis 2019;15(7):1104–12.

31. Conceicao EM, de Lourdes M, Pinto-Bastos A, et al. Problematic eating behaviors and psychopathology in patients undergoing bariatric surgery: the mediating role of loss of control eating. Int J Eat Disord 2018;51(6):507–17.

32. King WC, Belle SH, Hinerman AS, et al. Patient Behaviors and Characteristics Related to Weight Regain After Roux-en-Y gastric bypass: a multicenter prospective cohort study. Ann Surg 2020;272(6):1044–52.

33. Holsen LM, Davidson P, Cerit H, et al. Neural predictors of 12-month weight loss outcomes following bariatric surgery. Int J Obes (Lond) 2018;42(4):785–93.

34. Alamuddin N, Vetter ML, Ahima RS, et al. Changes in fasting and prandial gut and adiposity hormones following vertical sleeve gastrectomy or Roux-en-Y-Gastric bypass: an 18-month prospective study. Obes Surg 2017;27(6):1563–72.

35. Ivezaj V, Barnes RD, Cooper Z, et al. Loss-of-control eating after bariatric/sleeve gastrectomy surgery: similar to binge-eating disorder despite differences in quantities. Gen Hosp Psychiatry 2018;54:25–30.

36. Conceicao EM, Mitchell JE, Pinto-Bastos A, et al. Stability of problematic eating behaviors and weight loss trajectories after bariatric surgery: a longitudinal observational study. Surg Obes Relat Dis 2017;13(6):1063–70.

37. Mitchell JE, Selzer F, Kalarchian MA, et al. Psychopathology before surgery in the longitudinal assessment of bariatric surgery-3 (LABS-3) psychosocial study. Surg Obes Relat Dis 2012;8(5):533–41.

38. Association AP, ed The Diagnostic and Statistical Manual of Mental Disorders (DSM-5). Arlington, VA: American Psychiatric Publishing; 2013.

39. Goldschmidt AB, Conceicao EM, Thomas JG, et al. Conceptualizing and studying binge and loss of control eating in bariatric surgery patients-time for a paradigm shift? Surg Obes Relat Dis 2016;12(8):1622–5.

40. Smith KE, Orcutt M, Steffen KJ, et al. Loss of control eating and binge eating in the 7 years following bariatric surgery. Obes Surg 2019;29(6):1773–80.

41. Colles SL, Dixon JB, O'Brien PE. Grazing and loss of control related to eating: two high-risk factors following bariatric surgery. Obesity (Silver Spring) 2008;16(3):615–22.

42. Goodpaster KPS, Marek RJ, Lavery ME, et al. Graze eating among bariatric surgery candidates: prevalence and psychosocial correlates. Surg Obes Relat Dis 2016;12(5):1091–7.

43. Schulte EM, Gearhardt AN. Development of the modified yale food addiction scale version 2.0. Eur Eat Disord Rev 2017;25(4):302–8.

44. Koball AM, Clark MM, Collazo-Clavell M, et al. The relationship among food addiction, negative mood, and eating-disordered behaviors in patients seeking to have bariatric surgery. Surg Obes Relat Dis 2016;12(1):165–70.

45. Ivezaj V, Wiedemann AA, Grilo CM. Food addiction and bariatric surgery: a systematic review of the literature. Obes Rev 2017;18(12):1386–97.

46. Schulte EM, Grilo CM, Gearhardt AN. Shared and unique mechanisms underlying binge eating disorder and addictive disorders. Clin Psychol Rev 2016;44:125–39.

47. Ivezaj V, Wiedemann AA, Grilo CM. Overvaluation of weight or shape and loss-of-control eating following bariatric surgery. Obesity (Silver Spring) 2019;27(8):1239–43.

48. Herring LY, Stevinson C, Davies MJ, et al. Changes in physical activity behaviour and physical function after bariatric surgery: a systematic review and meta-analysis. Obes Rev 2016;17(3):250–61.

49. Hansen D, Decroix L, Devos Y, et al. Towards optimized care after bariatric surgery by physical activity and exercise intervention: a review. Obes Surg 2020;30(3):1118–25.

50. Ouellette KA, Mabey JG, Eisenman PA, et al. Physical activity patterns among individuals before and soon after bariatric surgery. Obes Surg 2020;30(2):416–22.

51. King WC, Hsu JY, Belle SH, et al. Pre- to postoperative changes in physical activity: report from the longitudinal assessment of bariatric surgery-2 (LABS-2). Surg Obes Relat Dis 2012;8(5):522–32.

52. Konttinen H, Sjoholm K, Jacobson P, et al. Prediction of suicide and nonfatal self-harm after bariatric surgery: a risk score based on sociodemographic factors, lifestyle behavior, and mental health: a nonrandomized controlled trial. Ann Surg 2019. https://doi.org/10.1097/SLA.0000000000003742.

53. Morgan DJ, Ho KM. Incidence and risk factors for deliberate self-harm, mental illness, and suicide following bariatric surgery: a state-wide population-based linked-data cohort study. Ann Surg 2017;265(2):244–52.

54. Castaneda D, Popov VB, Wander P, et al. Risk of suicide and self-harm is increased after bariatric surgery-a systematic review and meta-analysis. Obes Surg 2019;29(1):322–33.

55. Belle SH, Berk PD, Chapman WH, et al. Baseline characteristics of participants in the Longitudinal Assessment of Bariatric Surgery-2 (LABS-2) study. Surg Obes Relat Dis 2013;9(6):926–35.

56. Sogg S, Lauretti J, West-Smith L. Recommendations for the presurgical psychosocial evaluation of bariatric surgery patients. Surg Obes Relat Dis 2016;12(4): 731–49.

57. Toussi R, Fujioka K, Coleman KJ. Pre- and postsurgery behavioral compliance, patient health, and postbariatric surgical weight loss. Obesity (Silver Spring) 2009;17(5):996–1002.

58. Jurgensen JA, Reidt W, Kellogg T, et al. Impact of patient attrition from bariatric surgery practice on clinical outcomes. Obes Surg 2019;29(2):579–84.

59. Himes SM, Grothe KB, Clark MM, et al. Stop regain: a pilot psychological intervention for bariatric patients experiencing weight regain. Obes Surg 2015; 25(5):922–7.

60. Mechanick JI, Youdim A, Jones DB, et al. Clinical practice guidelines for the perioperative nutritional, metabolic, and nonsurgical support of the bariatric surgery patient–2013 update: cosponsored by American Association of Clinical Endocrinologists, The Obesity Society, and American Society for Metabolic & Bariatric Surgery. Obesity (Silver Spring) 2013;21(Suppl 1):S1–27.

61. Orth WS, Madan AK, Taddeucci RJ, et al. Support group meeting attendance is associated with better weight loss. Obes Surg 2008;18(4):391–4.

62. Martins MP, Abreu-Rodrigues M, Souza JR. The use of the internet by the patient after bariatric surgery: contributions and obstacles for the follow-up of multidisciplinary monitoring. Arq Bras Cir Dig 2015;28(Suppl 1):46–51.

63. Koball AM, Jester DJ, Pruitt MA, et al. Content and accuracy of nutrition-related posts in bariatric surgery Facebook support groups. Surg Obes Relat Dis 2018; 14(12):1897–902.

64. Miller WR, Rollnick S. Helping people change. 3rd edition. New York: Guilford Press; 2013.

65. Armstrong MJ, Mottershead TA, Ronksley PE, et al. Motivational interviewing to improve weight loss in overweight and/or obese patients: a systematic review and meta-analysis of randomized controlled trials. Obes Rev 2011;12(9):709–23.

66. DiMarco ID, Klein DA, Clark VL, et al. The use of motivational interviewing techniques to enhance the efficacy of guided self-help behavioral weight loss treatment. Eat Behav 2009;10(2):134–6.

67. Ekong G, Kavookjian J. Motivational interviewing and outcomes in adults with type 2 diabetes: a systematic review. Patient Educ Couns 2016;99(6):944–52.

68. Teixeira PJ, Palmeira AL, Vansteenkiste M. The role of self-determination theory and motivational interviewing in behavioral nutrition, physical activity, and health: an introduction to the IJBNPA special series. Int J Behav Nutr Phys Act 2012;9:17.

69. Martins RK, McNeil DW. Review of Motivational Interviewing in promoting health behaviors. Clin Psychol Rev 2009;29(4):283–93.
70. Goldberg JH, Kiernan M. Innovative techniques to address retention in a behavioral weight-loss trial. Health Educ Res 2005;20(4):439–47.
71. Kaly P, Orellana S, Torrella T, et al. Unrealistic weight loss expectations in candidates for bariatric surgery. Surg Obes Relat Dis 2008;4(1):6–10.
72. Ames G, Clark MM, Grothe KB, et al. Talking to patients about bariatric surgery: guiding meaningful conversations and evoking commitment to change. Bariatric Times 2015;11:16–24.

Emerging Procedures in Bariatric Metabolic Surgery

Mohit Bhandari, MS*, Susmit Kosta, PhD, Manoj Khurana, MS,
Winni Mathur, BPT, MBA(HA), Manoj Kumar Reddy, MS, Mathias Fobi, MD

KEYWORDS

- Emerging procedures • Bariatric metabolic surgery • Obesity • Weight-loss
- Type 2 diabetes mellitus

KEY POINTS

- Bariatric/metabolic surgery is a viable option for long-term treatment of obesity and its related metabolic disorders.
- Many new procedures have been developed and changed the face of modern bariatric surgery.
- There is a need for prospective randomized comparative clinical studies of emerging surgical procedures.

INTRODUCTION

Metabolic surgery includes a variety of procedures performed on individuals who are obese and have associated obesity-related metabolic diseases.[1] The procedure also is extended to treat severely diabetic individuals where medical therapy is not as effective.[2,3] Because it is a recalcitrant disease, however, the treatment options and paradigm are ever-changing. Recently, metabolic diabetes surgery has become a viable option for long-term treatment of type 2 diabetes mellitus (T2D). This branch of medicine was referred to as *bariatric* (from the Greek, *baros*, for weight), but recent awareness that these procedures can treat concomitant obesity-related metabolic diseases effectively has given rise to a new specialty of bariatric metabolic surgery.[4]

It is understood that there is an independent weight mechanism for the treatment of diabetes. The least efficient bariatric surgical treatment is many times more effective than medical treatment. There is a massive growth in the number of bariatric procedures because the need for one most effective and least complicated procedure still goes on. There are emerging bariatric procedures that are created to address those

Mohak Bariatrics and Robotics Center, SAIMS Campus, Indore-Ujjain Highway, Indore, Madhya Pradesh, India
* Corresponding author.
E-mail address: drmohitbhandari@gmail.com

Surg Clin N Am 101 (2021) 335–353
https://doi.org/10.1016/j.suc.2020.12.001
0039-6109/21/© 2020 Elsevier Inc. All rights reserved.

surgical.theclinics.com

concerns. Emerging bariatric procedures can be defined, like the one that has been devised, in the past 5 years, which have reached a stage of randomized controlled trial to prove clinical efficacy over existent bariatric procedures.

In some cases, although emerging procedures have failed to establish a definitive clinical advantage, they are at least as compelling and less technically challenging than the existing bariatric procedures. There are certain racial, ethnic, and cultural differences that affect the food habits and living conditions in a given geographic area. It, therefore, is pertinent that the bariatric procedure is altered in accordance with the existent food habits. Like in areas in the world where the food is predominantly vegetarian, a more malabsorptive procedure creates more deficiencies and nutritional issues. Similarly, certain areas may have a propensity to prefer less invasive procedures for weight loss. Endoscopic procedures thus are the preferred procedures in these geographic areas. Many countries have a high incidence of T2D, and they develop diabetes at a lower body mass index (BMI). It makes sense to have a procedure with a robust metabolic effect in these countries. Some countries have a high incidence of endemic iron deficiency anemia and therefore need a robust procedure for metabolic effects but much less hypoabsorption. There has been new research in areas to understand how vagal stimulation has an impact on early satiety, and other full-sense devices have been tested to give a similar effect. Each bariatric procedure should be identified by a single set of precise anatomic measurements that characterize its final anatomic reconfiguration standard. Such identification of procedures facilitates accurate data collection and analysis of outcomes to improve the targeting of treatment of specific aspects of metabolic disease. To avoid the creation of confounding results, procedure variants, by definition, must vary from a single foundational standard procedure applied consistently by the field.

The article has inclusion and discussion of emerging procedures, a multitude of bariatric metabolic procedures from around the world enables surgeons to tailor treatment to the needs of the patient.

EMERGING PROCEDURAL APPROACHES

Roux-en-Y gastric bypass (RYGB), sleeve, gastric banding, and duodenal switch have been the traditional procedures performed for morbidly obese patients for a long time. Several newer procedures or emerging procedures have come to the fore.

- Banded sleeve gastrectomy (BSG)
- Sleeve gastrectomy (SG) with jejunojejunostomy/enteral bypass (SG-JJEB)
- SG with jejunoileostomy anastomosis (SG-JIA)
- SG with duodenojejunal bypass (SG-DJB)
- SG with loop duodenojejunal bypass (SG-LDJB)
- SG with transit bipartition (SG-TB)
- SG with jejunoileal interposition (SG-JII) and SG with duodenal, ileal interposition (SG-DII)
- Single-anastomosis sleeve with ileal bypass (SASI)
- One-anastomosis gastric bypass (OAGB) or mini–gastric bypass (MGB)
- Banded OAGB (BOAGB) or banded MGB (BMGB)
- Single-anastomosis gastroileal bypass (SAG-I)

The procedures presented are new, with limited knowledge of safety and long-term efficacy. Their places in the management of obesity and morbid obesity are discussed.

BANDED SLEEVE GASTRECTOMY

- Introduction
  Banding of the SG was initially was reported in 2009 to 2011 by Karcz and colleagues,[5] Agrawal and colleagues,[6] and Alexander and colleagues[7] as a response to intermediate-term issues with weight regain in SG.
- Surgical anatomy
  The BSG is an SG that is banded with a nonadjustable ring placed loosely around the proximal sleeve 3 cm to 5 cm from the gastroesophageal junction. This operation is based on the experience of banding the gastric bypass. The sleeve in the BSG is less narrow than the one used in the stand-alone SG because the ring serves as the restrictive mechanism, which creates a lower likelihood of stricture and leaks at the gastroesophageal junction[8] (**Fig. 1**).
- Advantages
  Reports indicate that banding the sleeve enhances weight loss and weight-loss maintenance, just as with the RYGB in the short term.[9,10] Better diabetes control has been reported with the BSG in the short term, related to the enhanced weight loss.
- Disadvantages
  Complications reported with the BSG include ring erosion, kinking at the site of the ring, and solid food intolerance. As with the BGBP, complications of band erosion are treated with outpatient endoscopic band removal. Solid food intolerance is treated by either band/ring removal or revision of the operation to an RYGB. Concerns about increased reflux when banding the sleeve are unconfirmed.
- Surgical outcomes
  BSG is indicated for obese patients with clear contraindications against RYGBP or biliopancreatic diversion (BPD) and for those on medication who need

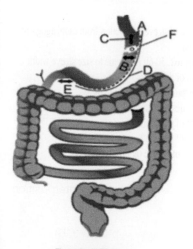

A = 1-2 cm	Distance of sleeve transection from esophagogastric junction
B = 3 cm	Use 32–40F bougie to size sleeve width
C = 3-4 cm	Length of proximal pouch
D = As is	Length of the sleeve
E = 2–6 cm	Antrectomy distance from pylorus
F = 7–7.5 cm	Ring size placed 3–4 cm from esophagogastric junction
V = <30 mL	Volume of proximal pouch

Banded Sleeve Gastrectomy (BSG)

Fig. 1. BSG. (*From* Bhandari M, Fobi MAL, Buchwald JN, et al. Standardization of bariatric metabolic procedures: world consensus meeting statement. Obes Surg.2019; 29(Suppl 4):309–345; with permission.)

strong intestinal resorption.[5] In a long-term comparative study of SG (n = 51) and BSG (n = 96) in obese and superobese patients, excess weight loss (EWL) increased at each point through longer-term follow-up, from 77.4% at year 1 to 86.7% at 5 years. No weight regain was seen in greater than 97% of the BSG group versus 80% of the SG group, and the SG group had less than 50% weight loss in 35.2% of patients at 5-year follow-up.[8,11]

- Future
  As with the BGBP, the absence of a Food and Drug Administration–approved ring device has limited the use of this operation in the United States.

SLEEVE GASTRECTOMY WITH JEJUNOJEJUNOSTOMY/ENTERAL BYPASS

- Introduction
  The SG-JJEB is an emerging operation, first described by Alamo and colleagues,[12] in 2006, and advanced by de Menezes Ettinger and colleagues.[13] Described by Alamo, in 2018, approximately 2000 cases have been performed worldwide. SG-JJEB is technically more straightforward than RYGBP.[14]

- Surgical anatomy
  Sleeve gastrectomy is done with a volume of 150 mL to 250 mL, and, after counting 100 cm from the duodenojejunal junction, the small bowel is divided, and jejunoileostomy is performed diameter of 3 cm, 200 cm from ileocecal junction (**Fig. 2**).

- Advantages
  This procedure offers advantages of restriction and reduced ghrelin secretion resulting from the sleeve element and hindgut mechanism of ileal stimulation.

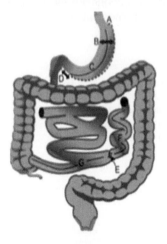

A = 2–3 cm	Distance of sleeve transection from esophagogastric junction
B = 3–4 cm	Use approx. 50-60 Fr bougie to size sleeve width
C = As is	Length of the sleeve
D = 2–6 cm	Antrectomy distance from pylorus
E = 3 cm	Jejuno-ileal anastomosis
F = 100 cm	Length of jejunal limb
G = 200 cm	Length of ileal limb
V = 150–250 mL	Volume of sleeve (approx.)

Sleeve Gastrectomy with Jejuno-Jejunostomy/Enteral Bypass (SG-JJEB)

Fig. 2. SG-JJEB. (*From* Bhandari M, Fobi MAL, Buchwald JN, et al. Standardization of bariatric metabolic procedures: world consensus meeting statement. Obes Surg.2019; 29(Suppl 4):309–345; with permission.)

There is no remnant stomach left, so it can be done in patients with high risk for malignancy of the stomach. It does not cause dumping.

- Disadvantages

    Blind loop syndrome with bacterial overgrowth can become a concern that sometimes can cause intractable diarrhea.

- Surgical outcomes

    Weight loss and T2DM resolution appear to be better with SG-JJEB than with SG and similar to RYGBP.[14] In a 2012 study of 49 SG-JJEB patients with BMI less than 35 kg/m², mean BMI at 18 months was 24.0 kg/m². Complete remission of T2DM was seen in 40/41 (97.5%) patients receiving oral hypoglycemic agents, and partial remission in 8/8 (100%) patients receiving insulin.[15]

- Future

    It can be done in high-risk areas for stomach cancer without the worry of remnant stomach.

SLEEVE GASTRECTOMY WITH JEJUNOILEOSTOMY ANASTOMOSIS

- Introduction

    The emerging SG variant, SG-JIA, developed by Melissas and colleagues,[16] offers the benefits of SG combined with an enhanced neuroendocrine response. It is thought that faster gastric emptying and reduced ghrelin combined with the shorter duodenum-to-cecum transit time enhance incretin effect.[16]

- Surgical anatomy

    Sleeve gastrectomy is done with a volume of 150 mL to 250 mL and, after counting 100 cm from the ligament of Treitz. Jejunoileostomy is performed with a diameter of 3 cm, 200 cm from IC junction[8](**Fig. 3**).

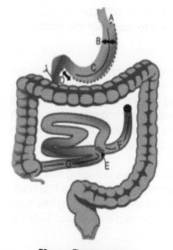

A = 2–3 cm	Distance of sleeve transection from esophagogastric junction
B = 3–4 cm	Use 50–60F bougie to size sleeve width
C = As is	Length of sleeve
D = 2-6 cm	Distance from pylorus
E = 3 cm	Width of jejuno-ileal anastomosis
F = 100 cm	Length of jejunal limb
G = 200 cm-	Length of ileal limb
V = 150-250 mL	Volume of sleeve (approx.)

Sleeve Gastrectomy with Jejuno-Ileostomy Anastomosis (SG-JIA)

Fig. 3. SG-JIA. (*From* Bhandari M, Fobi MAL, Buchwald JN, et al. Standardization of bariatric metabolic procedures: world consensus meeting statement. Obes Surg.2019; 29(Suppl 4):309–345; with permission.)

- Advantages

    It can be done in patients with failed sleeve. This procedure offers the advantage of restriction and reduced ghrelin secretion resulting from sleeve element and incretin effect because of the bypass. In cases of severe malabsorption, it can easily be reversed while leaving the sleeve component intact. There is no remnant stomach left, so it can be done in patients with higher risk for stomach cancer. It does not cause dumping.

- Disadvantages

    The blind loop syndrome is often due to an overgrowth and diarrhea of bacteria in the intestine. It cannot be offered to patients with liver cirrhosis.

- Surgical outcomes

    In a dual-center study (Crete and Istanbul), weight loss was compared in SG-JIA patients (n = 100, mean BMI 46.8; Crete and Istanbul) versus SG patients (n = 360, Crete only). Statistically significant mean EWL differences at 6 months and 12 months were found between SG-JIA versus SG patients, 59.9% versus 50.0% and 77.3% versus 61.4%, respectively. When comparing the SG-JIA group versus SG, at 6 months, resolution of T2DM (85.8% vs 50.0%, respectively), hypertension (100% vs 33.3%, respectively), and dyslipidemia (100% vs 44.4%, respectively) were found statistically significant, thus suggesting that SG-JIA is preferable in patients with obesity with comorbidities.[8]

- Future

    It can be preferred in failed SG.

SLEEVE GASTRECTOMY WITH DUODENOJEJUNAL BYPASS

- Introduction

    The SG-DJB was introduced by Kasama and colleagues[17] in 2009 to treat obesity and metabolic disorders as an alternative to RYGBP. In SG-DJB, the bypass of the duodenojejunal axis is believed to augment the metabolic effects of the SG.

- Surgical anatomy

    Sleeve gastrectomy is performed and dissection then is continued through the lower part and posterior wall of the duodenum above the gastroduodenal artery. The duodenum is divided by preserving the right gastric artery and supraduodenal vessels. Roux-en-Y loop is constructed with biliopancreatic limb of 100 cm and Roux limb of 150 cm, and hand-sewn gastrojejunostomy is performed with 2-cm to 3-cm diameter[8] (**Fig. 4**).

- Advantages

    Preservation of the physiologic pylorus in SG-DJB reduces dumping syndrome and marginal ulcer. SG-DJB is indicated for patients in areas with a high incidence of gastric cancer (the highest prevalence of which is in Asia) because the duodenojejunal bypass is accessible to endoscopic evaluation. There is no bile reflux into the sleeve.

- Disadvantages

    In cases of severe malabsorption, it is difficult to reverse the procedure.

    It could cause gastroesophageal reflux disease (GERD) higher than RYGB.

    It is a technically challenging operative procedure to perform laparoscopically, with a long learning curve and increased operative times.

    Relative contraindications include duodenal ulcer

- Surgical outcomes

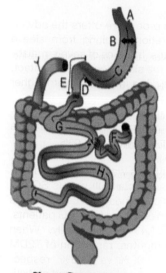

A = 1–2 cm   Distance of sleeve transection from esophagogastric junction
B = 2.5–3 cm   Use 32–40F bougie to size sleeve width
C = As is   Length of sleeve
D = 2–6 cm   Distance from pylorus
E = 2–3 cm   Length of duodenum from pylorus
F = 100 cm   Length of biliopancreatic limb
G = 150 cm   Length of Roux-en-Y limb
H = As is   Common limb
V = 75–90 mL   Volume of sleeve (approx.)

**Sleeve Gastrectomy
with Duodeno-Jejunal
Bypass (SG-DJB)**

Fig. 4. SG-DJB. (*From* Bhandari M, Fobi MAL, Buchwald JN, et al. Standardization of bariatric metabolic procedures: world consensus meeting statement. Obes Surg.2019; 29(Suppl 4):309–345; with permission.)

Reduction in mean BMI, from 39.0 kg/m₂ to 28.0 kg/m₂, was observed in a short-term study by Naitoh et al 2018 with year follow-up.[20] When comparing at 1 year, approximately equal weight loss was observed with SG-DJB with RYGBP and was reported by Praveen Raj and colleagues.[18] Lee and colleagues[19] published, in their study, that when SG is combined with DJB, EWL may increase by 20%. SG-DJB (n = 121) was found to be more effective for weight loss and T2DM resolution compared with SG (n 5 177) at 1- year follow-up in a multicenter comparative study done by Naitoh et al 2018. They also reported that in lower BMI patients (27.5–34.9 kg/m₂), SG-DJB was found more effective in resolving T2DM.[8,20]

- Future
  It can be done high-risk areas for stomach cancer without the worry of remnant stomach and can add metabolic effect to SG.

SLEEVE GASTRECTOMY WITH LOOP DUODENOJEJUNAL BYPASS

- Introduction
  In 2013, Huang and colleagues[21] introduced the SG-LDJB as a modification of single anastomosis duodenoileal bypass with sleeve (SADI-S).
- Surgical anatomy
  SG is performed using a 38F bougie with duodenal transection, 2 cm to 4 cm beyond the pylorus. A side-to-side duodenojejunal anastomosis (approximately 1.5 cm) is performed, hand-sewn with 3-0 absorbable sutures at 200 cm to 300 cm from the ligament of Treitz by bringing up the jejunal loop in an isoperistaltic and antecolic fashion (**Fig. 5**).

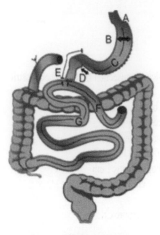

A = 1–2 cm	Distance of sleeve transection from esophagogastric junction
B = 2.5 cm	Use 32–40F bougie to size sleeve width
C = As is	Length of sleeve
D = 2–6 cm	Antrectomy distance from pylorus
E = 2–3 cm	Length of transected duodenum from pylorus
F = 200 cm	Length of biliopancreatic limb
G = ??? cm	Common limb
V = 75–150 mL	Volume of sleeve (approx.)

**Sleeve Gastrectomy
with Loop Duodenojejunal
Bypass (SG-
LDJB)**

Fig. 5. SG-LDJB. (*From* Bhandari M, Fobi MAL, Buchwald JN, et al. Standardization of bariatric metabolic procedures: world consensus meeting statement. Obes Surg.2019; 29(Suppl 4):309–345; with permission.)

- Advantages

  Because of the preservation of pylorus, there is a very low chance of marginal ulcer and dumping syndrome. Because there is no remnant stomach, it can be done in high-risk patients for stomach cancer.

- Disadvantages

  In cases of severe malabsorption, it is difficult to reverse the procedure.

  It could cause GERD higher than RYGB.

  It is a technically challenging operative procedure to perform laparoscopically.

  Contraindicated in patients with duodenal ulcer.

- Surgical outcomes

  Huang and colleagues[21] studied 22 diabetic patients (mean duration 8 years) with mean BMI 28.4 kg/m^2, where all patients were on oral hypoglycemic agents, and 3 (14%) also were on insulin. Eleven patients (50%) had complete remission of T2DM whereas 20 (91%) achieved glycemic control with hemoglobin (Hb)A$_{1c}$ less than 7% without medication. Mean HbA$_{1c}$ dropped from 8.6% to 6.2%, fasting blood sugar (FBS) from 147 mg/dL to 110 mg/dL, and C-peptide from 2.4 ng/mL to 1.3 ng/mL at 6 months.[21] In a group-matched study by the same investigators comparing RYGB and LDJB-SG (n = 30 in each group), both procedures proved equally effective with respect to mean BMI, FBS, and HbA$_{1c}$ at 1 year, both showing a significant reduction in those parameters from their preoperative levels ($P<.01$). Both groups had similar comorbidity resolution; however, the LDJB-SG group had better β-cell function (estimated by Homeostatic model assessment [HOMA2]) compared with the RYGB group ($P = .004$); morbidity was higher in the RYGB group ($P = .08$).[22]

- Future

  In a case report of 2 T2DM patients, SG-LDJB was performed as revisional surgery after RYGB to overcome intractable dumping syndrome. Six months postsurgery, the Sigstad score decreased to 2 points.[23] This procedure is like a shorter Duodenal Switch (DS), where malabsorption is expected to be much less, and efficacy is likely to be much lower; biliary access is lost even in LDJB-SG.

SLEEVE GASTRECTOMY WITH TRANSIT BIPARTITION

- Introduction

  Santoro and colleagues[24] first described SG-TB. This later was modified by Mui and colleagues,[25] from Hongkong, into SG with loop bipartition (SG-LB) (also known as SASI, as reported by Mahdy).[31]

- Surgical anatomy

  After performing an SG, the ileum is transected at 250 cm proximal to ileocecal junction. The distal ileal end is anastomosed to the antrum in an antecolic fashion, with a stapler or completely hand sewn (anastomosis up to 3 cm is advocated to avoid excess food transit and malabsorption). This creates 2 potential routes for the transit of food: through the gastroileal anastomosis into distal ileum and also through the intact duodenum, thus minimizing malnutrition and malabsorption. The proximal ileal end of the transection is anastomosed side to side at 80 cm to 130 cm proximal to the ileocecal junction (depending on the length of common channel required), to create the ileoileal anastomosis (**Fig. 6**).

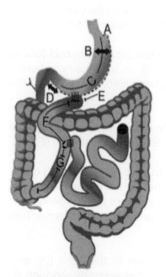

A = 2–3 cm	Distance of sleeve transection from esophagogastric junction	
B = 3–4 cm	Use 50–60F bougie to size sleeve width	
C = As is	Length of sleeve	
D = 5–6 cm	Antrectomy distance from pylorus	
E = 3 cm	Gastroileal anastomosis	
F = 50 cm	Roux gastroileal limb length	
G = 200 cm	Common limb	
V = 150–250 mL	Volume of sleeve (approx.)	

**Sleeve Gastrectomy
with Transit Bipartition
(SG-TB)**

Fig. 6. SG-TB. (*From* Bhandari M, Fobi MAL, Buchwald JN, et al. Standardization of bariatric metabolic procedures: world consensus meeting statement. Obes Surg.2019; 29(Suppl 4):309–345; with permission.)

- Advantages

    It adds metabolic effect to sleeve component.

    It does not have remnant stomach and risk of cancer.

- Disadvantages

    It has fewer chances of malnutrition as duodenal transit are also maintained.

- Surgical outcomes

    SG-TB is indicated for obese patients with T2DM. In a study by Santoro and colleagues[26] of 1020 patients (mean BMI 41.0 kg/m^2) undergoing SG-TB, mean excess BMI loss (EBMIL) was 91.0% at 1 year and 74.0% at 5 years (59.1% follow-up). SG-TB resolution of hypertension was 62.0%, hypertriglyceridemia 85.0%, and respiratory problems 91.0%. T2DM was resolved in 86.0% of patients, a rate superior to that reported in a 2016 meta-analysis for RYGBP, 56.8%.[27] In a 2018, 24-month, parallel-group, randomized controlled trial of the metabolic effects of SG-TB, 20 low-BMI patients with T2DM were randomized to SG-TB or standard medical therapy. At 24 months, HbA$_{1C}$ was statistically significantly reduced from baseline in the SG-TB group (9.3% ± 2.1% vs 5.5% ± 1.1%, respectively; $P<.05$) relative to the medical therapy group (8.0% ± 1.5% vs 8.3% ± 1.1%, respectively, P = NS).[28]

- Future

    It can be used in patients with diabetes in areas of increased stomach cancer.

SLEEVE GASTRECTOMY WITH JEJUNOILEAL INTERPOSITION AND SLEEVE GASTRECTOMY WITH DUODENAL, ILEAL INTERPOSITION

- Introduction

    This procedure has gained a lot of popularity as diabetes surgery or metabolic surgery, having been introduced by DePaula from Brazil in 2003.[29]

- Surgical anatomy

    BMI-adjusted SG is performed either completely laparoscopic, hybrid (SG by laparoscopy and interposition by open approach), or robotically, where a 170-cm segment of the terminal ileum is interposed into the jejunal or the duodenal area.

    SG-JII

    After SG, the ileal segment is interposed into the proximal jejunum, at 20 cm to 50 cm from the ligament of Treitz, without any bowel exclusion (**Fig. 7**).

    SG-DII

    After SG, the ileal segment is interposed between the divided first part of duodenum proximally, with the distal end attached to the jejunum at 50 cm from duodenojejunal flexure. This results in a bypass of the duodenumand proximal 50 cm of jejunum, liminating the foregut anti-incretin factor (see **Fig. 7**).

- Advantages

    o Type 1 diabetes mellitus, latent autoimmune diabetes of the adult (by estimating glutamic acid decarboxylase antibody, islet cell antibody, and insulin auto-antibody)

    o Beta-cell burn out, indicated by fasting C-peptide less than 0.5 ng/mL and/or stimulated C-peptide less than 1 ng/mL

- Disadvantages

    o Complex surgical anatomy and long learning curve

- Surgical outcomes

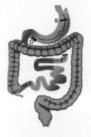
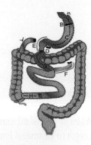

A = 1–2 cm	Distance of sleeve transection from esophagogastric junction
B = 2.5–3 cm	Use 32–40 F bougie to size sleeve width
C = As is	Length of sleeve
D = 2–6 cm	Antrectomy distance from pylorus
E = 3–4 cm	Length of duodenum from pylorus
F = 50 cm	Length of biliopancreatic limb
G = 150–170 cm	Length of ileal interposed limb
H = 30 cm	Distance of ileal transection from ileocecal junction
V = 75–150 mL	Volume of sleeve

Sleeve Gastrectomy w/Jejunoileal Interposition (SG-II) & Duodenal Ileal Interposition (SG-DII)

Fig. 7. SG-JII and SG-DII. (*From* Bhandari M, Fobi MAL, Buchwald JN, et al. Standardization of bariatric metabolic procedures: world consensus meeting statement. Obes Surg.2019; 29(Suppl 4):309–345; with permission.)

In a study conducted by the authors, 490 patients underwent II (SG-JII 10.2% and SG-DII 89.8%) at 2 different centers; 63% of the patients had BMI less than 35 kg/m² (mean BMI 29.5 kg/m²), mean HbA$_{1c}$ was 9.8%, and duration of T2DM 9.5 years. With a mean follow-up of 24 months (range, 10–72 months), complete remission was observed in 72% of patients and partial remission in 81.5%. Similar results supported these findings by different investigators in their respective study.[30]

- Future
  Uncontrolled diabetes despite optimal medical treatment; gradually worsening T2DM with a family history of diabetes-related complications, and stimulated C-peptide greater than 1 ng/mL

SINGLE-ANASTOMOSIS SLEEVE WITH ILEAL BYPASS

- Introduction
  The SASI bypass is a modification of the SG-TB of Santoro popularized by Mahdy and colleagues. 31 It combines an SG and loop transit bipartition rather than Roux-en-Y gastroileostomy 300 cm from the ileocecal junction.[8]
- Surgical anatomy
  SG is performed keeping sufficient length of the antrum (approximately 6 cm proximal to pylorus) with a loop gastroileostomy at 250 cm proximal to the ileocecal valve, using 2 layers of hand-sewn sutures/stapled anastomosis. In SASI bypass, compared with SADI-S, the duodenum is not transected, and the anastomosis is gastroileal instead of duodenoileal (**Fig. 8**).
- Advantages
  Duodenum is endoscopically accessible.
  Metabolic effect added to the sleeve component gives better resolution of metabolic syndrome.
  It has less chance of protein energy malnutrition.
  It is easily reversible leaving sleeve intact.
- Disadvantages
  o It can have marginal ulcer in transit bypass and ileal contents in the stomach, in loop bipartition.
- Surgical outcomes

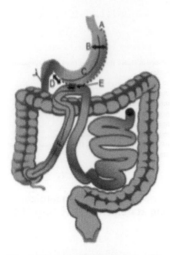

A = 2–3 cm	Distance of sleeve transection from esophagogastric junction
B = 3–4 cm	Use 50–60F bougie to size sleeve width
C = As is	Length of sleeve
D = 2–6 cm	Distance from pylorus
E = 3 cm	Width of gastroileal anastomosis
F = 300 cm	Length of gastroileal limb
V = 150–250 mL	Volume of sleeve (approx.)

Single-Anastomosis Sleeve with Ileal Bypass (SASI)

Fig. 8. SASI. (*From* Bhandari M, Fobi MAL, Buchwald JN, et al. Standardization of bariatric metabolic procedures: world consensus meeting statement. Obes Surg.2019; 29(Suppl 4):309–345; with permission.)

Santoro and colleagues[26] studied 1020 obese patients (BMI 33–72 kg/m^2), with a follow-up rate of 59.1% (range, 4 months to 5 years) and reported excellent weight loss (91% EBMIL at 1 year; 94% at 2 years, 85% at 3 years, 78% at 4 years, and 74% at 5 years). Partial diabetes remission was seen in 86%, with a complication rate of 6%, including 2 deaths (0.2%).[26]

- Mui and colleagues[25] published a case report of SG-LB, with 97% EWL at 12 months' follow-up in a 46-year-old obese diabetic patient who achieved normoglycemia without medication within 2 months. Mahdy and colleagues[31] published results of SASI bypass in 50 patients suffering from obesity and diabetes. They have shown %EWL of 90% at 1 year, normoglycemia in 100% of patients at 3 months, and resolution of hypertension (86%), hypercholesterolemia (100%), and hypertriglyceridemia (97%).[31]

- Future
    It can have marginal ulcer in transit bypass and ileal contents in the stomach, in loop bipartition.

ONE-ANASTOMOSIS GASTRIC BYPASS OR MINI–GASTRIC BYPASS

- Introduction
    The OAGB/MGB was devised by Robert Rutledge in USA. The procedure essentially is a loop gastroenterostomy with a single large, nonobstructive anastomosis. The procedure has gained popularity due to technical ease, shorter learning curve, and similar results to a gastric bypass. Most studies have determined it as effective as gastric bypass. The procedure is done by making a long gastric tube and fashioning an anastomosis of 4.5-cm to 6-cm long between a bypassed loop of small bowel, 150-cm to 300-cm long. The gastroenterostomy is wide and nonrestrictive.[32,33]

- Surgical anatomy

  The procedure is done by making a long gastric tube and fashioning an anastomosis of 4.5-cm to 6-cm long between a bypassed loop of small bowel 150-cm to 300-cm long. The gastroenterostomy is wide and nonrestrictive (**Fig. 9**). The authors recommend 150 cm to 300 cm of BPL to avoid excessive malnutrition.

- Advantages
  - Good weight loss at 10 years
  - Higher or equally good resolution of type 2 diabetes than ____?
  - Technically less challenging
  - No internal hernia defects

- Disadvantages
  - Comparatively higher nutritional deficiencies
  - Marginal ulcers
  - Mild reflux esophagitis
  - More than 100% EWL

- Surgical outcome

  Weight loss: %EWL after 1 year is reported to be from 55% to 91%, maintained at 85% over 6 years.[34,35]

  Diabetes resolution/remission: diabetes remission was observed in 83% to 93% of patients. Long-term results, however, still are awaited.[36,37]

- Future

  The procedure has gained popularity in most parts of the world except for the United States. Most insurance companies in the states do not reimburse it. The procedure is used primarily as a secondary/revision procedure in the United States. Apart from the United States, the procedure has been used widely as a primary procedure in all other countries, especially India and major European countries.

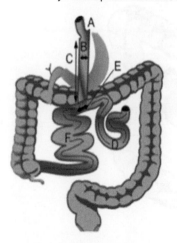

A = 1–1.5 cm	Distance from esophagogastric junction
B = 2.5–3 cm	Width of pouch
C = 15 cm	Length of pouch (12–19 cm)
D = 200 cm	Length of biliopancreatic limb BMI >50 kg/m^2
D = 150 cm	Length of biliopancreatic imb BMI <50 kg/m^2
E = 3–4 cm	Width of gastroenterostomy
F = As	Length of common channel
V = 50–75 mL	Volume of pouch (approx.)

One-Anastomosis Gastric Bypass or Mini Gastric Bypass (OAGB/MGB)

Fig. 9. OAGB/MGB. (*From* Bhandari M, Fobi MAL, Buchwald JN, et al. Standardization of bariatric metabolic procedures: world consensus meeting statement. Obes Surg.2019; 29(Suppl 4):309–345; with permission.)

BANDED ONE-ANASTOMOSIS GASTRIC BYPASS OR BANDED MINI-GASTRIC BYPASS

- Introduction

  Developed as an innovation to OAGB/MGB in morbidly obese patients to prevent weight regain
- Surgical anatomy

  Same as the procedure of OAGB, discussed previously, with a nonadjustable ring placed loosely around the proximal pouch 3 cm to 5 cm from the gastroesophageal junction (**Fig. 10**)
- Advantages

  With fixed bilioipancreatic limb of 180 cm and increased restriction by placing the band, it can prevent malnutrition and at the same time achieve desired weight loss without need for long bilioipancreatic limb.
- Disadvantages

  Comparatively higher nutritional deficiencies

  Marginal ulcers

  Reflux esophagitis

  More than 100% EWL in some patients

  Band erosion and band slippage
- Surgical outcomes

  At the authors' center, there is an ongoing prospective comparative study comparing banded versus nonbanded one-anastomosis gastric bypass patients. Results seen in 40 patients after 3 years of follow-up suggest 36.75%

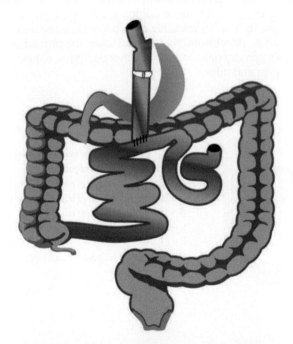

BANDED OAGB/MGB

Fig. 10. BOAGB/BMGB. (*From* Bhandari M, Fobi MAL, Buchwald JN, et al. Standardization of bariatric metabolic procedures: world consensus meeting statement. Obes Surg.2019; 29(Suppl 4):309–345; with permission.)

total body weight loss percentage (TWL%) in the banded group compared with 25.19% TWL% in the nonbanded group. There is a need for prospective and more extensive series studies to confirm these findings.

- Future

  It can be used in superobese patients with good results.

SINGLE-ANASTOMOSIS GASTROILEAL BYPASS

- Introduction

  The SAG-I technique is primarily that of OAGB; however, to address possible insufficient absorption of the efferent intestinal limb, de Luca and colleagues modified the OAGB technique, constructing the gastrointestinal anastomosis at a fixed distance (approximately 300 cm) from the ileocecal valve.[37,38]

- Surgical anatomy

  The procedure is done by making a long gastric tube and fashioning an anastomosis of 3-cm to 4-cm long with a common limb of 300 cm from the ileocecal junction (**Fig. 11**).

- Advantages

  SAG-I can be used as a revision procedure for insufficient weight loss or regain after LAGB, OAGB, or SG.

  It is easily reversible.

  The resolution of the metabolic syndrome is better.

- Disadvantages

  Marginal ulcer

  Protein energy malnutrition

  Loose stools and odor

- Surgical outcomes

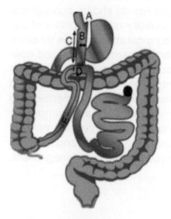

A = 1–1.5 cm	Distance of sleeve transection from esophagogastric junction
B = 2.5–3 cm	Width of pouch (approx.)
C = 12–18 cm	Length of pouch
D = 3–4 cm	Width of gastroenterostomy
E = 300 cm	Length of gastrocecal limb
V = 50–75 mL	Volume of gastric pouch

Single-Anastomosis Gastro-Ileal Bypass (SAG-I)

Fig. 11. SAG-I. (*From* Bhandari M, Fobi MAL, Buchwald JN, et al. Standardization of bariatric metabolic procedures: world consensus meeting statement. Obes Surg.2019; 29(Suppl 4):309–345; with permission.)

De Luca and colleagues[38] demonstrated mean EWL was 55.1% with BMI 34.3 at 3months (n 5 7) and 82.1%with BMI 27.8 kg/m2 at 6months (n 5 2). The patients reported 2 to 4 daily bowel movements of soft stool. The number and softness of bowel movements were related to oral fat intake.

- Future
  Can be used as a revision procedure for insufficient weight loss or regain after LAGB, OAGB, or SG

SUMMARY

There is now a worldwide epidemic of obesity. Metabolic bariatric surgery induces durable and sustainable weight loss. The role of metabolic surgery in the treatment of obesity is well established. The remission of obesity-related comorbidities, such as metabolic syndrome after bariatric surgery, is accompanied by increased longevity. And, emerging procedures in bariatric metabolic surgery are successful for achieving significant and sustainable weight loss; it is the resolution of metabolic conditions like diabetes that currently is getting the most attention. To understand the elements in each procedure that correlate with beneficial weight loss and metabolic effects, uniform measurement is a fundamental requirement. Yet, a variety of versions of bariatric metabolic procedure configurations exist, to say nothing of the range of variations in the sequence of steps involved to complete the procedure. The dramatic increase in demand for surgical remedies for severe obesity and other metabolic disorders has stimulated tremendous interest in developing new operative procedures. These emerging procedures are striving for less invasiveness, excellent safety, lack of permanent alterations of the gastrointestinal tract, lack of long-termconsequences, and even novel mechanisms of action. Although an exciting time in bariatric surgery is being entered, that is rich with rapid change and exciting innovations, it should be kept in mind that currently none of these new modalities has been adequately studied to warrant introduction into practice. Some of these innovations ultimately may be deemed worthy for use, whereas others likely will fail to achieve meaningful results and be abandoned.

Moreover, new metabolic surgical procedures reduce obesity-related costs and use of health care resources. It is estimated that the cost of surgical interventions for class II to class III obesity is offset by the subsequent reduction in pharmaceutical and hospitalization cost within the first 2 years after bariatric surgery. New surgical options should be reserved for weight loss and weight-loss maintenance, and further research into the biology and psychology of weight-loss maintenance should be undertaken to develop more effective approaches. Finally, more intensive public health campaigns and training opportunities on upcoming metabolic bariatric procedures are needed to better inform providers, industry stakeholders, insurers, policymakers, and the general public about the health impact of obesity and the need for optimal management.

CLINICS CARE POINTS

- There are many emerging surgical procedures in bariatric metabolic surgery.
- Some emerging surgical procedures are modifications of existing procedures and have advantages, such as less technically challenging, minimized inherent complications, better weight loss, and/or better metabolic effects over existing procedures.
- Some emerging surgical procedures are modifications of existing procedures that address geographic variances, such as racial, ethnic, and cultural differences.

- Most of the emerging surgical procedures have been used in a relatively limited number of patients and have had only short-term follow-up.
- There is need for prospective randomized comparative clinical studies of emerging surgical procedures.

DISCLOSURE

All authors have nothing to disclose.

REFERENCES

1. Wolfe BM, Kvach E, Eckel RH. Treatment of obesity: weight loss and bariatric surgery. Circ Res 2016;118(11):1844–55.
2. Rubino F, Nathan DM, Eckel RH, et al. Metabolic surgery in the treatment algorithm for type 2 diabetes: a joint statement by international diabetes organizations. Diabetes Care 2016;39(6):861–77.
3. Pareek M, Schauer PR, Kaplan LM, et al. Metabolic Surgery. J Am Coll Cardiol 2018;71(6):670–87.
4. Pasupathy S, Tham KW. Metabolic-Bariatric surgery: an emerging specialty. Proceedings of Singapore Healthcare 2012;21(3):194–8.
5. Karcz WK, Marjanovic G, Grueneberger J, et al. Banded sleeve gastrectomy using the GaBP ring—surgical technique. Obes Facts 2011;4(1):77–80.
6. Agrawal S, Van DE, Akin F, et al. Laparoscopic adjustable banded sleeve gastrectomy as a primary procedure for the super-super obese (body mass index > 60 kg/m²). Obes Surg 2010;20:1161–3.
7. Alexander JW, Martin Hawver LR, Goodman HR. Banded sleeve gastrectomy—initial experience. Obes Surg 2009;19:1591–6.
8. Bhandari M, Fobi MAL, Buchwald JN, et al. Standardization of Bariatric Metabolic Procedures: World Consensus Meeting Statement. Obes Surg 2019;29(Suppl4): 309–45.
9. Gentileschi P, Bianciardi E, Siragusa L, et al. Banded sleeve gastrectomy improves weight loss compared to nonbanded sleeve: midterm results from a prospective randomized study. J Obes 2020;2020:1–7.
10. Fink JM, Hoffmann N, Kuesters S, et al. Banding the Sleeve Improves Weight Loss in Midterm Follow-up. OBES SURG 2017;27:1098–103.
11. Lemmens L, Van Den Bossche J, Zaveri H, et al. Banded sleeve gastrectomy: better long-term results? A long-term cohort study until 5 years follow-up in obese and superobese patients. Obes Surg 2018;28(9):2687–95.
12. Alamo M, Torres CS, Peez LZ. Vertical isolated gastroplasty with gastro-enteral bypass: Preliminary results. Obes Surg 2006;16(3):353–8.
13. de Menezes Ettinger JE, Azaro E, Mello CA, et al. analysis of the vertical isolated gastroplasty: a new bariatric operation. Obes Surg 2006;16:1261–3.
14. Sepulveda M, Alamo M, Lynch R, et al. Comparison of long-term weight loss between sleeve gastrectomy and sleeve gastrectomy with jejunal bypass. A case-control study. Obes Surg 2018;28(11):3466–73.
15. Alamo M, Sepulveda M, Gellona J, et al. Sleeve gastrectomy with jejunal bypass for the treatment of type 2 diabetes mellitus in patients with BMI <35 kg/m²: a cohort study. Obes Surg 2012;22(7):1097–103.
16. Melissas J, Peppe A, Askoxilakis J, et al. Sleeve gastrectomy plus side-to-side jejunoileal anastomosis for the treatment of morbid obesity and metabolic diseases: a promising operation. Obes Surg 2012;22(7):1104–9.

17. Kasama K, Tagaya N, Kanehira E, et al. Laparoscopic sleeve gastrectomy with duodeno-jejunal bypass: technique and preliminary results. Obes Surg 2009; 19:1341–2.
18. Praveen Raj P, Kumaravel R, Chandramaliteeswanran C, et al. Is laparoscopic duodenojejunal bypass with sleeve an effective alternative to Roux en Y gastric bypass in morbidly obese patients: preliminary results of a randomized trial. Obes Surg 2012;22:422–6.
19. Lee WJ, Almulaifi AM, Tsou JJ, et al. Duodenal-jejunal bypass with sleeve gastrectomy versus the sleeve gastrectomy procedure alone: the role of duodenal exclusion. Surg Obes Relat Dis 2015;11(4):765–70.
20. Naitoh T, Kasama K, Seki Y, et al. Efficacy of sleeve gastrectomy with duodenal-jejunal bypass for the treatment of obese severe diabetes patients in Japan: a retrospective multicenter study. Obes Surg 2018;28(2):497–505.
21. Huang CK, Goel R, Tai CM, et al. Novel metabolic surgery for type II diabetes mellitus: loop duodenojejunal bypass with sleeve gastrectomy. Surg Laparosc Endosc Percutan Tech 2013;23:481–5.
22. Huang CK, Tai CM, Chang PC, et al. Loop Duodenojejunal Bypass with Sleeve Gastrectomy: Comparative Study with Roux-en-Y Gastric Bypass in Type 2 Diabetic Patients with a BMI <35 kg/m(2), First Year Results. Obes Surg 2016;26: 2291–301.
23. Ugale S, Vennapusa A, Katakwar A, et al. Laparoscopic bariatric surgery current trends and controversies. Ann Laparosc Endosc Surg 2017;2:154.
24. Santoro S, Castro LC, Velhote MC, et al. Sleeve gastrectomy with transit bipartition: a potent intervention for metabolic syndrome and obesity. Ann Surg 2012; 256:104–10.
25. Mui WL, Lee DW, Lam KK. Laparoscopic sleeve gastrectomy with loop bipartition: A novel metabolic operation in treating obese type II diabetes mellitus. Int J Surg Case Rep 2014;5:56–8.
26. Santoro S, Castro LC, Velhote MC, et al. Sleeve gastrectomy with transit bipartition: a potent operation for metabolic syndrome and obesity. Ann Surg 2012; 256(1):104–10.
27. Yan Y, Sha Y, Gao G, et al. Roux-en-Y gastric bypass vs medical treatment for type 2 diabetes mellitus in obese patients: a systematic review and meta-analysis of randomized controlled trials. Medicine (Baltimore) 2016;95(17):e3462.
28. Azevedo FR, Santoro S, Correa-Giannella ML, et al. A prospective randomized controlled trial of the metabolic effects of sleeve gastrectomy with transit bipartition. Obes Surg 2018;28(10):3012–9.
29. DePaula AL, Macedo AL, Mota BR, et al. Laparoscopic ileal interposition associated to a diverted sleeve gastrectomy is an effective operation for the treatment of type 2 diabetes mellitus patients with BMI 21-29. Surg Endosc 2009;23: 1313–20.
30. De Paula AL, Stival AR, Macedo A, et al. Prospective randomized controlled trial comparing 2 versions of laparoscopic ileal interposition associated with sleeve gastrectomy for patients with type 2 diabetes with BMI 21–34 kg/m2. Surg Obes Relat Dis 2010;6:296–304.
31. Mahdy T, Al Wahedi A, Schou C. Efficacy of single anastomosis sleeve ileal (SASI) bypass for type-2 diabetic morbid obese patients: Gastric bipartition, a novel metabolic surgery procedure: A retrospective cohort study. Int J Surg 2016;34:28–34.
32. Rutledge R. The mini-gastric bypass: experience with first 1,274 cases. Obes Surg 2001;11:276–80.

33. Rutledge R, Walsh TR. Continued excellent results with the mini-gastric bypass: six-year study in 2,410 patients. Obes Surg 2005;15:1304–8.
34. Kular KS, Manchanda N, Rutledge R. A 6-year experience with 1,054 mini-gastric bypasses-first study from the Indian subcontinent. Obes Surg 2014;24:1430–5.
35. Georgiadou D, Sergentanis TN, Nixon A, et al. Efficacy and safety of laparoscopic mini-gastric bypass. Surg Obes Relat Dis 2014;10:984–91.
36. Shivakumar S, Tantia O, Goyal G, et al. LSG vs MGB-OAGB-3 year follow-up data: a randomised control trial. Obes Surg 2018;28(9):2820–8.
37. De Luca M, Tie T, Ooi G, et al. Mini gastric bypass-one anastomosis gastric bypass (MGB-OAGB)-IFSO position statement. OBES SURG 2018;28:1188–206.
38. De Luca M, Himpens J, Angrisani L, et al. A new concept in bariatric surgery. single anastomosis gastro-ileal (SAGI): technical details and preliminary results. Obes Surg 2016;27(1):143–7.

Endoscopic Balloon Therapy

Michael J. Klingler, MD[a],*, Matthew Kroh, MD[b]

KEYWORDS

- Intragastric balloon • Endoluminal bariatrics • Endoscopic bariatrics

KEY POINTS

- Intragastric balloon (IGB) therapy is a low-morbidity, easily reversible treatment of obesity.
- IGB therapy promotes a range of weight loss and comorbidity resolution in between lifestyle/pharmacotherapies and more invasive bariatric procedures, such as sleeve gastrectomy or Roux-en-Y gastric bypass.
- Intragastric balloons may help to bridge the gap between lifestyle modification and bariatric surgery in patients with moderate obesity (BMI, 30–35 kg/m²).

INTRODUCTION

Bariatric surgery is an effective and durable treatment of morbid obesity and its related comorbidities, although few effective therapies are available for the more than 130 million Americans with moderate obesity who are not candidates for, or do not wish to undergo surgery.[1] Currently, lifestyle modification and pharmacotherapy are the mainstay of treatment of obesity in this group, neither of which promote similar weight loss or comorbidity resolution when compared with bariatric surgery.[2,3] There is a significant demand for low-risk, minimally invasive therapies to help bridge the gap between the current standard of care and bariatric surgery in patients with class I and class II obesity.

As outlined in Winder and Rodriguez's article, "Emerging Endoscopic Interventions in Bariatric Surgery," in this issue, new endoluminal obesity therapies, such as endoscopic gastric plication, offer a minimally invasive treatment option for the moderately obese, although outcomes data are limited and these procedures account for less than 5% of all bariatric procedures performed worldwide.[4] Intragastric balloons (IGBs), which occupy space in the stomach promoting satiety and weight loss, have been used internationally for more than 20 years with sufficient data to support their efficacy and safety. IGBs are particularly appealing to patients who are hesitant to undergo bariatric surgery because they have a low associated morbidity, are easily removable, and treatment can be repeated in cases of weight regain. Originally with extensive use limited to Europe, South America, Asia, and the Middle East, IGBs

[a] Cleveland Clinic, 9500 Euclid Avenue, Mail Code H18, Cleveland, OH 44195-0001, USA;
[b] Cleveland Clinic Abu Dhabi, PO Box 112412, Al Maryah Island, Abu Dhabi, United Arab Emirates
* Corresponding author.
E-mail address: Klinglm@ccf.org

Surg Clin N Am 101 (2021) 355–371
https://doi.org/10.1016/j.suc.2020.12.009
0039-6109/21/© 2020 Elsevier Inc. All rights reserved.

are gaining popularity in the United States as more devices are approved by the Food and Drug Administration (FDA). As global rates of obesity continue to increase, the international market size for IGBs is predicted to double by the year 2025.[5]

THE EVOLUTION OF INTRAGASTRIC BALLOON THERAPY

The Garren-Edwards Gastric Bubble (GEGB) was the first IGB that was brought to the market, in 1985, as a treatment of morbid obesity in those who were unsuccessful with lifestyle changes and who were averse to surgery. A high rate of complications and device malfunctions, along with a failure to show added benefit to diet and exercise in a double-blinded, sham-controlled trial led to its removal from the market in 1992 (**Fig. 1**).[6]

In 1987, a working group of expert gastroenterologists, surgeons, and behavioral medicine physicians convened in Florida to evaluate the available evidence for IGBs. They developed guidelines for patient selection and outlined characteristics of the ideal IGB, which provided a blueprint for the devices available on the market today. They proposed all balloons should have a radiopaque marker to easily locate the device in cases of migration; be composed of durable material with the ability to stretch, which may allow the volume to be individualized to the patient; and be filled with fluid rather than air, which may better prohibit food intake.[7] Subsequent devices with these attributes would prove to be safer and more effective than the GEGB predecessor, although several effective air-filled IGBs have also been brought to market. The Bio-Enterics Intragastric Balloon (BIB) was the first successful balloon, introduced in 1991, which had substantial international use before its FDA approval as the Orbera balloon (Apollo Endosurgery, Austin, TX) in 2015.

The goal of this article is to familiarize the surgeon with commercially available IGBs, the indications for their use, general guidelines for balloon insertion and removal, and to summarize the available outcomes data for FDA-approved IGBs and those currently under review for FDA approval. At the time of this publication there are three FDA-approved balloons on the market in the United States and several balloons approved in Europe (Conformité Européenne mark) that are undergoing clinical trials in the United States. Balloons are either fluid-filled (saline) or gas-filled (nitrogen mixture) and have implantation durations ranging from 4 to 12 months. Currently, most US

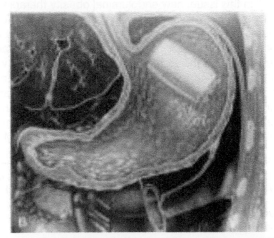

Fig. 1. The first IGB, the Garren-Edwards Gastric Balloon. (*From* Velchik MG, Kramer FM, Stunkard AJ, et al. Effect of the Garren-Edwards gastric bubble on gastric emptying. J Nucl Med. 1989;30(5):692-6; with permission.)

insurance companies do not cover IGBs and patients in the United States should expect to pay out-of-pocket for treatment. A description of the most common commercially available IGBs in the United States and Europe are listed in **Table 1**.

MECHANISM OF WEIGHT LOSS IN INTRAGASTRIC BALLOON THERAPY

IGBs promote weight loss through a combination of mechanical and neurohormonal effects that are still being elucidated. Stretching of gastric wall mechanoreceptors by ingested food activates vagal afferent fibers, leading to centrally mediated feelings of satiety. Abnormal signaling of this vagal pathway has been implicated in the development and maintenance of obesity, and therapies targeting the vagus nerve have been shown to promote weight loss.[8,9] In normal individuals, the gastric fundus relaxes to accommodate an incoming food bolus, reducing intragastric pressure and mechanical stretch of the gastric wall.[10] IGBs are thought to act as an "artificial bezoar," occupying space in the stomach that leads to an earlier stretch of the gastric wall during meals, promoting early satiety.

There is mounting evidence that fluid-filled IGBs may also promote weight loss by delaying gastric emptying. In a meta-analysis of five studies (n = 66), gastric emptying times were delayed by nearly 2 hours after placement of a fluid-filled IGB but not in those who received a gas-filled balloon.[11] The gas-filled IGB used as a comparison was the GEGB, which was proven ineffective for weight loss and occupies less than half the volume of the current FDA-approved gas-filled balloons. In a randomized prospective study of 29 subjects randomized to either IGB (n = 15) or to control (n = 14), subjects in the treatment arm had significantly greater delays in gastric emptying at 8 weeks, and greater delays were associated with higher percent total body weight loss (TBWL).[12] Gastric emptying returned to baseline after balloons were removed.

Balloon volume may be of greater importance in terms of weight loss in gas-filled compared with fluid-filled balloons. The placement of two additional gas-filled balloons between weeks 9 and 12 in a randomized controlled trial (RCT) of the gas-filled Obalon balloon (Obalon Therapeutics Inc, Carlsbad, CA) promoted more weight loss.[13] No correlation between filling volume and weight loss was demonstrated in a meta-analysis of 44 studies (n = 5549) of the single fluid-filled Orbera balloon, although lower rates of migration were noted at higher volumes.[14]

Although alterations in neurohormonal regulation of hunger and satiety are well-known consequences of anatomy altering bariatric surgery procedures, such as the Roux-en-Y gastric bypass, the effects of IGB on hormones regulating energy balance are less well understood.[15] The hunger-inducing hormone, ghrelin, has been the most extensively studied in IGB therapy, although results have been mixed. Mion and colleagues[16] observed significantly lower ghrelin levels in 17 subjects after initiation of IGB therapy, and greater fluctuations in ghrelin levels were associated with more weight loss. No changes in fasting or meal-suppressed ghrelin concentration were found in a randomized, sham-controlled study of the BIB, although ghrelin levels did not increase as would be expected in subjects who are in a state of negative energy balance.[17] In contrast, a transient elevation in serum ghrelin levels was reported in a RCT of morbidly obese patients with a single fluid-filled IGB, which returned to baseline 3 months after the balloon was removed.[18,19] Changes in levels of the hormones leptin, adiponectin, and cholecystokinin have also been observed in patients undergoing IGB therapy.[17,18]

INDICATIONS

In the United States, IGB therapy is indicated for adults with class I and II obesity (body mass index [BMI], 30–40 kg/m^2) who have been unsuccessful in achieving weight loss

Table 1
Most common FDA and non-FDA approved intragastric balloons available in the US and worldwide

Intragastric Balloon	Balloon Design	Filling Substance	Placement Duration	Placement Method	Extraction Method	FDA Approval	Notes
Orbera™ (Apollo Endosurgery, Austin, TX, USA)	Single silicone balloon, silicone	Saline 400–700 mL	6–12 mo	Endoscopic, transoral catheter	Endoscopic	Yes	Largest market share, 12-mo version (Orbera™ 365) in development
Courtesy of Apollo Endosurgery, Austin, TX; with permission.							
ReShape Duo™ (Apollo Endosurgery; Austin TX, USA) sale discontinued in 2018	Double silicone non-communicating balloons	Saline 900 mL	6 mo	Endoscopic, transoral catheter	Endoscopic	Yes	Second balloon may prevent migration in the instance of single balloon deflation, no longer on the market
Courtesy of Apollo Endosurgery, Austin, TX; with permission.							
Obalon™ Gastric Balloon (Obalon Therapeutics Inc; Carlsbad, CA, USA)	Up to three individual polyethylene blend balloons	Gas (nitrogen mix) 250 mL per balloon (up to 3 balloons)	6 mo	Swallowed in a capsule (no endoscopy, verified by imaging)	Endoscopic	Yes	Second balloon is typically placed at week 3, third balloon placed between weeks 9–12

Spatz3™ Adjustable Balloon (Spatz Medical; NY, USA)	Single, adjustable silicone balloon	Saline	12 mo	Endoscopic	Endoscopic	No (CE mark)	Downward adjustments for excessive accommodative symptoms, upward adjustments made for plateaus in weight loss, possible higher cost due to need for multiple endoscopies
Courtesy of Spatz Medical, Great Neck NY; with permission.							
Ellipse™ balloon (Allurion Technologies, Natick, MA, USA)	Single, swallowable silicone balloon	Saline 550 mL	4 mo	Swallowed in a capsule (no endoscopy, verified by imaging)	Excreted naturally through GI tract	No (CE mark)	Only balloon that does not require endoscopy for either placement or removal
Courtesy of Allurion Technologies, Natick, MA; with permission.							

Courtesy of Spatz Medical (https://spatzmedical.com/), Great Neck, NY; with permission.

with lifestyle modification. Similar to bariatric surgery, patients should be evaluated by a multidisciplinary team including a bariatric physician, dietician, and psychologist. It is important to address comorbid psychosocial issues that may contribute to the development of obesity and may also interfere with IGB therapy. After implant, patients should be willing to undergo a supervised 12-month diet and exercise plan and should follow up monthly with members of the multidisciplinary team during treatment.

IGB therapy may also be used to promote weight loss as a bridge to bariatric surgery in patients with morbid or supermorbid obesity.[20] Several studies have demonstrated IGBs can promote weight loss and reduce liver volume in supermorbidly obese patients before bariatric surgery, which may make the operation safer.[21–23] The timing of bariatric surgery in patients who underwent IGB therapy beforehand is important, because significant gastric wall hypertrophy can occur during fluid-filled IGB therapy, which may interfere with gastric stapling.[24] In a randomized trial comparing standard medical care and 6 months of IGB therapy before laparoscopic Roux-en-Y gastric bypass, superobese (average BMI, 54.7 kg/m^2) patients lost significantly more preoperative weight in the treatment arm, but suffered a higher postoperative complication rate.[25] Patients underwent gastric bypass at an average of 9 days after IGB therapy, which may have contributed to the higher complication rate. Gastric wall width has been shown to return to baseline 30 days after balloon removal, which is likely the appropriate interval between IGB therapy and bariatric surgery.[24] In addition to bariatric surgery, IGBs have also been shown to promote weight loss before nonbariatric operations, such as heart and liver transplantation, hernia repair, and orthopedic surgery.[26–29]

CONTRAINDICATIONS

The contraindications to IGB therapy are those that preclude safe endoscopic placement and removal of the balloon, the presence of comorbidities that may be exacerbated by the balloon, or psychosocial issues that may interfere with surveillance or participation in a supervised weight loss program.[30] These contraindications are outlined in **Box 1**. Relative contraindications that may require additional testing or surveillance are eosinophilic esophagitis, nonbleeding gastric angioectasias, or the anticipated need for endoscopic procedures during the time of balloon therapy. The presence of mild gastritis, benign hyperplastic gastric polyps, and a positive *Helicobacter pylori* status without signs of malignancy or ulceration are not considered contraindications, although treatment of *H pylori* infection is recommended.[30]

A diagnostic upper endoscopy evaluating the entire esophagus, stomach, and duodenum should be done before or at the time of IGB placement to identify any gastric pathology or undisclosed gastric surgery that may prohibit placement of a balloon. A nuclear gastric emptying study should be ordered in patients with suspected gastroparesis, because the additional delay in gastric emptying caused by fluid-filled IGBs may cause intolerable nausea and vomiting, leading to early balloon removal.[11] Gas-filled balloons, or other procedures that increase gastric emptying, such as sleeve gastrectomy, may be better options for these patients.

BALLOON PLACEMENT

IGB placement is device dependent and should be performed using the manufacturers guidelines. Generally, patients should be *nil per os* per hospital endoscopy protocol and should be given antiemetics before the procedure. For endoscopically

---

Box 1
Contraindications to IGB therapy

- History of gastric or esophageal surgery
- Inflammatory bowel disease
- History of gastric or esophageal malignancy
- Presence of a large hiatal hernia (>5 cm)
- Presence of gastric or esophageal ulcers
- History of cirrhosis, liver failure, or esophageal varices
- Coagulopathy or known clotting/bleeding disorder
- Chronic nonsteroidal anti-inflammatory drug use
- Allergy to materials, such as silicone
- Active substance abuse disorder
- Uncontrolled psychiatric disease
- Inability to participate in a medically supervised weight loss program or to undergo routine follow-up
- Pregnancy or active breastfeeding

---

placed balloons the procedure is performed safely in most cases under conscious sedation (Orbera, ReShape Duo [Apollo Endosurgery], and Spatz3 [Spatz Medical, Great Neck, NY]). A preliminary upper endoscopy should be performed with a standard adult gastroscope before passing the balloon catheter into the stomach. This is done under direct endoscopic vision to ensure appropriate positioning below the gastroesophageal junction to prevent esophageal or gastric injury.

For swallowable, capsule-type balloons (Obalon and Elipse [Allurion Technologies, Natick, MA]), patients do not require sedation and the balloon capsule is consumed with a small cup of water while in the upright position. The long filling catheter is used to inflate the balloon after confirmation of the position below the gastroesophageal junction is confirmed with fluoroscopy or abdominal radiograph. Although these balloons may be placed by practitioners not experienced in endoscopy, swallowable balloon placement should be performed in a facility with access to endoscopy if the need for emergent balloon removal arises.

Fluid-filled balloons are often filled with a small amount of methylene blue dye, which alerts the patient to possible balloon rupture by a change in urine color.

POST-PROCEDURE MANAGEMENT AND MONITORING

A period of adaptation directly following IGB placement is anticipated, and symptoms of nausea, vomiting, abdominal discomfort/cramping, and reflux are common but are generally self-limited and typically resolve within 14 days. Patients should be instructed to call the clinic if there are changes in urine color, possibly indicating balloon rupture. Antiemetic/antispasmodic prescriptions should be filled before the procedure and taken on a scheduled basis, along with a mandatory proton pump inhibitor, which should be taken as long as the balloon is in place. Patients should be instructed to avoid all nonsteroidal anti-inflammatory drug (NSAID) medications for the duration of treatment. Diet should be advanced slowly from liquids to solid foods, and patients should be seen within a week of placement to assess for improvement in accommodative symptoms and to assess for dehydration. Severe nausea and vomiting or symptoms lasting longer than 14 days should prompt a visit with the clinician to evaluate proper balloon position and may necessitate early balloon removal in some cases. Patients may follow up with members of the multidisciplinary team on a monthly basis thereafter.

INTRAGASTRIC BALLOON REMOVAL

Balloon removal can be performed at an outpatient endoscopy center with access to anesthesia personnel. Aspiration is a greater concern during balloon removal and many endoscopists recommend general anesthesia and intubation in all cases of balloon removal. To lower the risk of aspiration, a liquid diet is recommended for 1 to 2 days before removal, in addition to a period of *nil per os* immediately before the procedure.

Balloon removal is also device dependent and should be performed using the manufacturer's instructions, although in emergent situations all balloons can be removed by aspirating the balloon contents with an endoscopic injection needle and removing the balloon with an endoscopic grasper. The Elipse balloon is unique in that it is designed to self-empty at approximately 4 months and pass through the gastrointestinal (GI) tract before being naturally excreted without need for endoscopic removal.

DISCUSSION
Weight Loss and Safety Outcomes of Food and Drug Administration–Approved Balloons

A summary of the weight loss and safety outcomes of IGB therapy from the major US RCTs and clinical studies are listed in **Tables 2** and **3** and are outlined in greater detail next.

Orbera
The single fluid-filled Orbera IGB, formerly the BIB, has been used for more than 20 years internationally and makes up most of the global market share for all IGBs.[31] Results from the pivotal, open-label, RCT of the Orbera IGB demonstrated the efficacy and safety of the balloon, leading to its approval by the FDA in 2016.[32] In this trial, 255 patients with a mean BMI of 35 kg/m^2 underwent either a 12-month behavioral and diet modification program alone (n = 130), or underwent the same program with the Orbera IGB placed for the first 6 months (n = 125). Subjects in the treatment arm had a TBWL of 10.2% at the time of balloon removal compared with 3.3% in the control arm (P<.001). Total weight loss was 7.6% in the balloon group at 12 months, and 32% of subjects in the treatment group maintained greater than 10% TBWL from their baseline. Weight loss at balloon removal was higher in this open-label trial of the Orbera when compared with the sham-controlled pivotal trials of the gas-filled Obalon and dual fluid-filled ReShape Duo balloon **Table 2**.[32,33] Outcome comparisons between these trials should be interpreted with caution, as knowledge of treatment group in open-label RCTs has been shown to impact weight loss when compared to trials of blinded subjects.[13] Weight loss at balloon removal in the retrospective postregulatory trial of the Orbera was 11.8%, similar to those reported in the postregulatory trials of the ReShape Duo (11.4%) and Obalon (10.0)% balloons (see **Table 3**).[34–36]

Accommodative symptoms were common after balloon placement in the pivotal RCT, because 75% to 80% of patients experienced nausea and vomiting that was generally self-limited, although dehydration occurred in 14.4% of IGB patients. Early balloon removal occurred in 18.8% of patients mainly caused by device intolerance or subject request. Serious adverse events occurred in 10% of patients and included two cases of severe dehydration, one gastric outlet obstruction, and one gastric perforation with sepsis.[32] In the postregulatory study, there were no cases of balloon migration, obstruction, or perforation and early balloon removal occurred in 16.5% of patients, similar to the RCT.[34]

In a meta-analysis of 17 studies (n = 1638) that evaluated the Orbera balloon as a primary treatment of obesity over a range of baseline BMIs (including those with BMI >40 kg/m^2), the pooled TBWL was 13.2% (55 studies) at 6 months and 11.3% (three studies) at 12 months. A meta-regression demonstrated that the balloon also performed well in patients with BMI greater than 40 kg/m^2, surpassing the weight loss threshold set by the American Society for Gastrointestinal Endoscopy Bariatric Endoscopy Taskforce for use as a bridge to other bariatric procedures. Early balloon removal was less than those of the FDA trials at 7%. Balloon migration occurred in 1.4% of patients and gastric perforation occurred in 0.1% (n = 8) patients, 50% of which had a history of prior gastric surgery.[20]

There are limited data on long-term outcomes in IGB therapy, although several studies reporting outcomes greater than 12 months have been published using the BIB, which is the precursor to the Orbera. In a study of 100 consecutive patients with a mean BMI of 35 kg/m^2 who underwent BIB placement for weight loss, 24% were able to maintain greater than or equal to 10% TBWL from baseline at 2.5 years. At the final follow-up at an average of 4.8 years, mean weights were similar to those at baseline and 35% patients had undergone bariatric surgery.[37] High rates of bariatric surgery (32%) were also reported in a retrospective study of 140 BIB patients with a mean follow-up of 18.3 months.[38] All patients in this cohort initially refused bariatric surgery, which led the authors to conclude that IGBs may serve as a gateway to bariatric surgery in patients who are initially hesitant.

A total of four deaths have been reported with Orbera in the United States since 2016, all of which were related to gastric perforation or aspiration events.[20,39] A trial update listed by the FDA in April 2020 cited six cases (2.3%) of balloon hyperinflation of unknown cause, which led to early balloon removal in four of six cases.[39]

ReShape Duo

The dual fluid-filled balloon ReShape Duo was evaluated in a pivotal, sham-controlled, double-blinded, multicenter RCT (the REDUCE trial), which was published in 2015.[33] Patients were enrolled in a lifestyle-modification program and were randomized to either IGB (n = 187) or to sham endoscopy (n = 139) and followed for a total of 12 months. The mean TBWL at 6 months was 7.6% compared with 3.6% in the control arm (P<.001). Mean TBWL was 4.8% at 12 months, and subjects maintained 66% of the weight lost at the time of balloon removal. Significant improvements in hemoglobulin A$_{1c}$, lipid profiles, and systolic blood pressure were reported at the time of balloon removal in the treatment group. Early balloon removal for intolerance occurred in 9.1% of patients, which was reduced to 7.7% when the fill volume was decreased for short stature patients. Serious adverse events occurred in 7.5% of patients, most (60%) of which were related to GI symptoms, such as vomiting and abdominal pain, but also included one contained esophageal perforation and one upper GI hemorrhage. Two cases of acute pancreatitis early in balloon placement were reported in an FDA update of the trial.[39] There were no balloon migrations or obstructions, even in the event of single balloon deflation. There was initially a remarkably high gastric ulceration rate of 35%, which improved to 10% when the tip was modified, and only one ulcer required clinical intervention. Weight loss in the postregulatory trial was 11.4% at 6 months and 13.3% at 9 months, similar to those reported in the Orbera postregulatory trial. Early balloon removal occurred in 6.4% of cases.[34,35] Sale of the ReShape Duo balloon was discontinued in January 2019 after the company's acquisition by Apollo Endosurgery, who will now solely focus on the Orbera balloon.

Obalon

The pivotal trial for the gas-filled Obalon balloon was a double-blind, randomized sham-controlled trial (the SMART trial) where 387 subjects were randomized to either 6 months of (three balloon) IGB treatment (n = 198) or to three sham sugar capsules (n = 189).[40] Subjects in the treatment arm had significantly greater percent TBWL compared with the control group (6.6% vs 3.6%) at the time of balloon removal, and subjects maintained 88.5% of the weight lost at 1-year follow-up. Subjects continued to lose weight after the placement of the third balloon between weeks 9 and 12. Modest but significant improvements in systolic blood pressure, blood glucose, cholesterol, and triglyceride concentrations were observed at the time of balloon removal. Serious adverse events were rare (0.3%) and included one bleeding ulcer that required transfusion in a patient taking NSAIDS and one balloon deflation with no cases of migration or obstruction. Early removal because of balloon intolerance only occurred in 3.3% of patients, which is lower than the fluid-filled Orbera (18.8%) and the ReShape Duo (9%) balloons.[13,32,33]

Retrospective data published from the largest IGB registry of 1343 patients receiving the Obalon balloon from 108 centers were published in 2018. Similar to the postregulatory studies of the ReShape Duo and Orbera IGBs, the reported percent TBWL at balloon removal was higher in this retrospective study (10%) than those reported in the pivotal RCT (7.1%). This trial also evaluated weight loss in patients outside the typical BMI range for intended use and reported a 10.3% TBWL for patients with a BMI of 25 to 29.9 kg/m^2 and 9.3% TBWL for patients with BMI greater than 40 kg/m^2. Serious adverse events only occurred in one patient (0.15%) who was not compliant with proton-pump inhibitor treatment and suffered a perforated ulcer. A total of seven device deflations were reported, five were removed endoscopically and two were excreted naturally without intervention.[36] The rate of dehydration requiring intravenous fluids was reported much less frequently in the Obalon postregulatory trial (0.07%) compared with the fluid-filled Orbera (8%).[34,36]

Outcomes in Non–Food and Drug Administration–Approved Balloons

Spatz3 adjustable balloon

The Spatz3 balloon is currently under FDA review in the United States, and is the most recent generation of the device, which was modified by removing an anchoring device from original design, which was implicated in a high incidence of balloon impaction necessitating surgical retrieval.[41,42] The device has a 12-month dwelling time and the balloon volume is adjusted endoscopically to relieve initial accommodative symptoms or to promote additional weight loss if the patient experiences a plateau in weight loss during treatment. The pivotal RCT of the balloon was completed in January of 2019, although the results have yet to be published.

In a retrospective review of 165 patients who underwent Spatz3 placement for 12 months, subjects with BMIs from 27 to 40 kg/m^2 had 15.8% TBWL.[43] In a subgroup

Table 2
Weight loss and safety outcomes from clinical studies of IGB therapy

	Balloon Trial Design	Number of Subjects		Mean BMI Treatment Group (kg/m²)	%TBWL at Balloon Removal		%TBWL at ~12 mo		Response Rate ≥5 % TBWL or >25% EWL	Early Removal Rate (%)	Serious Adverse Event Rate (%)
		Control	IGB		IGB Group	Control Group	IGB Group	Control Group			
Orbera US Pivotal Trial Courcoulas et al,[32] 2017	RCT, open label BMI 30–40	125	130	35.2 ± 3.2	10.2 ± 6.6	3.3 ± 5.0	7.6 ± 7.48	3.1 ± 5.9	79.2	18.8	10
ReShape US Pivotal Trial (REDUCE Trial) Ponce et al,[33] 2015	RCT, sham controlled, BMI 30–40	139	187	35.3 ± 2.8	6.8 / 7.6 ± 5.5 (completer analysis)	3.6 ± 6.3	NA	NA[b]	48.8	7.7[a]	7.5
Obalon US Pivotal Trial SMART (blinded) Sullivan et al,[40] 2018	RCT, double blind, sham-controlled BMI 25–>40[d]	189	198	35.2 ± 2.7	6.6 / 7.1 ± 5.3 (completer analysis)	3.4 ± 5.0	6.9 ± 6.5[c]	NA[b]	62.1 / 66.7 (completer analysis)	3.3	0.3

Results from RCTs of FDA-approved IGBs. All values reported as the modified intention-to-treat analysis if available.
[a] Reduced from 9.1% after volume was reduced for short-stature patients.
[b] Study allowed for crossover after 6 months so no control weight loss evaluated at 12 months.
[c] Obtained from patients that experienced any weight loss in the first 24 weeks.
[d] Reported results are from patients with BMI ranging from 30 to 40.
Data from Refs.[32,33,40]

Table 3
Results from clinical studies of FDA-approved and non–FDA approved IGBs

Device[a]	Study Design	Number of Subjects (n)	Mean Starting BMI (kg/m²)	%TBWL At Device Removal	%TBWL 9 Mo	%TBWL 12 Mo	Responder Rate at Balloon Removal (%) TBWL ≥5%	Responder Rate at Balloon Removal (%) TBWL >10%	Early Removal Rate	Serious Adverse Events
Orbera postregulatory approval study Vargas et al,[34] 2018	Retrospective, multicenter, BMI >30 kg/m²	321	37.9 ± 6.9	11.8 ± 7.5 (6 mo)	13.3 ± 9.5	NA	88	62	16.6	1 (1%) deflation 26 (8%) dehydration
ReShape Duo postregulatory study Agnihortri 2018	Retrospective, multicenter, BMI >30 kg/m²	202	36.8 ± 8.4	11.4 ± 6.7 (6 mo)	13.3 ± 7.8	14.7 ± 11.8 (12 patients)	82.2	60.4	6.4	1 (0.5%) deflation requiring surgical removal
Obalon postregulatory trial Moore et al,[36] 2019	Retrospective, multicenter, BMI ≥25 kg/m²	787	35.4 ± 5.4	10.0 ± 6.1[b] (6 mo)	NA	NA	75.4	46.1	NA	1 (0.07%) removal because of intractable pain/vomiting 1 (0.07%) gastric perforation requiring surgery[c]
Spatz3 Usuy and Brooks,[43] 2017	Retrospective, multicenter, BMI 27–40 kg/m²	136	34 ± 26.5–40	15.8 (range, 2–49) (12 mo)	NA	15.8 (2–49)	NA	91.2	12.7[d]	1 (0.7%) gastric perforation in patients not on PPI

| Elipse Ienca et al[48] 2020 | Retrospective, multicenter, BMI >27 | 1770 | 34.4 ± 5.3 | 14.2 ± 5.0 (4 mo) | NA | NA | NA | NA | 2.9 | 3 (0.17%) bowel obstructions requiring surgery
4 (0.02%) spontaneous hyperinflation
1 (0.06%) pancreatitis
1 (0.06%) gastric outlet obstruction
1 (0.06%) gastric perforation requiring surgery |

Abbreviations: NA, not available; PPI, proton pump inhibitor.

Study results from clinical trials of FDA-approved and non–FDA approved IGBs.

a Includes only patients who received all three balloons and includes patients outside the intended use range with BMIs from 25 to 29.9 and greater than 40.

b In patients with BMI 30–40 kg/m².

c Patient was not compliant with proton pump inhibitor therapy and had a perforated gastric ulcer.

d Number reported is for balloon removal after <4 months, 70.3% of patients completed at least 8 months of IGB therapy.

Data from Refs.[34,36,43,48]

analysis, 91.2% of subjects with BMI of 27 to 40 kg/m^2 achieved greater than 10% TBWL compared with 69% in the cohort with a BMI of 41 to 60 kg/m^2, suggesting a greater efficacy in patients with class 1 and 2 obesity than those with class 3 obesity. Volume adjustments were made in 51% of patients and decreasing balloon volume alleviated intolerance in 16 of 20 patients. Furthermore, upward adjustments seemed to promote additional weight loss when patients plateaued, yielding an additional mean weight loss of 5.7 kg in 64 patients. Similar to other fluid-filled IGBs, post-placement nausea and vomiting are common (70%–90%), although downward adjustments were shown to alleviate symptoms of intolerance in 80% of patients. Late gastric perforation, including those resulting in death, have been reported in case reports and may be the result of long-term pressure-induced ischemic changes of the gastric wall.[43–45]

Although the Spatz3 balloon has been shown to promote greater weight loss compared with other IGBs, further long-term data are needed to assess balloon results and safety. A cost-effectiveness assessment is also warranted, because the need for multiple endoscopies for volume adjustment may significantly increase the cost of treatment.

Elipse

The swallowable and naturally excreted fluid-filled Elipse balloon is currently under clinical investigation for use in the United States, although the safety and efficacy of the balloon has been investigated in several US and international studies. In a prospective, multicentered study of 34 patients, subjects had 10% TBWL at the time of balloon removal (4 months), with no serious adverse events and all balloons were uneventfully excreted by either defecation (88%) or by vomiting (12%).[46] Early balloon removal because of intolerance only occurred in two (6%) patients. Results were similar in a single-center prospective study of 106 patients, where patients had 10.9% TBWL at 6 months.[47] Most (85%) subjects followed up over a year, with a 7.9% TBWL at a mean follow-up of 19.6 months. There was one case of small bowel obstruction caused by incomplete deflation that was resolved via laparoscopic surgery. Six patients (5%) had balloons removed because of intolerance. The largest retrospective study of 1770 consecutive patients who underwent Elipse balloon placement at 19 international centers was recently published in April 2020. Subjects had a mean of 14.2% TBWL and significant improvements in subject lipid profiles and hemoglobulin A$_{1c}$ were reported at the time of balloon removal. Early removal only occurred in 2.9% of patients because of intolerance. There were three (0.17%) cases of small bowel obstruction and one (0.06%) case of gastric perforation, all requiring laparoscopic surgery for resolution. All three subjects with small bowel obstructions had an earlier design of the balloon. Most (95.6%) balloons were passed in stool, 11 empty balloons (0.6%) were excreted by vomiting, and 63 (3.6%) required endoscopic removal.[48]

SUMMARY

IGB therapy is a low-morbidity, reversible, and repeatable therapy that is used alongside diet and behavioral modification to promote weight loss in between that achieved with lifestyle and pharmacotherapy, and bariatric surgery. Serious adverse events are rare, and include intestinal obstruction, pancreatitis, gastric ulceration, and gastric perforation. Long-term outcomes data are lacking, although weight regain seems to occur in a significant amount of patients after balloon removal, which may necessitate a second IGB or bariatric surgery.

CLINICS CARE POINTS

- Patients undergoing IGB therapy must be able to participate in a supervised diet and exercise program managed by a multidisciplinary team.

- Mandatory proton-pump inhibitors and refraining from NSAID use during IGB therapy is critical in preventing pressure-related ulcer formation, and balloon removal should be performed using general anesthesia with endotracheal intubation to prevent aspiration.

- Percent total body weight loss after IGB therapy ranges from 6% to 12% at the time of device removal, although these are limited long-term outcomes data after 1 year of treatment.

DISCLOSURE

Nothing to disclose.

REFERENCES

1. Hales CM. Prevalence of obesity and severe obesity among adults: United States, 2017–2018. NCHS Data Brief 2020;(360):8.
2. Schauer PR, Bhatt DL, Kirwan JP, et al. Bariatric surgery versus intensive medical therapy for diabetes: 5-year outcomes. N Engl J Med 2017;376(7):641–51.
3. Gadde KM, Atkins KD. The limits and challenges of antiobesity pharmacotherapy. Expert Opin Pharmacother 2020;1–10. https://doi.org/10.1080/14656566.2020.1748599.
4. Angrisani L, Santonicola A, Iovino P, et al. Bariatric surgery and endoluminal procedures: IFSO worldwide survey 2014. Obes Surg 2017;27(9):2279–89.
5. Ugalmugle S, Swain R. "Intragastric balloons market share 2019-2025 | Industry Size Report." n.d. Global Market Insights, Inc. 2019. Available at: https://www.gminsights.com/industry-analysis/intragastric-balloon-market. Accessed June 1, 2020.
6. Hogan RB, Johnston JH, Long BW, et al. A double-blind, randomized, sham-controlled trial of the gastric bubble for obesity. Gastrointest Endosc 1989; 35(5):381–5.
7. Schapiro M, Benjamin S, Blackburn G, et al. Obesity and the gastric balloon: a comprehensive workshop. Gastrointest Endosc 1987;33(4):323–7.
8. Kentish SJ, Page AJ. The role of gastrointestinal vagal afferent fibres in obesity. J Physiol (Lond) 2015;593(4):775–86.
9. Camilleri M, Toouli J, Herrera MF, et al. Intra-abdominal vagal blocking (VBLOC therapy): clinical results with a new implantable medical device. Surgery 2008; 143(6):723–31.
10. Xing J, Chen JDZ. Alterations of gastrointestinal motility in obesity. Obes Res 2004;12(11):1723–32.
11. Vargas EJ, Bazerbachi F, Calderon G, et al. Changes in time of gastric emptying after surgical and endoscopic bariatrics and weight loss: a systematic review and meta-analysis. Clin Gastroenterol Hepatol 2020;18(1):57–68.e5.
12. Gómez V, Woodman G, Abu Dayyeh BK. Delayed gastric emptying as a proposed mechanism of action during intragastric balloon therapy: results of a prospective study. Obesity (Silver Spring) 2016;24(9):1849–53.
13. Sullivan S, Swain JM, Woodman G, et al. Randomized sham-controlled trial evaluating efficacy and safety of endoscopic gastric plication for primary obesity: the ESSENTIAL trial. Obesity (Silver Spring) 2017;25(2):294–301.

14. Kumar N, Bazerbachi F, Rustagi T, et al. The influence of the Orbera intragastric balloon filling volumes on weight loss, tolerability, and adverse events: a systematic review and meta-analysis. Obes Surg 2017;27(9):2272–8.
15. Cummings D, Weigle D, Frayo S, et al. Plasma ghrelin levels after diet-induced weight loss or gastric bypass surgery. N Engl J Med 2002;346:1623–32.
16. Mion F, Napoléon B, Roman S, et al. Effects of intragastric balloon on gastric emptying and plasma ghrelin levels in non-morbid obese patients. Obes Surg 2005;15(4):510–6.
17. Mathus-Vliegen EMH, Eichenberger RI. Fasting and meal-suppressed ghrelin levels before and after intragastric balloons and balloon-induced weight loss. Obes Surg 2014;24(1):85–94.
18. Konopko-Zubrzycka M, Baniukiewicz A, Wróblewski E, et al. The effect of intragastric balloon on plasma ghrelin, leptin, and adiponectin levels in patients with morbid obesity. J Clin Endocrinol Metab 2009;94(5):1644–9.
19. Mathus-Vliegen EM, de Groot GH. Fasting and meal-induced CCK and PP secretion following intragastric balloon treatment for obesity. Obes Surg 2013;23(5):622–33.
20. ASGE Bariatric Endoscopy Task Force and ASGE Technology Committee, Abu Dayyeh BK, Kumar N, et al. ASGE Bariatric Endoscopy Task Force systematic review and meta-analysis assessing the ASGE PIVI thresholds for adopting endoscopic bariatric therapies. Gastrointest Endosc 2015;82(3):425–38.e5.
21. Borges AC, Almeida PC, Furlani SMT, et al. Intragastric balloons in high-risk obese patients in a Brazilian center: initial experience. Rev Col Bras Cir 2018; 45(1). https://doi.org/10.1590/0100-6991e-20181448.
22. Ball W, Raza SS, Loy J, et al. Effectiveness of intra-gastric balloon as a bridge to definitive surgery in the super obese. OBES SURG 2019;29(6):1932–6.
23. Frutos MD, Morales MD, Luján J, et al. Intragastric balloon reduces liver volume in super-obese patients, facilitating subsequent laparoscopic gastric bypass. Obes Surg 2007;17(2):150–4.
24. Périssé LGS, Ecbc RJ, Ribeiro KF, Périssé LGS, Ecbc -Rj, Ribeiro KF. Gastric wall changes after intragastric balloon placement: a preliminary experience. Rev Col Bras Cir. 2016;43(4):286–8.
25. Coffin B, Maunoury V, Pattou F, et al. Impact of intragastric balloon before laparoscopic gastric bypass on patients with super obesity: a randomized multicenter study. OBES SURG 2017;27(4):902–9.
26. Patel NJ, Gómez V, Steidley DE, et al. Successful use of intragastric balloon therapy as a bridge to heart transplantation. Obes Surg 2020. https://doi.org/10.1007/s11695-020-04572-7.
27. Choudhary NS, Puri R, Saraf N, et al. Intragastric balloon as a novel modality for weight loss in patients with cirrhosis and morbid obesity awaiting liver transplantation. Indian J Gastroenterol 2016;35(2):113–6.
28. Storm AC, Lakdawala NK, Thompson CC. Intragastric balloon for management of morbid obesity in a candidate for heart transplantation. J Heart Lung Transplant 2017;36(7):820–1.
29. De Waele B, Reynaert H, Urbain D, et al. Intragastric balloons for preoperative weight reduction. Obes Surg 2000;10(1):58–60.
30. Neto MG, Silva LB, Grecco E, et al. Brazilian Intragastric Balloon Consensus Statement (BIBC): practical guidelines based on experience of over 40,000 cases. Surg Obes Relat Dis 2018;14(2):151–9.
31. Orbera non-surgical weight loss balloon. Available at: https://www.orbera.com/. Accessed June 13, 2020.

32. Courcoulas A, Abu Dayyeh BK, Eaton L, et al. Intragastric balloon as an adjunct to lifestyle intervention: a randomized controlled trial. Int J Obes 2017;41(3): 427–33.
33. Ponce J, Woodman G, Swain J, et al. The REDUCE pivotal trial: a prospective, randomized controlled pivotal trial of a dual intragastric balloon for the treatment of obesity. Surg Obes Relat Dis 2015;11(4):874–81.
34. Vargas EJ, Pesta CM, Bali A, et al. Single fluid-filled intragastric balloon safe and effective for inducing weight loss in a real-world population. Clin Gastroenterol Hepatol 2018;16(7):1073–80.e1.
35. Agnihotri A, Xie A, Bartalos C, et al. Real-world safety and efficacy of fluid-filled dual intragastric balloon for weight loss. Clin Gastroenterol Hepatol 2018;16(7): 1081–8.e1.
36. Moore RL, Seger MV, Garber SM, et al. Clinical safety and effectiveness of a swallowable gas-filled intragastric balloon system for weight loss: consecutively treated patients in the initial year of U.S. commercialization. Surg Obes Relat Dis 2019;15(3):417–23.
37. Dastis NS, Deviere EFJ, Hittelet A, et al. Intragastric balloon for weight loss: results in 100 individuals followed for at least 2.5 years. Endoscopy 2009;41(07): 575–80.
38. Melissas J, Mouzas J, Filis D, et al. The intragastric balloon: smoothing the path to bariatric surgery. Obes Surg 2006;16(7):897–902.
39. Health C for D and R. UPDATE: Potential Risks with Liquid-filled Intragastric Balloons - Letter to Health Care Providers. FDA. 2020. Available at: https://www.fda.gov/medical-devices/letters-health-care-providers/update-potential-risks-liquid-filled-intragastric-balloons-letter-health-care-providers-1. Accessed May 30, 2020.
40. Sullivan S, Swain J, Woodman G, et al. Randomized sham-controlled trial of the 6-month swallowable gas-filled intragastric balloon system for weight loss. Surg Obes Relat Dis 2018;14(12):1876–89.
41. Genco A, Dellepiane D, Baglio G, et al. Adjustable intragastric balloon vs nonadjustable intragastric balloon: case–control study on complications, tolerance, and efficacy. OBES SURG 2013;23(7):953–8.
42. Yap Kannan R, Nutt MR. Are intra-gastric adjustable balloon system safe? A case series. Int J Surg Case Rep 2013;4(10):936–8.
43. Usuy E, Brooks J. Response rates with the spatz3 adjustable balloon. Obes Surg 2018;28(5):1271–6.
44. Daniel F, Abou Fadel C, Houmani Z, et al. Spatz 3 adjustable intragastric balloon: long-term safety concerns. OBES SURG 2016;26(1):159–60.
45. Dayan D, Sagie B, Fishman S. Late intragastric balloon induced gastric perforation. Obes Surg 2016;26(5):1138–40.
46. Machytka E, Gaur S, Chuttani R, et al. Elipse, the first procedureless gastric balloon for weight loss: a prospective, observational, open-label, multicenter study. Endoscopy 2017;49(2):154–60.
47. Jamal MH, Almutairi R, Elabd R, et al. The safety and efficacy of procedureless gastric balloon: a study examining the effect of Elipse intragastric balloon safety, short and medium term effects on weight loss with 1-year follow-up post-removal. Obes Surg 2019;29(4):1236–41.
48. Ienca R, Al Jarallah M, Caballero A, et al. The procedureless Elipse gastric balloon program: multicenter experience in 1770 consecutive patients. OBES SURG 2020. https://doi.org/10.1007/s11695-020-04539-8.

Emerging Endoscopic Interventions in Bariatric Surgery

Joshua S. Winder, MD[1], John H. Rodriguez, MD*

KEYWORDS

- Endoscopy • Bariatric endoscopy • Endoscopic sleeve gastroplasty
- Gastric aspiration • Incisionless magnetic anastomosis • Endoluminal barrier sleeve

KEY POINTS

- Various endoscopic techniques have been developed to treat obesity and metabolic disease.
- These techniques vary widely from implantable devices to gastric remodeling.
- Endoscopic strategies for treatment include both malabsorptive and restrictive models.
- These interventions generally are well tolerated and provide improvement in both weight management and metabolic disease.

INTRODUCTION

Obesity continues to be a major health care issue, and, despite great efforts, it continues to affect a growing number of people in all age groups worldwide.[1] Bariatric surgery has shown an effective tool for weight loss and improvement of weight-related comorbidities and has an acceptable risk profile.[2] Despite the proven efficacy of metabolic surgery, only a small number of individuals have access to high quality surgical care. This trend likely is multifactorial, including issues with cost, access, morbidity, and patient preference. Although bariatric surgery is relatively safe, it is not without risk, with reported rates of morbidity ranging from 3% to 20% and mortality rates ranging from 0.1% to 0.5%.[3,4] Endoscopic options to treat obesity are compelling options for many reasons. Endoscopy generally is less invasive. Depending on the technique or device used, endoscopy may be less expensive. Endoscopic therapies can be used as a bridge to further therapies for patients who comorbidities may limit their surgical options. Conversely, many patients may not qualify for bariatric surgery (body mass index [BMI] >35 kg/m^2 with comorbidities or BMI >40 kg/m^2) but still be may interested or benefit from weight loss. Various techniques in endoscopic interventions

Section of Surgical Endoscopy, Department of General Surgery, Cleveland Clinic Lerner College of Medicine, 9500 Euclid Avenue, Mail Code A-100, Cleveland, OH 44195, USA
[1] Present address: 500 University Drive, Mail Code H149, Hershey, PA 17033.
* Corresponding author.
E-mail address: Rodrigj3@ccf.org

in bariatric surgery (EIBSs) have emerged and generally fall into 2 different categories: procedures, and devices. This review examines the procedure or device, its efficacy, and any risks or adverse events associated with its use. EIBS devices include intra-gastric space-occupying devices (discussed elsewhere), gastric aspiration devices, incisionless magnetic anastomotic systems, and endoluminal bypass barrier sleeves. EIBS procedures include primary obesity surgery endoluminal (POSE), endoscopic sleeve gastroplasty (ESG), and duodenal mucosal resurfacing (DMR).

DEVICES
Gastric Aspiration Devices

Aspiration therapy works by inserting a tube, similar to a percutaneous endoscopic gastrostomy tube, and then aspirating a portion of the ingested contents into an external reservoir, which then is disposed of. This lessens the amount of chime, and therefore calories, that then is transmitted downstream for digestion and absorption by the gut. The AspireAssist system (Aspire Bariatrics, King of Prussia, Pennsylvania) is inserted with a typical pull-technique under endoscopic guidance. After the tract is developed, approximately 1 week to 2 weeks postprocedure, the external tubing is trimmed short and connected to an external skin port. The AspireAssist has been approved in the United States for use in patients with BMI between 35 kg/m^2 and 55 kg/m^2. Multiple small studies have shown promising results with regards to weight loss using the AspireAssist device. Noren and colleagues[5] saw a mean percentage of excess weight loss (%EWL) of 54.5% $\pm$ 28.8% at 1 year and BMI dropped from a mean of 39.8 kg/m^2 at inclusion to 32.1 kg/m^2. Forssell and colleagues[6] showed a mean %EWL of 40.8 $\pm$ 19.8% at 6 months in patients with a starting mean BMI of 40.3 kg/m^2. In a 12-month multicenter US trial, 171 patients underwent lifestyle coun-seling and treatment with the AspireAssist device or lifestyle counseling alone.[7] The investigators found a significant difference in %EWL and improvement in weight-related comorbidities in the treatment group. The baseline mean BMI for patients treated with the device was 42.2 kg/m^2. The mean %EWL in the treatment group was 37.2% $\pm$ 27.5% compared with 13.0% $\pm$ 17.6% in the control group. Hemoglobin (Hgb)A$_{1c}$ levels decreased to an average of 0.36%, relative to 5.7% at baseline ($P<.0001$). High-density lipoprotein cholesterol increased by 8.1% ($P = .0001$), and tri-glycerides decreased by 9.9% ($P = .02$). The most common adverse events reported in the study included peristomal granulation tissue, postoperative abdominal pain, peristomal irritation, nausea, abdominal discomfort, and peristomal bacterial infection. Early removal rate during the first year was 26.1%.

Aspiration therapy benefits from at least 2 mechanisms for weight loss: aspiration of calories and behavior changes. In a pilot study examining the AspireAssist device, Sul-livan and colleagues[8] found that 25% to 30% of calories from a meal were aspirated if performed according to protocol. This means that only 80% of weight loss seen can be attributed to aspiration of the ingested meal. The remaining 20% likely was due to the patient-reported decrease in food intake and food particles that must be small in size (<5 mm) and in a slurry to be removed adequately. This factor requires the patient to chew more thoroughly and ingest adequate amounts of water for the catheter to work, with both of these practices leading to smaller portion sizes.

Incisionless Magnetic Anastomotic Systems

The Incisionless Magnetic Anastomotic System (GI Windows, West Bridgewater, Mas-sachusetts) takes advantage of a dual-path anastomotic enteral bypass, which allows nutrients to follow their normal path through the gastrointestinal (GI) tract or through the bypassing anastomosis created with opposing magnetic discs. In this way, it may be classified as a malabsorptive procedure. The coupling discs are deployed using pediatric colonoscopes in the jejunum and ileum, respectively. Once the magnets are coupled, they create an anastomosis by causing local tissue necrosis and remodeling between the 2 discs. In the first human pilot study of the device, 10 patients with a mean baseline BMI of 41 kg/m^2 underwent combined endoscopic and laparoscopic placement (to ensure proper coupling and limb length).[9] At 12 months, the patients had experienced a 40.2%EWL. Improvement in HgbA$_{1c}$ was 1.9% for diabetic patients and 1.0% for prediabetic patients. Most patients complained of transient nausea and all patients had diarrhea with the procedure, which resolved. Four patients had recurrent diarrhea that responded to diet modification.

ENDOLUMINAL BYPASS BARRIER SLEEVES
Duodenojejunal Bypass Sleeve

The first endoluminal implant used to induce weight loss by malabsorption was the duodenojejunal bypass sleeve (DJBS).[10] The EndoBarrier (GI Dynamics, Lexington, Massachusetts) is a DJBS that is covered with Polytetrafluoroethylene, making it impermeable to nutrients. The device is deployed endoscopically within the duodenal bulb with a nitinol anchor that works like a self-expanding metal stent, which is connected to a long sleeve that extends distally approximately 65 cm into the jejunum. The Teflon-coated tube transports the ingested food through the duodenum and proximal jejunum without allowing interaction with the mucosa, thus prohibiting absorption. The biliary and pancreatic secretions flow freely down the outside of the tube, eventually mixing with the ingested food further downstream. This system can stay in situ for 3 months to 12 months. It currently is approved for use in Europe for patients with type 2 diabetes mellitus and obesity for 12 months. It currently is not approved for sale in the United States.

In the first prospective trial of the device, 12 patients with a baseline mean BMI of 43 kg/m^2 had the device implanted for 12 weeks.[11] Mean %EWL was 23.6% at 12 weeks and, of the 4 diabetic patients included in the study, 3 discontinued their diabetic medications. The average baseline BMI was 43 kg/m^2 and the average ending BMI was 38.7 kg/m^2. Two patients had the device removed prior to the 12 weeks due to abdominal pain, and 2 injuries occurred during removal of the device (an oropharyngeal and esophageal mucosal tear), which did not require further intervention.

In a subsequent human trial of the device, 25 patients with a mean starting BMI of 42 kg/m^2 were randomized to either device implantation, or dietary modification for a 12-week period.[12] The investigators reported a 22%EWL for the device group versus 5%EWL for the controls. They did see 3 patients with upper GI bleeds, 1 anchor migration, and 1 stent obstruction.

In the first European trial of the device, 41 patients were randomized to either device implantation or a diet control group[13]; 30 patients were randomized to the device group and 11 to the control group. Of the 30 randomized to the device group, 26 devices were safely implanted and 4 were removed early due to migration, dislocation of the anchor, obstruction, or continuous epigastric pain. Mean %EWL for the device group was 19.0% whereas the control group was 6.9%EWL ($P<.002$). Mean BMI at inclusion for the device group was 48.9 kg/m^2 and mean absolute BMI reduction over the study period was 5.5 kg/m^2; 8 patients of the device group had diabetes at baseline and showed improvement in 7 patients during the study period (lower glucose levels, HgbA$_{1c}$, and medication requirements). All patients in the device group reported abdominal pain and nausea for the first week following implantation.

In a 52-week prospective, open-label clinical trial of the DJBS, 22 patients with obesity and type 2 diabetes mellitus were recruited.[14] Their mean BMI at the start of the study was 44.8 kg/m². Of the 22 patients, 13 completed the 52-week study period. At the end of 1 year, the investigators noted an impressive reduction in HgbA$_{1c}$ levels (-2.1% $\pm$ 0.3%). For those 9 patients who had the stent removed early, reasons for removal included device migration (n = 3), hemorrhage (n = 1), abdominal pain (n = 2), principal investigator request (n = 2), and discovery of an unrelated malignancy (n = 1). For those patients who completed the study, the most common device-related adverse events were upper abdominal pain (n = 11), back pain (n = 5), nausea (n = 7), and vomiting (n = 7).

Gastroduodenal-Jejunal Bypass Sleeve

The gastroduodenal-jejunal bypass sleeve is another form of endoscopic barrier bypass, which is anchored at the gastroesophageal junction using a combined endoscopic/laparoscopic approach (Endo Bypass System [ValenTx, Hopkins, Minnesota]). This device extends distally through the stomach and 120 cm into the small bowel, more closely mimicking traditional Roux-en-Y gastric bypass anatomy.

In the first series of patients with 1 year of implantation of this device, the results seemed favorable. In the study, 13 patients with a mean baseline BMI of 42 kg/m² were included. Of the 13 patients enrolled, 10 completed the study period (1 patient did not have the device implanted due to inflammation at the gastroesophageal junction at the time of attempted placement, and 2 patients had the device removed early due to intolerance).[15] Six of the 10 patients who had the device implanted had fully attached and functional devices throughout the study period (the remaining 4 had partial detachment). The mean %EWL was 35.9% for the entire group, but was even higher for patients who had fully attached devices (54%EWL).

PROCEDURES

Two main procedures have been developed for gastric body remodeling in an attempt to help restrict the distensibility of the stomach and reduce the amount of food ingested by creating a sensation of early satiety. These procedures are the POSE and the ESG. Both procedures do require a separate endoscopic device to complete the procedure and are considered restrictive.

Primary Obesity Surgery Endoluminal

POSE is accomplished with the Incisionless Operating Platform (USGI Medical, San Clemente, California). This is a stand-alone device with 4 working channels that accommodate tissue graspers, an ultraslim camera, and tissue anchors. It measures approximately 54F and is maneuvered like a typical endoscope. The procedure is accomplished by placing 8 to 10 plicating anchors along a double-ridge configuration to reduce the size and shape of the fundic apex down to the level of the gastroesophageal junction. This reduces the volume of the stomach, limiting the amount that can be ingested, and increased gastric emptying time.

In a prospective case series presented by Lopez-Nava and colleagues,[16] for patients who underwent POSE and were followed-up at 1 year, the mean %EWL was of 44.9% $\pm$ 24.4%. Their mean baseline BMI was 38.0 kg/m². In their series of 147 patients, they had no serious short-term or long-term adverse events associated with the procedure.

In a recent, multicenter, randomized, sham-controlled trial, 332 patients were randomized in a 2:1 ratio to the POSE procedure or sham, with both groups receiving low-intensity lifestyle therapy.[17] The baseline mean BMI for patients in the treatment arm was 36.0 kg/m². The procedure success rate was 99.5%, and the procedure time was 40.0 minutes ± 12.9 minutes. After 1 year, the investigators reported a mean %TBWL (total body weight loss) of 4.95 ± 7.04% in active and 1.38 ± 5.58% in sham groups, respectively. Significant adverse events included pain, nausea, vomiting, 1 patient with a hepatic abscess, and 1 patient with extraluminal bleeding.

Endoscopic Sleeve Gastroplasty

ESG is an endoscopic procedure using a device called the OverStitch (Apollo Endosurgery, Austin, Texas). This consists of a cap that is placed on the end of a double-channel therapeutic endoscope. The device has a handle that attaches to the shaft of the endoscope at the instrument channels. The cap consists of a curved needle that, when toggled, swings in and out. One of the working channels is used to pass a shuttle device that helps pass the needle back and forth within the device. By using the shuttle and swinging needle, the operator can take full-thickness bites of the target tissue. The OverStitch allows the endoscopist to make various suturing patterns, including running or interrupted, with absorbable or permanent sutures.

Initial techniques performing ESG achieved the desired configuration with 6 to 12 stitches, each placed in a triangular fashion at the anterior wall, greater curvature, and posterior wall. Sharaiha and colleagues[18] described placing a median of 8 sutures in a running fashion by starting in the antrum and moving proximally.[18] This included fundic reduction. They reported that in their series of 23 patients, after 1 year, the mean BMI fell from 34.2 kg/m² to 29.4 kg/m².

In the largest series of patients who underwent ESG, 1000 patients were followed out to 12 months.[19] Their baseline mean BMI was 33.3 kg/m² ± 4.5 kg/m² and age of 34.4 years ± 9.5 years. Mean percentages of total weight loss at 6 months, 12 months, and 18 months were 13.7% ± 6.8%, 15.0% ± 7.7%, and 14.8% ± 8.5%, respectively. Mean BMI fell from 33.3 kg/m² to 28.9 kg/m² at 18 months. Thirteen of 17 patients with diabetes, all patients with hypertension, and 18 of 32 patients with dyslipidemia were in complete remission by the third month of the study. During the first week following ESG, 92.4% of patients complained of nausea or abdominal pain, which was managed conservatively. Twenty-four patients were readmitted: 8 for severe abdominal pain, 3 of whom ultimately underwent ESG reversal; 7 for postprocedure bleeding, 2 of whom required transfusion; 4 for perigastric collections with pleural effusion, with 3 requiring percutaneous drainage; and 5 for postprocedure fever with no sequelae.

Duodenal Mucosal Resurfacing

DMR is accomplished by performing a saline lift of the duodenal mucosa distal to the ampulla of Vater to the desired point distally in the duodenum. The lifted mucosa then is hydrothermally ablated using the Revita DMR (Fractyl, Lexington, Massachusetts). The 2-cm long balloon is filled with heated water and the tissue ablated under direct visualization. These steps are repeated along the length of the desired duodenum.

An international multicenter study enrolled 46 patients to undergo DMR.[20] Inclusion criteria included patients with type 2 diabetes mellitus on at least 1 oral hypoglycemic agent with BMI of 20 kg/m² to 40 kg/m². In 37 patients, the procedure was completed successfully (the remaining were unsuccessful due to technical issues), with 36 completing the study protocol. Mean BMI at enrollment was 31.6 kg/m². Only 1 significant adverse event (a fever) was reported, which self-resolved. HgbA$_{1c}$ was reduced by 10 mmol/mol ± 2 mmol/mol (0.9% ± 0.2%) (mean ± SD) at 24 weeks ($P<.001$) compared with baseline, and this effect was preserved out to 12 months following

DMR. Weight loss was observed for the first 4 weeks post-DMR, which then stabilized. This weight loss did not correlate with the improvement in diabetes control.

SUMMARY

EIBSs include novel devices and techniques that provide various modes of both malabsorptive and constrictive changes to the GI tract. Improvements in weight and metabolic activity have been observed with these techniques, although weight loss and improvement in diabetic control vary between different EIBSs. Most reported studies of these techniques are small case series with short follow-up. More research is needed to fully understand the long-term effect of these modalities and in which populations they would be most beneficial. They do represent an ongoing trend, however, toward less-invasive management strategies that show promising results in this early and exciting period.

DISCLOSURE

J.S. Winder has nothing to disclose. J.H. Rodriguez has no conflict of interest relevant to this publication. Outside of the scope of this publication, he has received research funding from Pacira Pharmaceuticals and Intuitive Surgical.

CLINICS CARE POINTS

- Endoluminal bariatric interventions offer potential treatment for obesity in patients with class 1 obesity.
- These procedures and devices have been designed with safety as the top priority to offer patients additional alternatives in the treatment of obesity and related medical conditions.
- Compared to metabolic surgery, these procedures should offer a safer profile despite decreased effectiveness and durability.
- Endoluminal procedures can be utilized as primary intervention, adjuvant therapy, or as a bridge to metabolic surgery in high risk cases.

REFERENCES

1. Obesity: preventing and managing the global epidemic. Report of a WHO consultation. World Health Organ Tech Rep Ser 2000;894(i-xii):1–253.
2. Schauer PR, Kashyap SR, Wolski K, et al. Bariatric surgery versus intensive medical therapy in obese patients with diabetes. N Engl J Med 2012;366(17):1567–76.
3. Morino M, Toppino M, Forestieri P, et al. Mortality after bariatric surgery: analysis of 13,871 morbidly obese patients from a national registry. Ann Surg 2007;246(6):1002–7 [discussion 7–9].
4. Buchwald H, Estok R, Fahrbach K, et al. Trends in mortality in bariatric surgery: a systematic review and meta-analysis. Surgery 2007;142(4):621–32 [discussion 32–5].
5. Noren E, Forssell H. Aspiration therapy for obesity; a safe and effective treatment. BMC Obes 2016;3:56.
6. Forssell H, Noren E. A novel endoscopic weight loss therapy using gastric aspiration: results after 6 months. Endoscopy 2015;47(1):68–71.
7. Thompson CC, Abu Dayyeh BK, Kushner R, et al. Percutaneous gastrostomy device for the treatment of class II and class III obesity: results of a randomized controlled trial. Am J Gastroenterol 2017;112(3):447–57.

8. Sullivan S, Stein R, Jonnalagadda S, et al. Aspiration therapy leads to weight loss in obese subjects: a pilot study. Gastroenterology 2013;145(6):1245–12452 e1-5.

9. Machytka E, Buzga M, Zonca P, et al. Partial jejunal diversion using an incisionless magnetic anastomosis system: 1-year interim results in patients with obesity and diabetes. Gastrointest Endosc 2017;86(5):904–12.

10. Patel SR, Mason J, Hakim N. The duodenal-jejunal bypass sleeve (EndoBarrier Gastrointestinal Liner) for weight loss and treatment of type II diabetes. Indian J Surg 2012;74(4):275–7.

11. Rodriguez-Grunert L, Galvao Neto MP, Alamo M, et al. First human experience with endoscopically delivered and retrieved duodenal-jejunal bypass sleeve. Surg Obes Relat Dis 2008;4(1):55–9.

12. Tarnoff M, Rodriguez L, Escalona A, et al. Open label, prospective, randomized controlled trial of an endoscopic duodenal-jejunal bypass sleeve versus low calorie diet for pre-operative weight loss in bariatric surgery. Surg Endosc 2009; 23(3):650–6.

13. Schouten R, Rijs CS, Bouvy ND, et al. A multicenter, randomized efficacy study of the EndoBarrier gastrointestinal liner for presurgical weight loss prior to bariatric surgery. Ann Surg 2010;251(2):236–43.

14. de Moura EG, Martins BC, Lopes GS, et al. Metabolic improvements in obese type 2 diabetes subjects implanted for 1 year with an endoscopically deployed duodenal-jejunal bypass liner. Diabetes Technol Ther 2012;14(2):183–9.

15. Sandler BJ, Rumbaut R, Swain CP, et al. One-year human experience with a novel endoluminal, endoscopic gastric bypass sleeve for morbid obesity. Surg Endosc 2015;29(11):3298–303.

16. Lopez-Nava G, Bautista-Castano I, Jimenez A, et al. The primary obesity surgery endolumenal (POSE) procedure: one-year patient weight loss and safety outcomes. Surg Obes Relat Dis 2015;11(4):861–5.

17. Sullivan S, Swain JM, Woodman G, et al. Randomized sham-controlled trial evaluating efficacy and safety of endoscopic gastric plication for primary obesity: The ESSENTIAL trial. Obesity (Silver Spring) 2017;25(2):294–301.

18. Sharaiha RZ, Kumta NA, Saumoy M, et al. Endoscopic sleeve gastroplasty significantly reduces body mass index and metabolic complications in obese patients. Clin Gastroenterol Hepatol 2017;15(4):504–10.

19. Alqahtani A, Al-Darwish A, Mahmoud AE, et al. Short-term outcomes of endoscopic sleeve gastroplasty in 1000 consecutive patients. Gastrointest Endosc 2019;89(6):1132–8.

20. van Baar ACG, Holleman F, Crenier L, et al. Endoscopic duodenal mucosal resurfacing for the treatment of type 2 diabetes mellitus: one year results from the first international, open-label, prospective, multicentre study. Gut 2020;69(2): 295–303.

Moving?

Make sure your subscription moves with you!

To notify us of your new address, find your **Clinics Account Number** (located on your mailing label above your name), and contact customer service at:

Email: journalscustomerservice-usa@elsevier.com

800-654-2452 (subscribers in the U.S. & Canada)
314-447-8871 (subscribers outside of the U.S. & Canada)

Fax number: 314-447-8029

**Elsevier Health Sciences Division
Subscription Customer Service
3251 Riverport Lane
Maryland Heights, MO 63043**

*To ensure uninterrupted delivery of your subscription, please notify us at least 4 weeks in advance of move.

Printed and bound by CPI Group (UK) Ltd, Croydon, CR0 4YY

03/10/2024

01040401-0004